EVERYTHING YOUR DOCTOR WOULD TELL YOU IF HE HAD THE TIME

EVERYTHING YOUR DOCTOR WOULD TELL YOU IF HE HAD THE TIME

Claire Rayner

Pan Books Ltd London and Sydney

Contents

Edited and designed by
Marshall Editions Ltd
71 Eccleston Square
London SW1V 1PJ

Editors
Sonya Larkin
Penny David
John Blackett-Ord
Christopher Cooper

Designers
Peter Saag
Piers Evelegh
Mark Pearson
Sue Buchanan

Printed and bound by
Printer Industria Gráfica SA
Barcelona, Spain

First published in
Great Britain in 1980 by
Pan Books Ltd
Cavaye Place
London SW10 9PG

ISBN 0 330 26038 3

This book is not intended as a substitute for the medical advice of physicians. The reader should regularly consult a physician in all matters relating to his health and particularly in respect of any symptoms which may require diagnosis or medical attention.

Brain and nerves

Mind and emotions

Eyes

Ear, nose and throat

Lungs

Rectum and anus

Genitals, kidneys and bladder

Women's disorders and childbirth

Pills and potions

Anaesthetics and pain-killers

Surgery

Tests and checks

Medical puzzles

Patients' problems

Index

Introduction

It is supposed to be children who spend all their time peppering their parents and teachers with question marks. 'Why?'; 'Who?'; 'When?'; 'How?'; 'What?' and so on . . . and on and on.

But we are all children, however long we live. Our questions may not come as thick and fast as the years go on, but this does not mean that they are not there bursting to be asked. Some adults don't ask questions because they have been able to find all the answers. There are very few of those. Some don't ask because they are ashamed to display their ignorance. There are a great many of those. Some don't ask because they don't know who to ask. There are quite a lot of them. And some don't ask even though they know who has the answers, for fear of 'being a nuisance', 'looking foolish' 'or wasting time'. And there are a great many of those, too.

This book is mainly for people in the last category. Most of us know we should ask our doctors any questions we may have about how our bodies and minds work but most of us really don't want to impose on them. We see our doctors as busy people who are much too occupied with life-saving to waste their precious time in telling us why we get gooseflesh, or what makes a bruise go blue and yellow and why we wake with a great jump sometimes just as we're falling asleep. In fact, most of the doctors I know would gladly answer such questions. They would make an agreeable change from listening to lists of symptoms. But still, most people won't ask. That is why this book was written – to answer the questions doctors would answer, given the chance.

Throughout this book, I have simplified my task by using the personal pronoun 'he' for both the doctor and patient (except, of course, when dealing with questions on obstetrics and gynaecology). This will no doubt infuriate those feminists who seek for – and constantly find – signs of covert anti-woman bias, but that can't be helped. The form was used for convenience and certainly not as a statement of the 'proper' roles of men and women. Of course there are women doctors (although more are men) and of course there are men patients. But it would be boringly trendy to deliberately reverse the pronouns to 'she' for the doctor and 'he' for the patient – and just as so-called sexist, anyway.

This book is not designed to be an alternative to a doctor's advice and care. Each patient is an individual and needs individual diagnosis, advice and treatment. But a patient who is informed, and who has some understanding of medical matters, is a happier patient than one who is ignorant and therefore more alarmed than he need be. Most doctors prefer dealing with patients who have some correct medical facts, and few today will trot out the boring old adage about a little knowledge being dangerous. Knowledge is always good. This book, I hope, adds some to your store.

Claire Rayner

Brain and nerves

The brain is the control centre of the human organism and the nerves which travel to and from it all over the body make up the nervous system. The word 'nerves' has been somewhat misused in recent years by many patients; symptoms of tension, anxiety and depression have been ascribed to 'bad' or 'weak' nerves. But this is in fact not the case. Nerves have precise and measurable functions, and the creation of anxiety is not among them. Such symptoms are more to do with the function of the mind than with the nerves. Neurology deals with the activity of the brain and nerves and, although a neurologist may be interested in the symptoms of emotional or psychological distress, he will not necessarily be involved with treating them. This is the province of psychiatrists.

The brain and nervous system

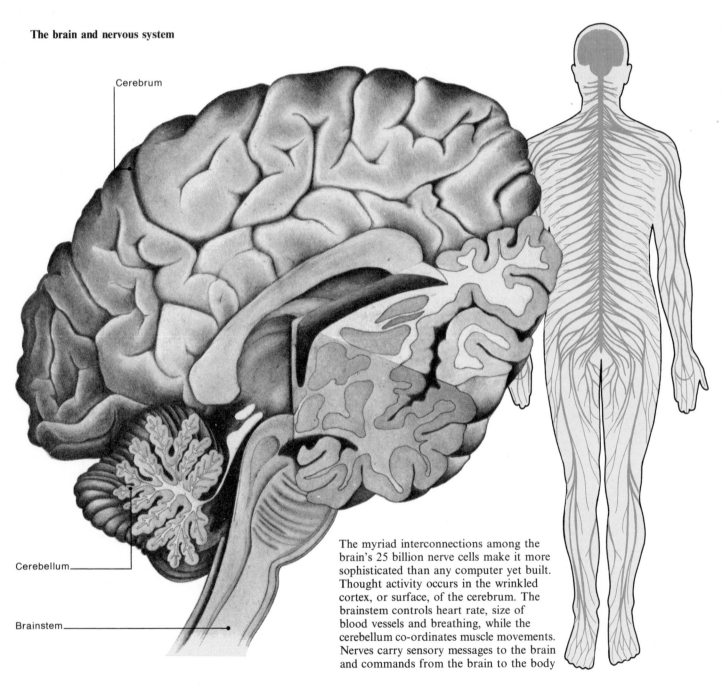

Cerebrum

Cerebellum

Brainstem

The myriad interconnections among the brain's 25 billion nerve cells make it more sophisticated than any computer yet built. Thought activity occurs in the wrinkled cortex, or surface, of the cerebrum. The brainstem controls heart rate, size of blood vessels and breathing, while the cerebellum co-ordinates muscle movements. Nerves carry sensory messages to the brain and commands from the brain to the body

Why are there so many different kinds of pain?

Actually, there are only two kinds of pain messages which are sent from different parts of the body to the brain, where pain is really experienced – fast ones and slow ones. You can check this when you next stub your toe. You will get a sharp, immediate pain followed by a much heftier one that comes after a distinct interval – in fact, you tend to stand tensed, waiting for the second pain to get through to you.

But, of course, we all know that we get many different sorts of sensation which we generally describe as pain. 'Splitting' headaches and 'burning' indigestion and 'stabbing' backache and 'gripping' cramp and so on. All of these descriptions prove one of the oddest facts about pain; it is, in a sense, entirely imaginary.

Pain comes from inside ourselves. It isn't like something we see or touch or smell or hear, so, in a way, it is non-existent. We can only interpret these strange messages that come to our brains from outlying parts of the body in images, comparing them to what we think might be going on inside us. Hence a headache is called 'splitting' although none of us who uses the term are ever likely to have actually felt our skulls split, just as few people who claim

to have a stabbing pain have ever actually had a knife in their vital parts (those who have report that it feels more like a heavy kick than a cut).

This is why emotional distress can result in real pain. When someone who

is deeply unhappy, and therefore has a bellyache is told dismissively, 'it's all in your mind', it is really unfair. The pain of an actual gastric ulcer is also 'all in the mind' and yet both kinds of pain can be equally disagreeable.

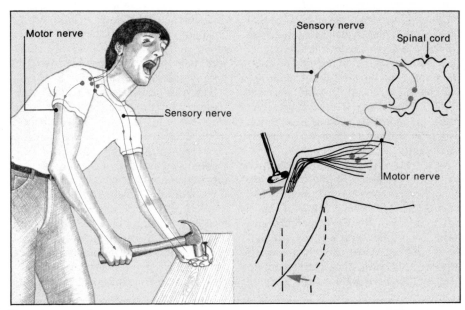

Responses to pain
When pain signals reach the spinal cord, they trigger a reflex signal to withdraw the left hand. Meanwhile, a message is passed to the brain which commands the right hand to withdraw. Another automatic response (*right*) is the knee jerk triggered by a gentle blow – this is checked as part of a routine examination

Why can't pain be remembered? Obviously it isn't, or women, for example, would never have more than one baby.

Although pain itself cannot be remembered, in the sense that it cannot be felt again after it has stopped, the emotions aroused by it are certainly memorable. This is well known by the sort of disciplinarian who thinks that the best way to rear a child in the way you want him to go is to inflict pain by beating. (In some cases it works. The child remembers the unhappiness the pain caused and the feeling of desolation and illness, because pain can make you feel nauseated and weak. If pain is severe enough it leads to shock, which is collapse of the circulation, and the child avoids the behaviour which caused the feeling. In other cases, however, the pain creates such resentment and anger that the child becomes hostile and aggressive and starts hitting out on his own behalf.)

And, of course, we all learn from pain, which proves that we do remember it. Once you have burned your fingers in a fire you are unlikely in the future to touch flame. If you have been hit on the head by walking through a low doorway, you are then inclined to stoop as you go through every other doorway that you come to, however lofty it may be.

The point about women having more than one child when labour is so painful begs the question, however, since it makes the assumption that childbirth is always dire agony. It isn't. Many women say that although the contractions of the uterus and the expulsive movements needed are extremely powerful and exhausting, they are not always registered as disagreeable pain. It can be an intense but pleasant experi-

ence. (This can happen in other sexual activities, too. Some forms of extra vigorous sex play can be painful but they are often regarded as pleasurable because of the associated experience.) So, there is seldom fear of repeating a painful experience when giving birth to another child.

Also, the question of reward comes into it. The woman who really wants a child will probably want it intensely enough to be prepared to tolerate the pain of producing it. It is usually the woman who really does not want a child who rejects a pregnancy, ostensibly for fear of the pain.

Brain and nerves

Why can some people put up with so much more pain than others?
Is it that they are really more brave, or do they feel it less?

Not only is our perception of pain affected by what we imagine is going on inside our bodies, but also our interpretation of what those happenings might mean. We have lively imaginations, and can frighten ourselves stiff just by thinking. For example, a person who feels a dull ache in her belly and who fears it is a sign of cancer will interpret that pain as being much more severe than someone who thinks it is due to swallowing green apples, and so is not at all worried. Fear, in other words, can cause an agonizing pain to one person which by another is regarded as merely mildly unpleasant.

Everyone differs in their reaction to pain. Some people – about five per cent of the world's population – hardly feel pain at all. A classic example of this is described by a British researcher into pain. He found that a small girl had been walking on a broken ankle for days without complaint. The same child also bit her forefinger to the bone in excitement while watching a film, and didn't feel a thing. And, on another occasion, in a rage, she bit pieces out of her tongue and made it bleed like a fountain, although she felt no pain at all.

Most of us are more fortunate than this (fortunate because an inability to feel pain exposes us to the risk of severe injury and illness for which we don't seek help when we should). We feel pain in different degrees.

Try this experiment. Catch your tongue between your teeth, and begin to bite down. At first you will feel no more than a slight 'pricking'; then a mild sensation which you may even regard as pleasant; then, as you increase the pressure, it will feel unpleasant, and, if you keep on, which you shouldn't, or you'll end up like the unfeeling child who bled like a fountain, it will be a hard and exceedingly disagreeable sensation.

This variation in the pain experience accounts for many everyday experiences. Consider for example the difference between getting into a cold bath, registered as unpleasant and even painful, a warm bath, which is felt as very agreeable indeed, and a too hot bath, which hurts horribly.

There are other factors which affect the way people react to pain, apart from their basic sensitivity. There is the cultural factor, for a start. In some parts of the world, stoicism is admired, so a Britisher brought up in the old way will grit his teeth and say nothing in the face of quite severe pain, while a more outgoing Italian, coming from a society where any kind of 'sensitivity' is admired, will roll around and shriek and not lose any of his machismo. This difference shows powerfully in women during childbirth; those reared within the classic northern European puritan ethic will be likely to make little fuss, while the more ebullient Mediterranean women will protest alarmingly. (Probably the latter emerge from the experience in better psychological

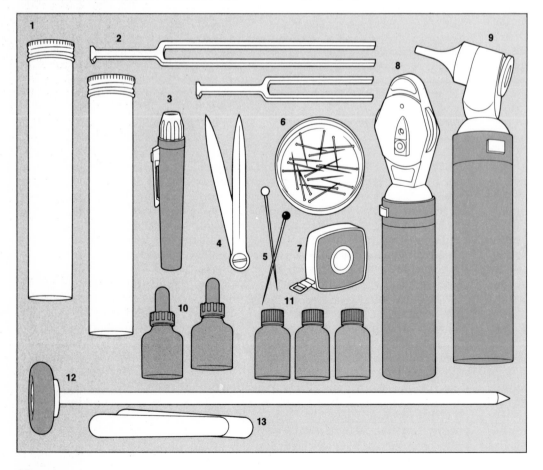

Instruments for testing the nervous system
The skin's sensitivity can be judged simply by brushing a cotton swab over it. The instruments shown here may also be used. **1** Metal cylinders, filled with hot and cold water when testing temperature perception. **2** Tuning forks for testing hearing. **3** Pen torch for examination of throat and eyes. **4** Calipers for measuring the ability to distinguish two points touching the skin. **5** Large pins to act as targets when finding limits of visual field. **6** Pins for testing sensation. **7** Tape measure to check for limb-wasting due to nerve defects. **8** Ophthalmoscope to examine eyes. **9** Otoscope to examine ears. **10** Eye drops. **11** Bottles containing oil of cloves, peppermint etc., to test the sense of smell. **12** Rubber hammer for testing knee jerk and other reflexes. **13** Tongue depressors

condition because repression is not always healthy behaviour.)

Personality differences matter, too. Research has shown that extroverts – lively, cheerful, outgoing types – seem to have a higher pain threshold (they can suffer more unpleasant stimuli before they feel pain) than introverts, who have low pain thresholds. However, the extroverts tend to complain sooner than the more stoical introverts, so both kinds of people, when they are hospital patients and in pain, are likely to get help for their pain at about the same time, though one group clearly suffers more than the other.

There is also the effect of concurrent experience. For example, a soldier in a battle or a football player in the heat of the game may go on functioning at top level, unaware of the fact that he has a bullet in his leg, or a broken ankle from that last tackle. Often it is only when the excitement is over that the pain registers.

Counter-irritants – sensation of another sort – help as well. That is why a mother will rub a child's hurt place to soothe it, and why applying heat or cold or an irritant reduces the pain. The pain hasn't actually been lessened; something else has been put in its way. And then there is the effect of possible reward. It has been noticed that people who have been injured and who may be entitled to legal damages experience more pain than those with similar injuries who have no hope of any reward for their sufferings. The former people are not 'putting on' the agony (well, not always) – they genuinely do feel their pain, because it is being encouraged.

Children may suffer a lot of pain because they have mothers who only react positively to them when they complain of pain. Many people, reared by such negative mothering to enjoy ill health, go through a lot of misery as a result.

___

Why is it that unimportant things like a hangnail can hurt dreadfully, but really dangerous illness, like cancer in its early stages, does not hurt at all?

Not all parts of the body are sensitive to pain. The bones are not, although their outer coatings are intensely so. The interior of solid organs such as the liver and kidneys are insensitive although structures near them are sensitive (which is why you don't get pain from a kidney stone while it is in the kidney, but you do when the stone moves into the tube leading to the bladder, which does have sensation). And the brain, although it is the organ where pain from everywhere else in the body is registered, is itself insensitive. It is possible to operate painlessly on the brain of a fully conscious person, as long as local anaesthetics are used on the scalp and the periosteum (bone covering) of the skull, which are very sensitive.

The fingertips are particularly sensitive, which is why we are such a dextrous species. This means that the fingertips are also more sensitive to pain, so fairly minor injury to the finger can be excruciatingly painful while a more severe injury in a less sensitive place, for example the skin of the middle of the back, is much less disturbing.

Early cancer is painless, unless it occurs in tissues which are sensitive, because the cells themselves have no nerve fibres to carry messages to the brain. It is only when a growth is large enough to press on adjacent sensitive structures or invade them, that it registers its presence with pain.

___

I am expecting my first baby in a month's time, and everything is going well, except for one problem – I have developed weakness and tingling of the first two fingers and thumb of my right hand, together with pain in my wrist, and it really drives me mad sometimes – the tingling wakes me in the night. The doctor says it will get better by itself after the baby is born, but I am very puzzled about this.

It is called 'carpal tunnel syndrome' and it can indeed be tiresome. It tends to be worse in the mornings, when you first get up, and it is the classic reason why pregnant women drop things. It is caused by the nerve supply and tendons that serve the hand having to pass from the forearm through a narrow tunnel made of bone and fibrous tissue. If there is any swelling of the hand and the wrist, the tunnel is, naturally enough, narrowed, so the nerves and tendons in it are pinched. There is weakness and tingling – the nerves' response to their constriction. The condition – called edema – is common in pregnancy. You were wise to tell your doctor because the symptom can be a warning that there is the sort of edema which may indicate the condition called pre-eclampsia. However, clearly, you have none of the other symptoms of this condition, such as raised blood pressure or traces of protein in your urine (these checks are made regularly through pregnancy) so you need not worry. And it is true – the symptom nearly always disappears completely soon after delivery.

Hangnail

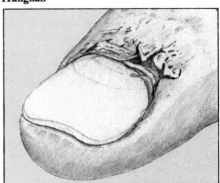

Brain and nerves

Why does a blow on the head cause concussion? And what is concussion?

The brain does not fit inside the skull as tightly as toothpaste in a full tube. There is a small amount of space which allows the brain to enlarge a little from time to time. This is necessary because brain cells, like other body cells, are flexible and respond to the body's internal climate, which changes all the time.

So, sometimes cells are a little saggy and sometimes they are plump with extra fluid, and the space between the skull and brain allows for this.

If the skull is moved rapidly – say, as you shake your head from side to side – the brain within it is not affected unduly. But if the speed of skull movement is rapid, like the sudden violent hitting of the head on the windshield in a car crash, with the possible force in excess of about 28 feet per second, then the brain is definitely affected. There may be minute damage to some of the tiniest blood vessels (the capillaries). There also may be some damage to the walls of some of the cells. And, as is common after any sort of injury, there is likely to be an increase of fluid (edema) in the cells. All of which results in loss of consciousness, which can be so short as to be almost unnoticed or so long that there is great anxiety about whether the sufferer will ever come round; some loss of memory, usually for the period immediately before the injury which caused the concussion; headache, nausea, and vomiting, and unsteadiness of gait and depression.

It must be said that some people who have suffered concussion show few or none of these symptoms. But of one thing you can be certain; those scenes which you see in films, or read about in novels, in which someone is felled with a wallop on the back of the neck or a swift right to the jaw (both of which can cause the brain shaking which leads to concussion, in the same way as a direct head blow) and comes round after a few minutes of unconsciousness with no further symptoms at all and is immediately able to return to the fray, are so much nonsense.

Concussion severe enough to cause unconsciousness of more than a minute or so leaves someone far from fit to recover the king's jewels or clobber the wicked foreign spy the moment he comes round. However, it is true that some people are less ill immediately after being concussed than they are some time later. Symptoms can increase in severity over succeeding hours and even days, which is why it is essential to keep a close watch on people who have experienced the condition.

Incidentally, frequent episodes of concussion, of the sort suffered by boxers and over-eager players of other sports in which the head may be hit, can cause progressive brain damage so that the person ends up 'punch drunk' – permanently limited in intellect and other brain functions.

Brain damage from a blow
Concussion results when the head receives a blow. The brain is thrown against the inner surface of the skull and some of its cells are damaged, perhaps irreversibly

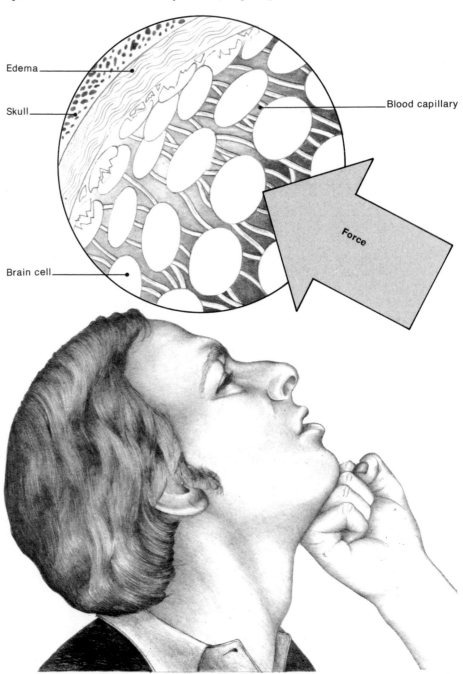

Edema

Skull

Blood capillary

Force

Brain cell

Is it true that women taste things differently from men?

Gender does indeed make a difference. There seems to be a link between taste sensitivity and female hormone levels and when these levels change dramatically, as in pregnancy, taste demands vary equally remarkably. This is part of the reason why pregnant women get cravings for some foods, especially sour ones (the other probable cause is the need for extra supplies of certain food substances that the brain recognizes and signals as cravings).

And, of course, culture has an effect. If you are an Asian child of either gender, weaned on spicy curry, you will grow up with a desire for powerful flavours and find the more bland tastes of some Western foods tedious.

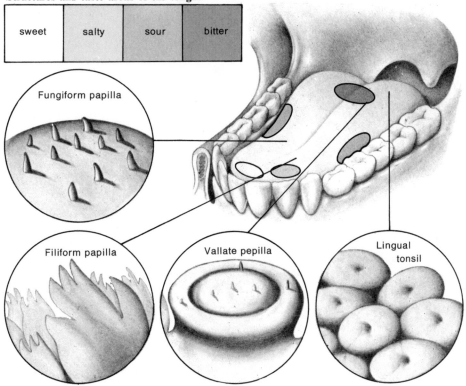

Structures and taste areas of the tongue

sweet	salty	sour	bitter

Fungiform papilla

Filiform papilla

Vallate pepilla

Lingual tonsil

When I was a child I loathed bitter tastes and loved sweet tastes. Now I'm completely the other way round. Does taste sensation go on changing with age?

Taste certainly does vary with age.

We recognize flavours via small structures in the tongue, called taste buds, of which we have about 10,000. They respond to four different flavours. Those at the tip of the tongue register sweetness; those at the sides, sourness; those at the back, bitterness; and all of them respond to saltiness.

Children have more taste buds than adults and tend to greatly prefer sweetness, partly because of their larger number of responsive buds, and partly because they use up great amounts of energy, and their blood sugar tends to be more volatile – children need extra replenishment more often than adults. The brain signals a sugar hunger when energy needs topping up; hence the 'childish' delight in lollipops.

In adult life, however, the bitterness taste buds seem to become more dominant, and account for the 'sophisticated' desire for dry sherry and olives. But as people get older still their tip-of-the-tongue taste buds become less sensitive and they need more of a substance to be able to recognize its flavour. So, 70-year-olds may want more sweetness than they did when they were 40.

When I run a lot and get breathless, especially in cold weather all my lower teeth hurt. Why is this?

This is partly due to referred sensation and partly due to direct stimulation of pain nerves in the teeth themselves. When you need extra air, you always open your mouth to take it in because the nose does not allow enough of an entry for you. The teeth, usually kept warm inside the mouth, are then exposed to the bite of the cold air and may respond by hurting. This, as a rule, is not because there is anything wrong with the teeth but is just that teeth are sensitive, being well supplied with nerves. It's the same sort of response that you get from eating ice cream.

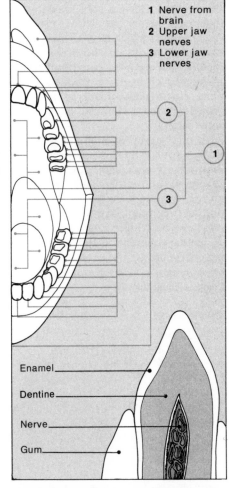

1 Nerve from brain
2 Upper jaw nerves
3 Lower jaw nerves

Enamel
Dentine
Nerve
Gum

Nerve supply to the teeth and mouth
Two nerves lead to each molar, but only one to each of the other teeth. Enamel, the hardest substance of the body, protects the bonelike dentine of the teeth

Brain and nerves

Why does eating cheese give me a migraine headache, though I know other migraine sufferers who are not bothered by cheese.

Migraine – the headache which affects half of the head rather than the whole of it – is a complex and disagreeable affliction which troubles about five per cent of the population, three-quarters of the sufferers being women.

It is known that it is associated with considerable dilation of the blood vessels on the affected side of the head; that the dilation is the probable cause of the banging pain, the flashing lights before the eyes, the nausea and vomiting and all the other disagreeable symptoms that go with it.

The causes of the blood vessel dilation are many, and one is an error of brain metabolism. Certain substances, when digested, throw out waste products (metabolites) which have a direct effect on blood vessels in the brain. These metabolites are most commonly found in foods such as dairy products, chocolate, citrus foods such as oranges and grapefruit, tea and coffee, alcohol and some others.

In one survey of migraine sufferers it was found that 74 per cent were sensitive to chocolate, four per cent to cheese and other dairy products, and 32 per cent to citrus fruits. So different people have different food allergies, or trigger causes which are altogether different, as the accompanying chart shows.

Causes of migraine

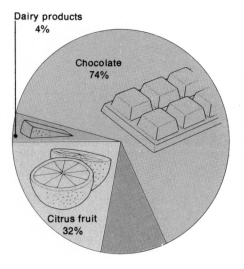

Dairy products 4%

Chocolate 74%

Citrus fruit 32%

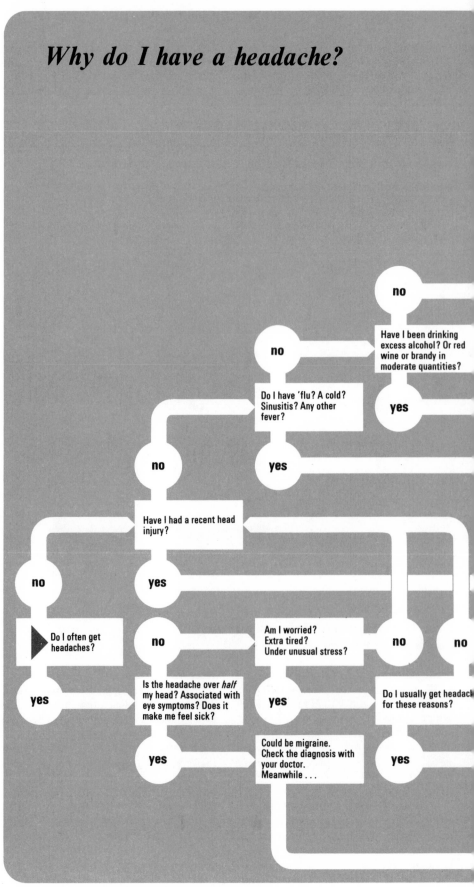

Why do I have a headache?

no — Have I been drinking excess alcohol? Or red wine or brandy in moderate quantities? — yes

no — Do I have 'flu? A cold? Sinusitis? Any other fever? — yes

no

Have I had a recent head injury? — yes

no

Do I often get headaches? — yes

no — Am I worried? Extra tired? Under unusual stress? — yes — no — no

Is the headache over *half* my head? Associated with eye symptoms? Does it make me feel sick? — yes

Do I usually get headache for these reasons? — yes

Could be migraine. Check the diagnosis with your doctor. Meanwhile . . .

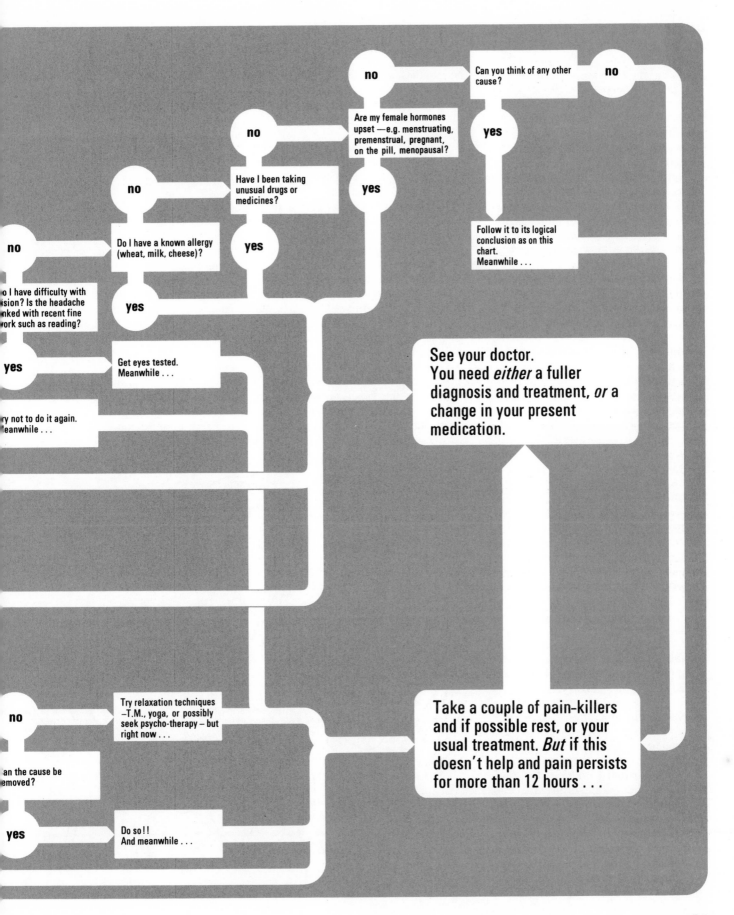

no

Can you think of any other cause?

no

no

Are my female hormones upset —e.g. menstruating, premenstrual, pregnant, on the pill, menopausal?

yes

no

Have I been taking unusual drugs or medicines?

yes

yes

Follow it to its logical conclusion as on this chart. Meanwhile . . .

no

Do I have a known allergy (wheat, milk, cheese)?

yes

no

o I have difficulty with ision? Is the headache nked with recent fine work such as reading?

yes

Get eyes tested. Meanwhile . . .

See your doctor. You need *either* a fuller diagnosis and treatment, *or* a change in your present medication.

ry not to do it again. eanwhile . . .

no

Try relaxation techniques –T.M., yoga, or possibly seek psycho-therapy – but right now . . .

Take a couple of pain-killers and if possible rest, or your usual treatment. *But* if this doesn't help and pain persists for more than 12 hours . . .

an the cause be emoved?

yes

Do so!! And meanwhile . . .

Brain and nerves

What causes trembling? Why does it happen more in some diseases, for example in Parkinson's disease?

Muscles operate in a complex way. They are made of many bundles of elastic fibres which can tighten up, and also become fatter and shorter. When they are fat and short, they are like a steel spring, storing up energy. When they flatten, they release the energy.

A muscle does not contract all at once. Different fibre bundles contract at different times, micro-seconds apart, to give smooth and continuous action. To do this, the muscles need stimulation from a nerve, which carries messages to and from the brain.

Nerves operate like electro-chemical machines. They convert molecules of body chemicals into electric impulses which go along the nerves from the brain – which is also an electro-chemical machine – to trigger muscle action, and then also back the other way to keep the brain informed of the fact that the work demanded is being done. So there is a complex control system involving the brain, and also another control system – the endocrine glands. A hormone made in one of these glands, adrenalin, has a powerful direct effect on the muscles. If a person is alarmed by any sort of threat, his adrenal glands, themselves stimulated by the brain, shoot out large quantities of adrenalin. This immediately moves around the body in the bloodstream and acts on a large number of structures, including the muscles. It tenses the bundles of fibres, making them store up energy ready to cope with the outside threat and it makes them do it at great speed. In other words, it primes the person to either deal directly with the threat or to escape from it. It has been called the 'fight or flight' response.

There are lots of other effects of adrenalin but this muscle tensing is important, because it is one of the first effects of adrenalin. However, adrenalin does not instruct the muscles in what to do; the brain must do that. But both brain and adrenalin ensure that the muscles are bombarded with messages with impulses to act.

It is this bombardment which probably causes the effect of trembling that is a part of fear. The tense muscles, responding to both adrenalin and brain messages by contracting and relaxing the bundles of fibres at great speed, ripple with activity, and unless the person is using the energy to run away or stand and fight, it is registered as a fine shaking.

Later, as the first wave of adrenalin wears off and the tensing effect is lost, the muscles respond fairly slowly, not relaxing smoothly but jerkily. Which is why trembling can be worse after a threat has subsided than at its height. A person who narrowly avoids a road accident will cope well while he has to, and then will dissolve into a shaking jelly once the danger is past.

There is another kind of muscular shaking that is due to cold. In this, the section of the brain which acts as the body's thermostat registers a dangerous chill, and needs more heat.

When muscles burn up sugar and oxygen to do work, heat is a by-product and so, for this function, working the muscles warms the body. The body's thermostat sends messages to the muscles to contract and relax at speed, thus creating extra heat. The effect is shivering – the teeth-chattering shaking that happens automatically when the outside temperature drops sharply and affects our inner temperature.

The trembling due to conditions such as Parkinson's disease is something quite different. This happens because there is failure of the parts of the brain and the nerves which carry the contract-relax messages to the muscles. The messages come through unevenly, and the result is uneven contraction and relaxation – trembling. There can be trembling in other illnesses which is not due to brain or nervous system damage. For example, trembling is a feature of an overactive thyroid. When one endocrine gland is overactive, the others are put out of harmony too; the cause in this case is extra adrenalin.

The trembling of old age is probably due to a gradual loss both of the ability of the brain and nerves to transmit impulses smoothly, and of the aging muscles to respond smoothly.

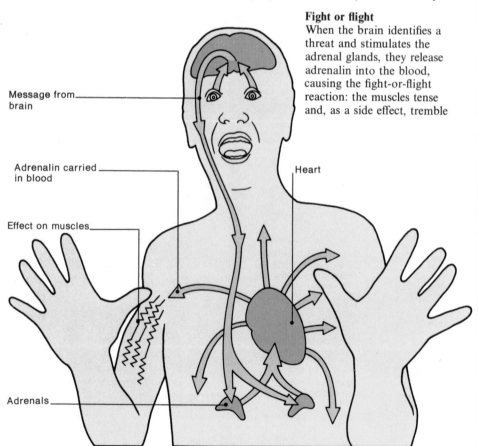

Fight or flight
When the brain identifies a threat and stimulates the adrenal glands, they release adrenalin into the blood, causing the fight-or-flight reaction: the muscles tense and, as a side effect, tremble

Message from brain

Adrenalin carried in blood

Effect on muscles

Adrenals

Heart

Can the damage from strokes be cured?

That depends on the cause of the original accident, and on the degree of damage.

For example, if the problem is a widespread narrowing of the blood vessels due to loss of elasticity in the walls of the blood vessels (arteriosclerosis) associated with high blood pressure, then all that can be done is to try to keep the blood pressure at a safely low level to encourage as rich a blood supply as possible to the brain. If, on the other hand, the cause is a blockage of one vessel, which can be identified by the use of modern X-ray techniques, it may be possible to remove the block, or to replace the useless vessel with a graft.

If the stroke is caused by a brain haemorrhage which is pressing on the brain tissue, then an operation to remove the clotted blood will relieve the pressure and, with it, its effects.

Usually, it has to be said, it is not possible to do much by means of surgery. The majority of stroke patients (and in Britain alone this is a total of 125,000 a year) need help to cope with the effects of the stroke rather than dramatic surgery to reverse the original accident. And a great deal can be done. The human brain is resilient and underused; there are large areas which, as far as researchers can tell at present, have no obvious function and which appear to be available for use if other sections fail. It has been found that, with devoted care and patient retraining, people who seem to have lost the use of legs and arms and speech can be rehabilitated to a remarkable degree, as other brain cells take over the work of the lost ones. A famous case was that of the actress Patricia Neal, who was left paralyzed and unconscious and speechless after a stroke and yet, with skilled physiotherapy and medical treatment as well as the untiring encouragement of her husband and the help of lots of her friends and neighbours, became a fully functioning and successful person again.

What causes a stroke?

Strokes – which were so-called because they seem to happen so suddenly – result when a portion of the brain is starved of its vital blood supply because of some sort of accident involving the blood vessels in the area. In fact, a stroke is not all that sudden; there will usually have been weeks, even years of disorder leading up to it.

Perhaps the blood vessels silt up with a fatty material which deposits plaques on their walls. This narrows the space through which blood can travel and one day, as a little more plaque is laid down, the blockage is complete.

Perhaps small clots form on the plaques, and are swept off and onwards into a smaller blood vessel which they can then block.

Perhaps the walls of the vessels lose some of their elasticity with advancing age, and fail to enlarge sufficiently in response to a need for extra blood, and so block the supply, and possibly the hardened walls have tiny weakened areas which break down and allow blood to escape and cause pressure on the surrounding brain tissue.

Whatever the accident – and the modern medical label for a stroke is CVA (cerebro-vascular accident) – the effect of quite a small stroke can sometimes be catastrophic and it's not surprising that people used to blame Providence for striking them so heavy a blow. However, many sufferers from strokes manage very well indeed.

Why do some people who have had strokes become half paralyzed?

The brain, comparatively small though it is – the liver is much larger – controls a great deal of the body's activities. Certainly, it controls motor activity (movement) and sensory experience (feelings of touch and pressure) and it does this in clearly defined areas of the brain. The larger part of the brain (the cerebrum) is divided in half, and each half has areas which control different sections of their own half of the body. But, and this is important, the body halves which are controlled by the brain halves are opposite to each other. The right brain controls the left leg, arm and so on, and the left brain looks after the right side.

When a CVA results in starvation or damage of a section of the right brain, and if it is the section which is involved with movement and sensation from the left arm and leg, the result will be failure of their activities – paralysis of the muscles which control movement, and loss of feeling.

Sometimes the paralysis involves only some muscles, so there may be movement of part of the leg or arm, but it is sluggish and awkward. Sometimes, there may be involvement of only some of the sensory pathways, so the result is only partly impaired sensation. The degree of loss is directly linked with the degree of damage in the brain, and expert doctors can map the situation in the brain by careful study of the effects on the body, and sometimes suggest surgery.

Why do people who have had strokes lose the ability to talk?

Not all of them do. It depends on which side of the brain has been affected by the interruption in a normal blood supply. If it is the right side, with left-sided paralysis, then speech patterns will usually not be affected, because it is the left brain which has the control of speech.

But note that word 'usually' because there are some people who are actually different. About 15 per cent of left-handed people and two per cent of right-handed people (and handedness is also controlled by opposite brain halves) have speech centres in both halves of the brain. And about half of all left-handed people have their speech centres on the left, not on the right, as might be expected. So there can be considerable variation from case to case.

Brain and nerves

What causes itching? And why does scratching relieve it?

An itch is really a minor pain. It is a sensory response to stimulation, and if it is intense enough it is registered as pain. It can be caused by the same things as pain although obviously to a much lesser degree – where a soft rub from a finger tip on your hand makes you itch, a hard scraping can hurt. The reason for this is that itching is the result of stimulation of the top surface of the skin (the epidermis) while pain results from stimulation of the deeper layers (the dermis).

Other causes are psychogenic – the brain is a sensitive and subtle organ which can respond in many different ways, and one of these is by translating an observed experience into a felt one. Nothing is as likely to make you itch as seeing someone else scratch. Even reading about itching can stimulate it. An account of a man sitting tied to a chair, with several soft-footed butterflies walking on his bare arms or fluttering their wings in his face, while feathers drift lazily around his bare legs and feet, can be enough to make a sensitive, imaginative reader break into an orgy of scratching. (Did it happen to you reading this?)

As for the reason for scratching – this is done to overwhelm the delicate sensation of itching with a more powerful one. Scratching can hurt if it goes on too long, as we all know. Over-stimulating the nerves by causing a small scratch pain is enough to cancel out the itch sensation. It may also be linked with the production of endorphins, the natural pain-killing substances which the body creates in response to painful stimuli.

When my brother had his heart attack he got pain in his left shoulder. Why does it hurt in this place?

Firstly, remember that pain is not felt at the site where it seems to be, but in the brain. And the messages the brain registers may not always be precisely accurate as to the location of the original stimulus.

Development of the body organs

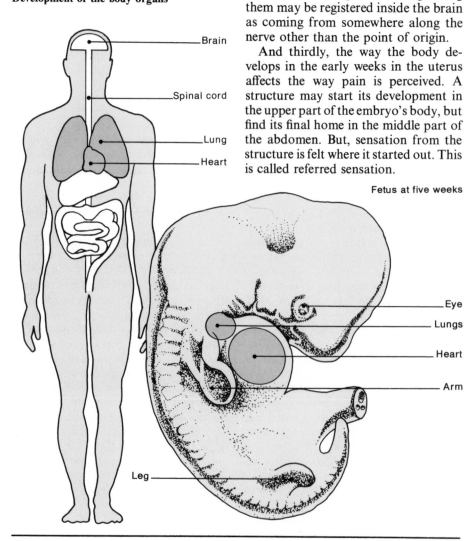

Fetus at five weeks

Secondly, the nerves which carry pain messages are complex and often very long; some important nerves from the base of the chest up towards the inner nerve sections of the spinal column and the brain have many branches going off them. So, messages travelling along them may be registered inside the brain as coming from somewhere along the nerve other than the point of origin.

And thirdly, the way the body develops in the early weeks in the uterus affects the way pain is perceived. A structure may start its development in the upper part of the embryo's body, but find its final home in the middle part of the abdomen. But, sensation from the structure is felt where it started out. This is called referred sensation.

Why do I get pins and needles in my hand in the morning, if I've been sleeping with my arm under me?

When your muscles are not being instructed to work to do a particular job their bundles of fibres are still contracting and relaxing in a fairly regular pattern. This is what maintains muscle tone; none of us are ever completely flaccid. To ensure this tone, the nerves must carry messages in a steady stream and if the nerve is compressed in any way, those messages cannot get through.

Also, the muscle needs a steady supply of blood carried to it by the blood vessels. If a weight is put on a limb so that the message and the blood cannot get through, the result is numbness of the limb and often pain. As soon as the pressure is released, the messages and blood start to come through again but it takes a little time for the rhythmic contraction and relaxation of the various fibres to be restored, and it is this period of restoration that is experienced as tingling – pins and needles – as numbness gives way to complete sensation once more.

Why do I get hiccups? What can I do to get rid of them?

This is one of those oddities of human experience which are not entirely explicable. We do know that irritation of the stomach can stimulate the nerve (the phrenic nerve) that supplies this area and this then transmits rhythmic extra impulses, causing the diaphragm (the huge muscle sheet that lies between stomach and chest) to go into rhythmic spasm. The muscles between the ribs (the intercostals) are also affected and they, too, produce these rhythmic spasms.

But the initial irritation is not always in the stomach. It may occur in the 'hiccuping centre' in the brain, an area which seems to control this sort of reflex movement; or it may be linked with disorders in the neck and chest, ranging from enlarged glands via tumours, both benign and malignant,

to coronary thrombosis. It can happen as a result of abdominal disorders, too, such as peritonitis, following an operation, or kidney failure. It can also be triggered by emotional experiences such as sudden shock or prolonged stress.

So, to sort out your hiccups you have to know the cause – and unless they are linked with another illness (in which case your doctor's treatment would be aimed at the hiccups as well as the illness) the likelihood is that the problem is in your stomach. Eating too much can give you hiccups. So can eating unusually spicy foods, or drinking alcohol (a common and well-known cause), or swallowing foods which are too hot or too cold.

Once you have identified a possible cause for your attacks you are better able to control the problem by avoiding

the cause in future. But if you can't, and an attack starts, just try the different folk remedies which are all aimed at altering the nerve response, until you find one that works.

For some people, breathing in carbon dioxide helps because it suppresses the brain's hiccuping centre. The easiest way to do that is to keep breathing the same air in and out of a paper bag.

Or, try breath-holding, which sometimes breaks into the hiccuping rhythm and so stops it; or try applying sudden cold or noise as a shock, which again can break the rhythm.

Only if the problem persists for a long time, and you begin to feel exhausted and tense, need you see your doctor for more complex treatment, which can include the use of special drugs or even giving a light anaesthetic.

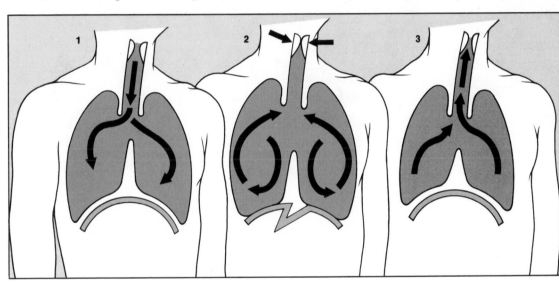

What causes hiccups
1 As a normal breath is drawn in, the sheet of muscle (the diaphragm) at the floor of the chest moves down, causing the lungs to expand and suck in air. **2** Then the diaphragm twitches and air is gulped in; but the glottis snaps shut, cutting off the air flow and making the typical hiccup sound. **3** Finally the glottis opens, the diaphragm relaxes and air is breathed out

What causes twitching? My eyelids sometimes twitch and my son has a frequent twitch which pulls up the corners of his mouth.

A muscular movement happens in response to messages from the brain, along nerve pathways, telling the fibres to contract and relax. Sometimes the message starts on its way because the conscious mind decides it wants to do something, to wink, for example, and sometimes because it is a necessary and routine movement such as blinking. Sometimes, however, there is a message sent for no immediate reason – as in the case of your eyelid twitch. For some reason of which you are unaware, the

nerve is stimulated and the muscle responds. It is usually a short-lived experience, and ends as the unknown stimulation switches itself off.

However, the sort of twitch your son has is different. This is called a tic and it starts out as a series of conscious movements. A worried or nervous person may, out of embarrassment and tension, operate a series of muscles, perhaps those lifting the corner of the mouth, or those turning the head to one side, as a form of something-to-do-

activity, rather as a cat suddenly pretends to wash itself when in fact it isn't at all serious about settling down to the job. In time, this trick, which provides a sort of emotional comfort, becomes almost unconscious; the person does it without realizing it, and so cannot control it, and this can become a distressing problem. Your son may need psychological help to overcome his tic, but it is exceedingly unlikely to be due to any basic malfunction of either muscle or nerve supply.

Mind and emotions

We know a great deal about the way the human body works. Over the past few hundred years men have studied its structure (anatomy) and activities (physiology) so that today although we by no means know all there is to know we have a fairly clear picture of what happens to our physical selves.

Our psychological selves, however, are far less well understood. Some of the workings of the psyche, the human mind, are as mysterious to us as they were to our forbears in Biblical times. But, slowly, researchers are unravelling its convolutions, and giving all of us more insights into our behaviour.

Depression is a problem that affects almost everyone at some time. It can often be a natural consequence of money worries, rows with the boss at work, the responsibility of caring for children or old people, alcohol abuse, and grief. Occasionally depression occurs spontaneously, without an obvious outside trigger

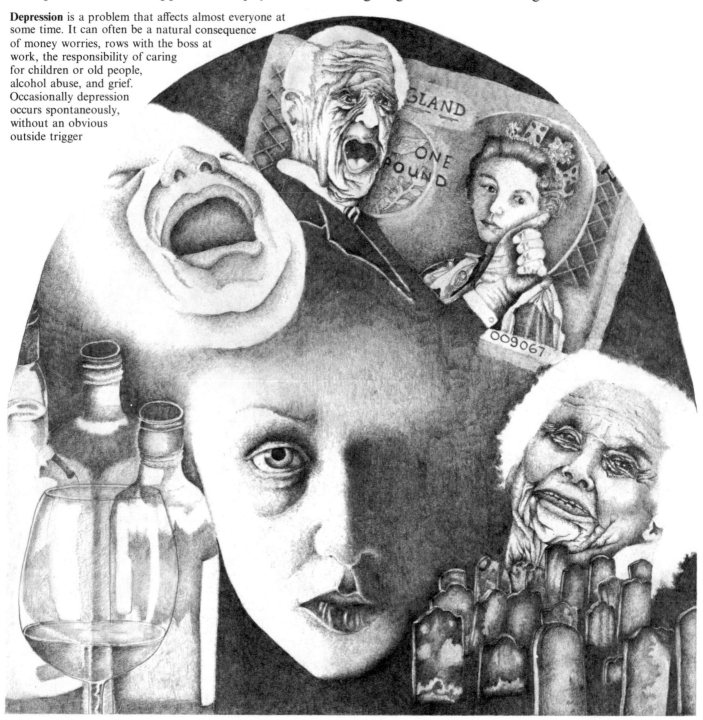

Why do some people suffer from depression for no apparent reason?

Depression is a horrid illness. It has a range of some of the nastiest symptoms anyone can ever suffer – feelings of flatness, worthlessness and deep unhappiness; sleep and appetite disturbance; and, in many cases, suicidal thoughts. This is why depression is a potentially fatal illness. Sometimes, sufferers from acute depression actually do succeed in committing suicide.

It used to be thought by doctors that there were two kinds of depression – exogenous and endogenous. The first kind, they said, was due to some outside trigger – a bereavement, a loss of any kind, such as a finished love affair, a broken home, an examination which someone wants to pass but fails, money problems – and was a normal healthy reaction to unhappy experiences. A person who did not lose his appetite, become sleepless for a while, and find himself unable to concentrate on work after the death of a beloved wife, would be regarded as very strange indeed.

It was the second kind of depression – endogenous – that doctors said was an illness; they saw it coming from inside, linked with no apparent outside trigger. They said it was similar to the sort of depression that afflicts people suffering from the severe mental illness of manic-depressive psychosis. This is a strange and distressing disorder in which a person swings from the depths of despair to the heights of excitement, often according to a rigid time structure. The illness is not yet fully understood, but is thought to be due to a fault in brain metabolism. Nowadays, it can be controlled by medicines but, in the past, sufferers often spent their entire lives incarcerated in mental hospitals because of it.

Endogenous depression was similar, the doctors said, to manic-depressive psychosis. It, too, is due to a fault in the brain chemistry. The doctors' views were supported by the fact that some forms of physical treatment gave dramatic relief to the afflicted person. It was noticed, for example, that people who suffered from epilepsy as well as 'endogenous' depression got over their depressive symptoms more quickly if they experienced fits. So experimenters deliberately induced fits in some of their depressed patients by using electric shocks and found that these often gave dramatic relief.

Then, certain medicines were discovered to have an effect on depression. Some of them, which were primarily used to treat TB (for example, isoniazid-INAH), were discovered to have the side effect of raising a patient's spirits, so chemically related medicines were developed from these. They seemed to act by altering the behaviour of an enzyme called monoamine oxidase – they were labelled monoamine oxidase inhibitors (MAOIs for short) – and they made the treatment of depressed people much simpler. Instead of months of misery waiting for the depression to lift by itself, which it eventually did, a course of tablets ended it.

Later, other medicines called the tricyclic compounds were developed which were simpler to use and more effective for some patients.

All of these medicines have their effect by altering brain chemistry, which raises the question – is depression caused by brain chemistry disorder, or does the depression itself cause the disorder? Psychiatrists are still arguing about this question, but more and more of them are coming round to the idea that there is no real difference between the endogenous and exogenous types of depression. The difference lies in the personality of the patient. One person is the phlegmatic coping kind who only suffers from symptoms when a really severe and recognizable blow such as a bereavement is inflicted. Another person is much more sensitive to emotional buffets and even one so small that the patient him or herself (let alone anyone else) cannot identify it, is enough to create a severe depressive attack.

Women appear to be more vulnerable to depression than men and their vulnerability is linked to their hormone status. They may become depressed around the time of the menstrual period as the progesterone–estrogen balance changes or after the birth of a baby (post-birth 'blues' are extremely common) and at the menopause (although the depression of this age group could be as much an effect of aging). Help for the hormone disorders can sometimes relieve the depression.

One thing is sure. No one today should ever struggle with the symptoms of depression without help. Medicines are available for the more distressing cases, and they can and should be used. Unfortunately, many depressed patients are so depressed that they do not even feel entitled to ask for help, and so they don't try to talk to their doctors about their problems. It is then up to their relatives to realize what is happening and to seek medical and perhaps psychiatric help for them.

What does a psychiatrist actually do? The patient just talks and the doctor just listens, after all.

There is more to psychiatry than the 'talking treatment', valuable though that is. Many psychiatrists use more physical methods such as medicines and ECT, while others are interested in 'behaviourism' in which a patient is taught to change his behaviour by means of reward and punishment, and also retraining of reflexes. An example of the latter is the treatment of bedwetting; a person can be trained to wake when his bladder is full by means of a system which causes a buzzer to sound when he starts to pass water in bed. This, used together with rewards given for every dry night, can remove the symptom in a matter of a few weeks. Similar techniques have been used for drug addicts and alcoholics and people with sexual problems.

Some psychiatrists use group treatments – encouraging patients to explore their problems by talking in a group with other patients. Others are wedded to a particular form of psychotherapy (the talking treatment) which seeks to analyze their patients' symptoms according to the ideas of Freud or Jung or Klein, or one of the other great fathers (or mothers) of psychiatry. Many psychiatrists, and probably they are the best, are eclectic, using different methods for different patients according to their particular needs.

Mind and emotions

Do children get depression?

Almost certainly, yes. First of all they are subject to as much stress as any adult – and very often more. There is a whole mythology that says that being a child is marvellous, that it is carefree and easy – the 'happiest days of life'. But if you think about it honestly you will see that it is anything but. Children are under constant pressure to change their natural attitudes and behaviour, to conform to a social norm which they do not fully understand or care about – all of which is called 'being raised'. They have to learn an enormous amount in terms of facts, concepts and skills – a process called education – and they have to learn to cope with their own powerful and often painful inner experiences.

The incredible thing is that so many children pass through these growing years with so little apparent difficulty and not that a few suffer from the response we call depression.

Depression rarely shows itself in the adult form in the child, which makes life difficult both for the child and the people caring for him. A baby, for example, does not get moody. But he may become fretful, refuse to feed, sleep badly, cry a great deal and be hard to pacify. Many causes will be suggested, ranging from 'wind' to 'teething', both of which are likely to be erroneous and are rarely the most likely cause, which is the mother's state of mind. A depressed mother passes on her condition to her baby. He is a most accurate barometer of the pressures she is experiencing. Since a large number of mothers suffer from post-birth depression, it is clear that a large number of babies do, too.

Childhood depression also rarely shows as a form of flattening and withdrawal, which is the adult symptom. It is more likely to appear as noisiness, aggressiveness, fretfulness, grizzling, food refusal, sleep difficulties, including pants wetting and soiling, stealing, lying, bullying, most of which forms of behaviour are regarded by adults as 'naughtiness' and are treated accordingly. The child responds to punishment and/or disapproval by becoming more depressed, shows more of the symptoms, gets more punishment, and is well on the way to becoming a 'problem child' unless he is fortunate enough to recover from his depression without help.

A most difficult time for depressive illness is adolescence. The process of metamorphosis from child to adult is almost as dramatic as that of a caterpillar to butterfly; yet adolescents get scant respect for the problems they face. Their depression – which may show as sulkiness, slatternliness, wild enthusiasm alternating with deep lethargy – tends to be seen as sheer villainy and not as the painful symptoms of a depressive episode.

It must be repeated: the remarkable thing is that so many young people grow into successful adults, not that a few have problems.

Should depressed children be given medicines like adults?

If depression is diagnosed, medicines may seem to be the best answer. Each child, in the same way as each adult, needs individual assessment. Many children do respond well to medicines and recover rapidly when they are used. But most children also benefit from counselling – the chance to talk out their anxieties and needs with a sympathetic but emotionally uninvolved outsider. Good school medical services these days frequently provide such help.

Does being highly strung run in families?

Yes, because the genes that affect the basic personality are handed on. So some children of a sensitive parent will be equally sensitive, though another child in the family may inherit a more phlegmatic nature from a grandparent.

Also, environments run in families, in that each member shares the same home. So they share the same nurture as well as some of the same nature.

Can you get addicted to tranquillizers?

Yes. There are some people who develop a physical dependence on tranquillizers. Others become habituated, that is, they don't become physically dependent, but emotionally so. They feel they cannot cope with life without the buffer of their pills and go to great lengths to get them – even trying to forge prescriptions if their doctors refuse to prescribe them.

Whether a person has become addicted or habituated, they have a problem that needs expert psychiatric help.

Drug	Effect	Possible side effects	Period of use
Antidepressants Anafranil Ludiomil Surmontil Tofranil Tryptizol	Relieve depression, sleep disturbances, anxiety, agitation and phobias	Drowsiness; dry mouth; constipation; urinary retention; blurred vision; alertness may be impaired	Relief of symptoms may take up to four weeks to develop. Dosage is gradually reduced once a satisfactory response is achieved. Treatment may be continued for several months
Tranquillizers Ativan Librium Nobrium Tranxene Valium	Reduce anxiety, tension and agitation	Drowsiness; light-headedness; headache; confusion; change in sex drive; dependence	Should only be given long enough to help the patient over the period of the problem
Hypnotics Dalmane Euhypnos Mandrax Mogadon Tuinal	Induce sleep	Sleep may not be as restful as normal sleep; patient may remain sleepy the next day; dependence; insomnia and vivid dreams on withdrawal	Short-term use only

Why do so many doctors give tranquillizing medicines?

When it was found in the early 1960s that anxiety could be controlled by the swallowing of a medicine, it offered a human revolution. Anxiety has always been one of the most powerful and painful of human experiences; it is probably an unpleasant by-product of our big brains. Animals with smaller brains and therefore less imagination only show signs of anxiety – which is the little brother of fear – when they have immediate cause to do so. Show a rabbit a dog and it gets anxious. Take the dog away and the rabbit forgets its anxiety.

We, on the other hand, can remember and also project. We can imagine ourselves facing the equivalent of a dog before it arrives, imagine ourselves still staring at it after it has gone, and so keep our anxiety going all the time. For many of us, anxiety is a constant companion, because our imaginations are going full tilt, looking for something to be frightened of.

It is probably anxiety that has brought us to our present civilized state and I believe that it is certainly the major

ingredient in ambition, the inevitable spur to striving onwards and upwards. The more we 'progress', the more anxious we get, so the more we strive.

So a treatment that promised to remove anxiety from us when we didn't want it seemed marvellous and the world fell on the little soothing pills as though they were manna. Doctors were as grateful for these pills as their patients. Now they had something they could give to those people who came constantly seeking help with symptom after symptom after symptom, and who could not accept the fact that they felt as they did merely because of anxiety.

And once the doctors started prescribing these medicines it became hard for them to stop. Patients came to rely on them more, and demanded more. Now we seem to have something new to be anxious about; the amount of tranquillizers we use.

This does not mean that they do not have a value – they do, as a temporary crutch. A person stunned by a recent and sudden bereavement may need a

few days on a tranquillizer to help him to face up to the painful weeks of adaptation and mourning that lie ahead. Someone facing a highly stressful short-term experience can benefit greatly from a dose of tranquillizers to see him through. Many are the fearful travellers who have managed to get into a plane because they are bemused by a couple of little pills.

It is when these medicines are used for too long as a permanent treatment that they become threatening. Just as the bereaved have to face the truth of their loss and mourn it and recover from it, so does an anxious man need to dig out the root cause of his anxiety and deal with that, instead of seeking perpetual help in a pill box.

Only those who are suffering from psychoses – the schizophrenias and the manias – should have tranquillizers all the time. For them, the treatment is as vital as is insulin to a diabetic. Anyway, different types of tranquillizer are used for these sufferers. The rest of us, however, do not often need tranquillizers.

How do emotional problems – such as nervousness – cause physical symptoms? And how can you treat them?

People who are 'suffering from nerves' in fact have nothing wrong with their actual nerves. The nerves are precise body structures with a precise function. They carry messages about the body, telling the brain of the sensations and experiences collected by outlying parts. They then carry back the brain's instructions on what to do about the information collected. Nerves ensure that when you put your hand in a flame and burn it, your muscles contract so that you pull your fingers out of painful danger, fast.

If nerves are damaged the results are dramatic, involving a breakdown in communication. If a man damages his spinal cord – the main trunk road of the nervous system – then the part of his body below the point of damage is cut off from his awareness. He cannot feel anything there, or make any conscious use of that part, and he is paralyzed.

But when people suffer from 'nervousness', their nerves are in perfect

condition, carrying messages to and fro and generally doing their job well. So, what causes the symptoms?

The brain is involved in 'nervous' troubles, acting through another body system – the endocrine system. This is made up of a few scattered little knobs of tissue, some deep in the brain itself (the pituitary and hypothalamus), some deep in the root of the neck (the thyroid and parathyroids), some deep in the body (the adrenals, the gonads – ovaries and testicles – and the pancreas).

When the brain is alerted by fear, the endocrine system swings into action. Messages go to the hypothalamus deep in the brain, and from there to the nearby pituitary, which triggers the adrenal glands (the ones just over the kidneys). They produce a hormone called adrenalin. This acts on muscles, blood vessels, skin, sweat glands, the digestive system, in fact on almost every corner of the complex structure that is a human body.

Adrenalin causes muscles to tense up when you are faced with a frightening situation; whether you are going to stand up to the threat from outside, or run away from it, your muscles prepare to act. Both these reactions – fight or flight – will need muscular effort, so adrenalin makes sure they are all set to go. And that makes the muscles tremble and sometimes ache.

Adrenalin makes the blood vessels constrict in some places, and relax in others. Blood vessels to the muscles relax so that more fuel-carrying blood can get to them. To compensate, adrenalin causes other blood vessels to contract, so that other areas are comparatively starved of blood. And that makes the face whiten, and sometimes the whole skin area goes pale, as blood is drawn from the surface to the muscles.

Adrenalin causes the heart to take on an added burden because the extra blood that goes to the muscles has to be pumped there. That makes the heart beat faster. It increases the pulsating in arteries as well, of course, and this causes a sensation of heavy throbbing in the neck and head, sometimes, as well as in the chest.

Adrenalin increases the demand for oxygen because all this extra work it is creating needs extra fuel. So the breathing becomes much more rapid to provide the extra oxygen.

Adrenalin causes the digestive system to go into action, because adrenalin cannot be entirely selective. It affects all muscles, not only those needed for fight or flight. So the digestive system, plentifully supplied with muscle, reacts to the high levels of adrenalin. That causes nausea, diarrhoea and sometimes cramp.

Adrenalin affects the body's water balance because the change in blood flow to the muscles, together with all the extra work being done, makes heavy demands on the body's reservoirs. So the mouth gets dry and sweat appears on the skin, particularly the palms of the hands which have a plentiful supply of sweat glands.

This is quite a list of activities for one hormone, though it does act with others. For example, the pancreas pumps out different levels of insulin, the hormone vital to the way we burn up the sugar which gives us our energy, and which, as a side effect, alters the appetite. Adrenalin also reacts on the sex hormones, made in the gonads, which is why in a woman there can be changes in period rhythms or even, in a very few cases, direct effects on pregnancy, leading to miscarriage. In a man, there can be episodes of impotence.

All these effects are vital to a person in need of them. If you are faced with a threat such as that of a would-be mugger, being primed to run or to hit him into submission is clearly vital. It can make all the difference between survival and death.

But suppose you get all these reactions when you are simply out shopping or doing your housework at home? If you are an average sort of person you note all these physical symptoms, and you are alarmed by them. You suspect that maybe you have some sort of disease that is causing this rapid heartbeat, breathlessness, trembling, and the weariness that follows them. You can't imagine that you feel like this just be-cause you are worried about your husband, or your children, or money. So the symptoms frighten you. And when a person is frightened, the brain reacts by sending out messages to the adrenals to release adrenalin.

This is how a cycle of symptoms can be started and perpetuated. The original cause of the fear, married to the secondary fear created by the adrenalin-caused sensations together build up and become a pattern of misery, spoiling the ability to work, to live and even to love. Many people suffering from this sort of constant anxiety lose their sex drive as a side effect; the hormones reacting on each other damp down these hormones that create sexual appetite.

To know that it is a fear trigger that sets off these symptoms does not necessarily help, and it certainly doesn't get rid of the symptoms. What is needed is to remove the original fear.

So, what is it that makes so many people so frightened? Let's clear up one misconception first. This 'epidemic of fear' is nothing new. People may hark back to a Golden Age when no one suffered in this way, and no one needed tranquillizers and medicines to help them to cope with breathlessness, trembling, bellyaches and the rest. But in fact, mankind has always suffered from his efficient fear-fighting reactions. In the past people simply had different labels for what happened.

They said that anybody with these symptoms had 'neurasthenia' or 'debilitation of the nerves'. They misunderstood what was going on and the label made it sound like a 'respectable' disease.

There were some famous sufferers from this nervous disease, one of whom was Florence Nightingale. She took to her couch in 1857 just after her triumphant return from the Crimean War, because she and her doctors were convinced that she was dying. Her trembling, loss of appetite, weakness and rapid heartbeat alarmed them all. But she didn't die until more than 50 years later, and she did her best work from her sickbed. Another famous invalid of this type was Charles Darwin. After his return from his remarkable journey on *The Beagle*, he virtually became a recluse, avoiding almost all public activities because they made him so ill. But he was physically in perfect health.

What is it then, that makes so many people so fearful? This is hard to define. Some of us have been trained to be frightened from earliest childhood. Child-rearing practices have, in the past, emphasized the punishment of wrongdoing, and given minimal encouragement to 'good' behaviour. Even today, many children, long before they start school, are on the edge of fear all the time. 'Am I a good girl? Will Mummy be angry with me? Am I doing right?'

These children go on being fearful all their lives though they may manage, as years go by, to bury their anxiety. But they can never bury it completely. Every so often a sudden surge of anxiety will burst out, perhaps for a reason so slight that the person doesn't realize what it is; it may be connected with some long-forgotten episode in childhood.

For example, one patient suffering from a severe attack of anxiety told her doctor that she had smelled a whiff of disinfectant and that had started it all off. In her childhood she had been beaten hard for walking on her mother's newly disinfected kitchen floor. Although she was now 57, she was still that four-year-old inside, still literally frightened sick.

Some people who suffered dreadfully as children manage to outgrow their childhood experiences and do not experience nervousness in adult life. Yet others who had little obvious distress in childhood respond to the smallest threat with a full panic attack.

People who are excessively sensitive may become so unable to cope with their adrenalin reactions that they shut themselves away from life and become agoraphobic – unable to leave their own homes for sheer terror. (The word derives from the Greek and means literally 'a fear of public places or open spaces', but for most sufferers it usually means a fear of leaving home.)

Others try to block out their alarming feelings by turning to 'crutches' such as food and drink to give them temporary comfort. They try to eat themselves into calmness, or drink themselves into peace of mind. Their case is tragic because, far from soothing their fears and tensions, obesity or drunkenness adds to them.

But most people seek medical help for their 'nerves', and doctors can help if they listen. They can offer medicines to lessen the discomfort of those adrenalin reactions, but that is of limited value. A medicine can be helpful to get you over a bad patch, when there is just cause for the symptoms (taking a tranquillizer to get you through a plane journey, for example, can be a good idea) but it is not a long-term answer.

Is there a long-term answer? There is, and more and more doctors are recommending it – self-help. The only cure for the nervousness that comes from an over-discharge of adrenalin due to a minor trigger is to teach yourself how to accept the feelings that the first surge of adrenalin causes.

If you can let them happen to you, wash over you and then ebb away, without getting more alarmed, then each episode of nervousness is cut short. Remember, it is reacting to the feelings of fear with more fear that causes these long, drawn-out periods of nervousness. Many people find, once they really understand what is happening to their bodies as a result of their mind's activities, that they can relax. No longer do they fear they are ill, but know that they are basically well. This knowledge in itself can act as a powerful stop to tension.

It can help to admit to yourself the root causes of your anxiety and deal with them. It might be because of a tottering marriage, poor work relationships, or unhappy contacts with your growing children. Psychological help – the talking-it-out technique – has helped many people. Good doctors will always provide help, either themselves or by passing a patient on to a specialist.

Other people need a positive technique for relaxation. In recent years there have developed a number of groups of people who teach relaxation, which includes yoga, transcendental meditation, and other techniques. These can do no harm and may well do good for a tense and anxious person.

Fight or flight
The physiological responses to something alarming take place in three rapid stages. The frontal lobe of the cerebral cortex activates the hypothalamus, which in turn causes the adrenal medulla to release adrenalin into the bloodstream. This puts different parts of the body into the appropriate state of readiness (*right*)

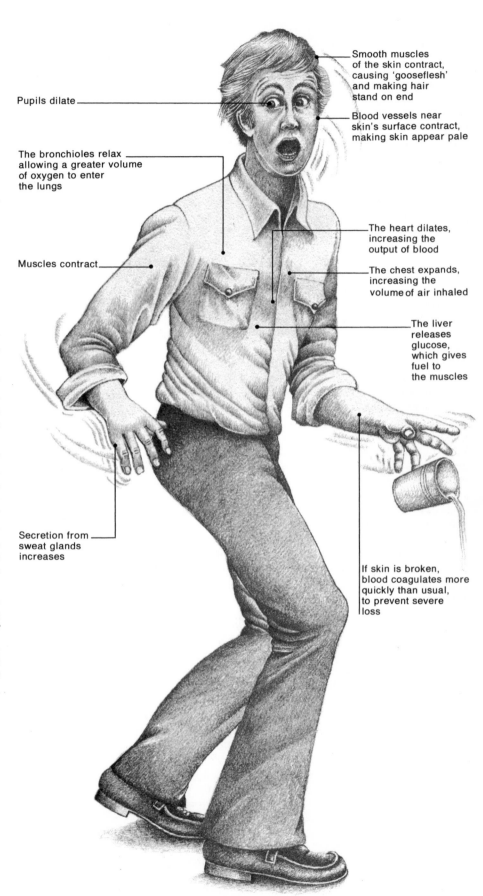

Pupils dilate

Smooth muscles of the skin contract, causing 'gooseflesh' and making hair stand on end

Blood vessels near skin's surface contract, making skin appear pale

The bronchioles relax allowing a greater volume of oxygen to enter the lungs

The heart dilates, increasing the output of blood

The chest expands, increasing the volume of air inhaled

Muscles contract

The liver releases glucose, which gives fuel to the muscles

Secretion from sweat glands increases

If skin is broken, blood coagulates more quickly than usual, to prevent severe loss

Mind and emotions

My doctor says I need electric shock treatment because tablets don't help my depression. I want so much to get well, but I'm scared because people say it's bad treatment. Is it? What does it do?

ECT – electroconvulsive therapy – has, over recent years, become a matter of great controversy among doctors. There are some who are violently opposed to it on the grounds that it might damage the brain. They say that in the past people suffered severe loss of memory as a result of ECT and some were injured. They also claim that because patients hate and fear the treatment it cannot be good for them. Efforts have been made in some parts of the world to make doctors ban the treatment.

On the other hand, there are doctors who defend the treatment with equal vehemence. They say that it is a method which brings relief to profoundly depressed people who do not respond to other methods. They say that the anxiety about its use stems not from rational thought but from emotional, misinformed people who lack understanding of the true facts of the case.

It is hard to pick out the truth from the two sides of the argument. It seems likely that the patients in the past did suffer distress because of ECT. It was given without anaesthetic, and to the whole brain. This could make it very alarming (suddenly losing consciousness is not pleasant) and also led to memory impairment, since the brain centres involved with memory were temporarily knocked out by the shock. Also some people suffered muscle and bone injuries when the treatment was badly controlled.

Today, however, patients are given a light general anaesthetic, which is much more pleasant, and feel and know nothing of what happens. They also are given a light muscle relaxant so there is no risk of bone or muscle injury. And the treatment is given to only one side of the brain which avoids the memory loss problem, while still having a good depression-lifting effect. But there are still patients who dislike the method.

So, there cannot be a simple answer to this question. Many patients today are deeply grateful for the help they receive from ECT and actively seek it again when they get another attack of depression. Others are so suspicious and fearful of it that they even refuse to see doctors for fear of experiencing it.

Most sensible people feel that the answer has to be an individual one. Find a doctor you can trust, and then trust him rather than haranguing an outsider. A qualified person who knows you and your illness is the only one, surely, who can give you useful advice.

(I will add one personal comment. If I were severely depressed and my doctor suggested the treatment I would accept it. I have cared for patients having it and have seen that it is neither frightening nor dangerous. And it works in many cases.)

Why do some people get cravings for drugs and alcohol while others don't? Is it a physical reason or are they just weak-willed and lazy?

It is impossible to measure the will for its strength and then award grades for success. It is as ridiculous as measuring people's height and then trying to say they are 'good' or 'bad' accordingly. Some people are vulnerable and succumb to pressure more rapidly than others. There is no sin nor virtue either way.

Is a tendency to get 'hooked' on a drug or alcohol physical? One school of opinion says that it is, and links it with the production in the brain of the natural pain-killers called endorphins. Others believe that some people have a complex brain chemistry that makes it difficult for them to obtain from their diet materials which they need, and this is why they seek them in bizarre substances.

We cannot know if this is true as yet, although research in the future may well find the answer. All we can know is that some people are vulnerable and easily become dependent, while others do not. It was ever thus; mankind has been looking upon the wine when it is red for millennia.

Why do doctors so often say, 'Oh it's just your nerves', when you have physical symptoms? How can they be so sure?

One of the most difficult things to explain to patients is that their minds and their bodies are not two separate things but an inextricably intertwined partnership. What happens in the mind has a profound effect on the body and vice versa. Physical symptoms such as pain, fever, nausea and vomiting can cause mental symptoms such as depression and irritability – whoever felt cheerful and happy when he had a bad attack of 'flu? – and mental experiences such as unhappiness, bereavement and fear can cause physical pains and physical reactions such as diarrhoea, nausea and vomiting, breathlessness, and changes in heart rhythms.

So, when a doctor sees a patient who complains of physical symptoms, and he has done all the necessary investigations and checks to identify physical disease – such as heart disease in someone who complains of attacks of palpitations (rapid heartbeat) – and finds no physical cause, then there is only one answer left. The symptoms are due to some sort of emotional and mental stress.

Unfortunately, too many doctors, and too many patients, dismiss such stress as unimportant. Both of them see physical illness as 'real' and emotional illness as 'false'. But if more doctors were more careful in their approach to the worried patient with functional symptoms (that is, symptoms for which no physical cause can be found) the patient would not feel his distress had been sneered at, and would be able to relax and accept help, which in itself would lead to some relief of the symptoms.

Anyone who has a doctor who makes him feel ashamed of having physical symptoms due to emotional stress and who gets no help from him with them needs to think seriously about changing to a different doctor. Neither of them are likely to benefit from the relationship. And a person who is affronted and suspicious when his doctor tries to tell him his disease is mostly emotional also needs to rethink his attitude. He has nothing to lose – except his symptoms – from trying the psychological approach.

Why are some people more highly strung than others?

The differences in the human personality are as many as those in the human physique. We are all a complex mixture of the genes of our forebears, and this governs our ability to respond to stress just as much as it governs the colour of our eyes. Some people are born with a tough personality, others with a vulnerable one.

But there is more than nature involved – there is nurture, too. Some people are made more sensitive to stress by their upbringing. A child reared by anxious parents who are always worried about him may be taught to be fearful, and taught to collapse under pressure. One reared by tougher more outgoing parents, who encourage self-reliance, may become tougher himself.

And then there is the effect of the environment. A constitutionally sensitive person living in a secure untroubled world, sure of his relationships, his employment and his comfort may seem very tough indeed, but be unable to cope with environmental changes. A less sensitive person in the same circumstances copes well. This shows most strongly in times of war; one man who seems quiet and retiring becomes a successful soldier while his neighbour, apparently bouncing and outgoing, collapses under the strain and cannot fit into the army.

What causes a nervous breakdown?

There is really no such thing. Nerves don't 'collapse'. However, as we all know, some people do have a fairly sudden and severe emotional illness in which they show a wide range of psychiatric symptoms and which makes them unable to go on living a normal life. This is what is popularly called a nervous breakdown.

But there can be so many different sorts of breakdown, and so many causes that it is impossible to classify them. One person will have a hysterical attack, that is, feel unable to cope with life and develop a range of bizarre uncontrolled behaviours ranging from violent weeping and/or laughing to apparent mania and spectacular suicide attempts. Another will become deeply depressed and withdraw from life entirely, just crawling into bed and staying there. Another will go on a wild 'bender', drinking or roistering around town until he or she is arrested. The possibilities are as varied as the human personality.

The basic cause is the same in all of them – an inability to cope any longer with an existing situation. And that can happen to someone who has never had any psychiatric problems or to someone who has a severe schizophrenic illness.

Brain waves
An electroencephalogram (EEG) records the brain's electrical activity, giving researchers information about different types of sleep and when dreaming occurs. An EEG gives a more accurate picture of a subject's sleep pattern throughout the night than simply observing body movements

How important are dreams?
Why do psychiatrists always ask about them?

Mankind has always been fascinated by the half-world of his own night. The images and emotions which flick across the screen of his closed eyelids seem fraught with meaning. The art of dream interpretation goes farther back than Joseph and the Pharoah in the Bible.

Many psychiatrists believe with Freud that dreams are loaded with symbols of underlying conflicts. Ideas and feelings we dare not express in our waking state we can cope with in an altered form in our dreams. So, for them, interpreting these symbols is a vital tool in psycho-analysis.

A more practical answer to the reasons for dreams has been offered by 20th-century researchers into sleep, who found that the essential component in sleep for humans is not rest, as most of us believe, but dreaming. In fact the body rests little during sleep, since all vital functions continue and our muscles are often active as we toss and turn our way through the night hours. A person deprived of dreaming time, but allowed to have all the non-dreaming sleep he needs, becomes disorientated and exhausted, and in this state is highly susceptible to suggestion. Anything a man is told when he is suffering from dream deprivation can alter his state of mind profoundly. This is one of the techniques used in 'brain washing' as it is said to be applied in some political regimes.

Why dreams are so vital to health is not clear. One theory is that the human brain operates like a computer. From time to time the circuits become overloaded and need 'clearing'. Dreams are the effect of the brain clearing itself of unwanted material, running over returned material and new information, and checking on its memory banks.

It is a pretty analogy, but not an entirely satisfying one. So far, in fact, no one has yet been able to prove just why dreaming is so vital to human psychological health – only that it is.

Psychiatrists who accept the computer analogy usually do not show much interest in the content of patients' dreams.

Alpha rhythms (**1**) are recorded when the eyes are closed but the subject is awake.

As sleep occurs, EEG waves become deeper and slower (**2**)

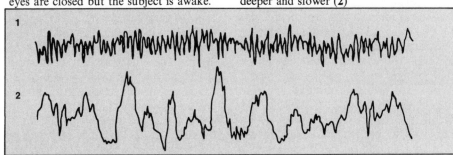

Mind and emotions

Does schizophrenia run in families? And just what is it?

Most people think the word schizophrenia means a 'split personality' and imagine a sort of 'Jekyll and Hyde' creature, sometimes 'normal' and sometimes 'mad'. This is quite inaccurate. There is no single disorder called schizophrenia. It is a label given to a number of as yet imperfectly understood mental illnesses which seem to have certain linking factors.

Schizophrenia attacks the young. Cases are usually diagnosed between the ages of 18 and 33, with a great many cases showing first symptoms in adolescence and certainly before the age of 25. It used to be called 'dementia praecox' which means 'the madness of the young'. And the younger the patient when the illness starts, the more severe and prolonged it is likely to be. There may be a pattern of attacks, followed by periods of remission, or the condition may be chronic and progressive.

The signs and symptoms are varied, and include loss of intellectual ability (a classic example is of the schoolchild, hitherto a satisfactory worker, seeming to be unable to concentrate or cope with studies any more); disturbance of thinking so that the patient talks nonsense, and shows signs of experiencing delusions; disturbed feelings, so that he seems to have no real emotions at all, being 'flattened' or having incongruous reactions – giggling at tragedies, weeping at jokes; withdrawal as the young person pulls away more and more from others, and turns into himself; and eventually disturbed behaviour in which there are odd mannerisms, strange rituals and other obviously bizarre activities – the classic 'madness' of which we have all heard. In severe untreated cases there may be catatonia, in which the patient goes into a rigid, trancelike state in which he is as still as a wax dummy, but this is rare these days.

If the patient is able to express his feelings at all, and this may be difficult for him to do, and even more difficult for outsiders to understand, he may say he feels that he is not himself any more, that others, either people or remote forces, are trying to control him. He may be deeply suspicious, thinking he is being watched or persecuted, even poisoned, or sent messages via the radio or television. He may develop a strong

desire for offbeat 'religious' cults, strange philosophical ideas, extrasensory perception theories and so on which he may express in strange 'poetry' which no one else can comprehend.

Psychiatrists suggest that these interests, together with the suspicion of being manipulated, are an attempt by the patient to explain why his feelings and thinking have gone haywire; he seeks an outside agent to blame for it.

As part of all this he may hear voices and have hallucinations, seeing, smelling, feeling and even tasting things that are not there. It seems very possible that many ghost stories are rooted in schizophrenic experiences and there is little doubt in the minds of many historians that the wave of fear of witches that marred so many countries in the Middle Ages and later were expressions of fear of schizophrenics. And possibly Joan of Arc with her 'voices' had the same illness.

One of the problems with schizophrenia is that mild forms of it are very like normal adolescent behaviour; withdrawal from and dislike of others, reticence and moodiness, sloppiness of dress, a curious sense of humour and an interest in weird cults, 'gibberish' poetry and art may all show themselves in perfectly normal adolescents. But when the young person's behaviour becomes more bizarre, or he becomes more withdrawn, the diagnosis is made.

The long-term effect of schizophrenia is variable. Some sufferers become 'dropouts' – many of the vagrants who inhabit the underside of our cities are schizophrenics. Prisons include a number of sufferers among their populations and, of course, our mental hospitals have many patients who have been there for years because of this tragic affliction.

What causes it? This is a difficult question to answer. With such a wide range of symptoms – ranging from the frankly 'mad' to the merely odd, it is difficult to know just what schizophrenia is and, therefore, even more difficult to know what causes it.

One group of psychiatrists believe that the symptoms and signs are due to errors in brain metabolism. They say that the brain cells are affected by chemicals which derive from the diet and

which in some people are not properly used in the body because they have an inherited inability to deal with them. Studies of the urine of schizophrenics were said to produce a characteristic 'pink spot' which was thought to point to this chemical imbalance. However, there is no scientific proof that this is so, although it is known that there are medicines which will help control schizophrenia – the phenothiazines – and which enable some sufferers to lead virtually normal lives, which again points to a chemical effect.

These medicines, which were hailed as the great breakthrough of our age, have revolutionized the treatment of schizophrenia. It has been estimated that about half of the patients using them lead normal lives, that about a quarter suffer recurrent attacks, and only the remainder fail to benefit from the treatment at present available.

Other research has suggested that the disease is due to eating the wrong foods; there are some who blame gluten, a constituent of cereals, others who point the finger at processed foods such as white sugar and flour. These theories again blame brain chemistry for the disorder but suggest that diet control rather than medicines is the best treatment.

But there is another school of psychiatric thought which says that schizophrenia is due entirely to the way a child is brought up. A mother who is at the same time demanding and rejecting, showing rage and/or giving punishment or coldness to her child whether he cuddles up to her and seeks her love, or keeps away from her, sets up in his mind a deep conflict. Whatever he does, he feels he is in the wrong and, these psychiatrists say, withdrawal and a search for reasons for the confusion created in his mind by his family life result in the symptoms. These psychiatrists deny that there is such an illness as schizophrenia at all. Their view is that it is society which is 'mad' and not the sensitive individual who reacts to the confusions and mixed-up attitudes to which he is exposed by showing what 'normal' people regard as crazy behaviour.

One factor which would seem to add weight to the chemical imbalance theory

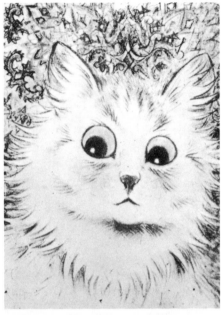
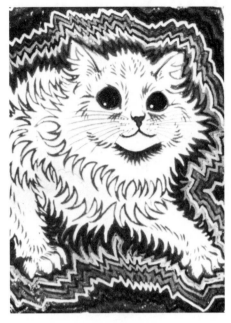
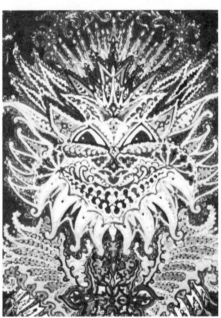
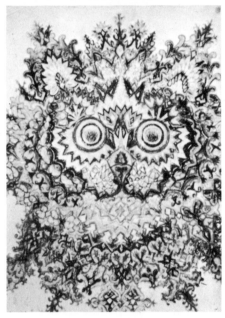

Illustrating schizophrenia
Psychiatrists may obtain useful information about the state of mind of schizophrenic patients from verbal discussions – or from a study of paintings done by patients who find this an alternative means of self-expression. These paintings of cats show the distortions of perception of the artist Louis Wain during a schizophrenic illness

is the way in which the illness runs in families. The children of a schizophrenic parent have a higher than average risk of the illness, which is greatly increased if both parents have the disorder. The 'bad family life' school of doctors retort that this fact supports their beliefs, since the child of such ill parents inevitably suffers from faulty mothering.

However, there is a fact that seems to add most strongly to the inborn chemical imbalance theory, and that is what happens with twins. If one of a pair of non-identical twins suffers from schizophrenia, then the risk to the other of developing it is the same as for ordinary brothers and sisters – a one-in-seven chance (14 per cent). But in identical twins, who have identical brain chemistry, the risk soars to well over 50 per cent – a one-in-two chance.

Furthermore, the most recent research suggests that prostaglandins may be involved. These are naturally occurring body substances which are now being discovered and studied and which seem to govern many of our body processes. A recent report suggests that schizophrenia may be due to a deficiency of certain prostaglandins. If this is so, then future treatment could be remarkably effective. Similarly, the endorphins are being considered as possibly involved in the causation of schizophrenic symptoms and, if they are, the use of the anti-endorphin treatment naloxone should help.

But these remain theoretical answers to this severe problem.

Glands and hormones

Endocrinology is the study of the disorders that affect the system of glands which produce the chemical messengers called hormones. Since hormones control such vital functions as growth, reproduction and metabolism – the rate at which the body burns food and oxygen – any malfunction of the endocrine system can have widespread effects. A child with a pituitary disorder, for example, may show marked excess of growth –

gigantism – or an equally marked lack of it – dwarfism. Fortunately, these are comparatively rare disorders. Most endocrinologists spend much more time in dealing with illnesses affecting, say, the thyroid gland, or the adrenal glands, than in dealing with such diseases of children. An important part of an endocrinologist's work may be in helping a childless woman to conceive; modern endocrinology has helped many couples to become parents.

The endocrine system

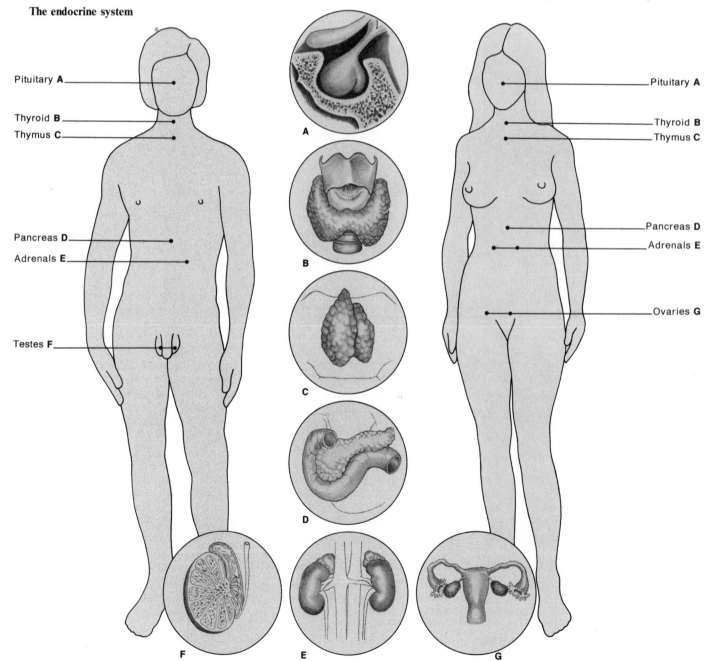

Pituitary **A**

Thyroid **B**
Thymus **C**

Pancreas **D**
Adrenals **E**

Testes **F**

Pituitary **A**

Thyroid **B**
Thymus **C**

Pancreas **D**
Adrenals **E**

Ovaries **G**

A

B

C

D

F

E

G

Why do women have so many more hormone disorders than men? Do they have more hormone glands?

Men and women have the same basic endocrine glands: the pituitary which is situated deep in the brain, the thyroid in the root of the neck, the pancreas tucked behind the stomach, the adrenals perched over the kidneys, and the gonads – the primary sex organs.

The only glands which differ between men and women, and actually look different, are the sex organs. Men have a pair of testes (in the scrotum, the loose bag of skin behind the penis) and women have a pair of ovaries (one for each side of the uterus situated low in the pelvis).

The testes operate in a pretty smooth way. Under the influence of the pituitary gland (which, in fact, governs all the endocrine glands – it's been called the 'leader of the orchestra') the testes produce their single hormone, testosterone, almost continuously, although there are peaks and troughs in the levels. For example, most men have high testosterone levels when they wake in the morning, which is why they are often at their most amorous then. It is testosterone which governs a man's sex drive and also gives him his sexual characteristics – deep voice, heavier muscles and a hairy body.

The ovaries, unlike the testes, produce two hormones – estrogen and progesterone. These are released into the blood in varying amounts during the month, with more estrogen than progesterone in the first two weeks of the cycle (counting from the start of the menstrual period) and more progesterone in the second two weeks. When a woman is pregnant the levels change again, with progesterone predominating. When she is going though the menopause, and the ovaries begin to falter and stop producing eggs that could develop into babies, the estrogen begins to diminish. And both hormones exert powerful effects on the breasts and the uterus, as well as affecting basic sex drive, and creating a woman's special characteristics – smooth skin and extra body fat, especially on the hips and breasts.

Obviously, with two ovarian hormones operating in a complicated interlocking way, and with a much bigger share of the human reproductive job to do, a woman's hormone rhythm is more likely to be disturbed than a man's. His is simpler and therefore less sensitive. But don't think that men have no hormone disorders. They can have thyroid, or pituitary, or adrenal problems in the same way as a woman, but it is true that they don't have as many sex hormone disorders.

Why do upset hormones make women bad tempered and depressed?

They don't always. Women with erratic hormone cycles sometimes find that they experience euphoria (abnormally high spirits) or are extraenergetic. But it is true that a lot of women find that they suffer from depression and irritability and headaches and fatigue when their hormone levels change.

There is a condition, labelled the 'premenstrual syndrome', in which women find that in the time just before the menstrual period, and perhaps for the first few days of the flow, they are tense, unhappy, often feel 'bloated' and know themselves to be hell to live with.

The reason is thought to be a fluid build-up in the woman's body. Her cells become plumped with extra water and this causes the bloated feeling. Lots of women say that their clothes are tight during this time, and they may need a full size larger in bras.

Feeling like that is in itself depressing, of course, but there is probably also a brain effect. The brain cells, too, share in this general rise in fluid, and this leads to the headaches, the anxiety, the sleep loss, the irritability and all the rest of the unpleasant symptoms.

That is one of the theories, anyway, but so far it has not been fully proven. If it were just excess fluid that was the cause, then the use of diuretics (drugs which make the kidneys extract extra water from the body) would relieve all symptoms. But diuretics do not do this in every case, although some women feel better if they take them. Another theory which many doctors think makes sense is that there is a too-low level of progesterone during the second half of the menstrual cycle. They say that this affects the cell fluid balance because it is well known that hormones have a considerable effect on the body's use of water and salt. These doctors give their patients progesterone in the form of pessaries or suppositories or implants (because progesterone is altered in the stomach and therefore cannot be swallowed) and find that this helps them to escape their bloated misery.

Pregnancy, while it is not a hormone disorder, does change hormone levels markedly, and many pregnant women find that they are usually more emotional, more weepy and more easily roused to anger, and that they return to their normal selves only several weeks after giving birth, when their hormone levels are restored. And the menopause, too, is known to make some women more tense and edgy.

But the question remains to be asked, – are these emotional changes due to hormones, or to the normal anxiety and excitement of being pregnant, or to the inevitable regrets of time passing that accompany the menopause? We do not know and it is a bit too easy to glibly blame hormones – that makes it sound as though taking extra hormones will cure the emotional problem. This is not usually the case: other treatment is frequently needed.

It is not only upset sex hormones that make women tense and unhappy. Any hormone disorder can do that, to both men and women, because the hormones are all closely linked with each other, and all have a profound effect on the brain and on the emotions. For example, people with an overactive thyroid become anxious and nervous, and those with an underactive one become lethargic and dull.

Glands and hormones

Does eating a lot of sugar cause diabetes?

You need first to understand what diabetes is. Healthy people, when they eat carbohydrate foods – the sugars and starches such as cakes, biscuits, candy, and potatoes and sweetcorn – digest them in the stomach and turn them into glucose. In this form, the food can go into the bloodstream and be carried about the body to be used as fuel to make the muscles work.

The amount of glucose in the bloodstream is governed by a hormone called insulin. It is made in the pancreas (the 'sweetbread' which lies behind the stomach, on the left of the belly, under the ribs). Insulin acts as a sort of controller; when more glucose is available than is needed by the muscles, it is shunted to the liver to be stored. When there is not enough glucose available, a further supply is called up from the storage depots, and pours into the blood. Thus insulin is involved in ensuring that blood glucose levels are finely adjusted to the individual body's needs, which change with the day's activities.

But in some people the insulin fails to do the job. It may not be produced at all, or there may be faults in the complicated pathways which govern the way insulin is produced.

Whatever the cause the results can be distressing indeed. The diabetic patient's blood is loaded with sugar. The kidneys, themselves programmed to help in keeping blood sugar levels as they should be, struggle to remove the excess, and the result is the production of large quantities of urine, often associated with itching of the genital regions, and an intense thirst. The undiagnosed or untreated diabetic spends a great deal of time just drinking and urinating.

Side by side with these distressing symptoms go others. The muscles get insufficient fuel to do their work, because insulin is not carrying the glucose from the blood to their cells, so there is intense weariness. There is also loss of weight because the body fails to store extra fuel. Injuries such as cuts fail to heal, because the blood sugar levels are so high that they interfere with normal healing processes. Similarly, there may be large painful boils that don't resolve – altogether very unpleasant. The brain is also affected because the sugar-laden blood fails to provide blood cells with other vital substances and there is confusion and sleepiness. If the condition goes on the result is coma and, ultimately, death.

What causes the problem? Why does the insulin supply fail? There can be a number of reasons. In children and young people there may be an inherited tendency to failure of the insulin-making cells in the pancreas (these cells are called the Islet cells of the Langerhans) though this is by no means the only cause. In recent studies of children who developed the illness, only one-in-ten showed a family history of diabetes.

Some researchers suspect that there may be viruses which attack and damage the pancreas and cause the disease, and other theories of all kinds are still being investigated.

There is another kind of diabetes, however, which is called 'maturity' or 'late-onset' diabetes. It usually happens to middle-aged and older people and is often diagnosed by accident. When some people go into hospital, for reasons other than diabetes, and have a routine urine test, the excess sugar, which has been thrown out by the kidneys, is discovered in the urine.

The causes of this sort of diabetes are still not fully understood, but one interesting fact has been noticed. People who are overweight tend to have high

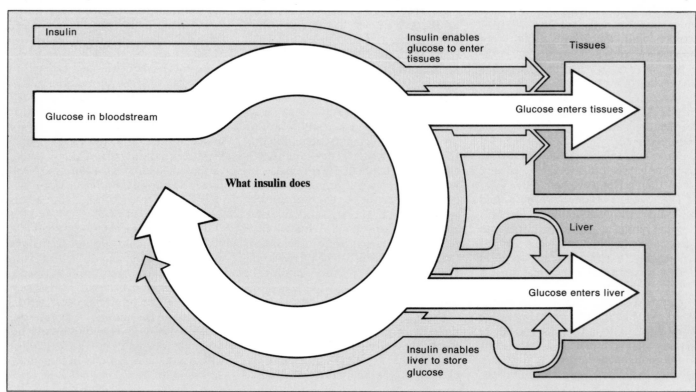

Why do some people with diabetes have to have injections while others just take tablets?

blood sugar levels, but they produce more insulin to compensate. But – and this is important – not all overweight people can produce this compensating extra supply of insulin and so they show mild diabetic symptoms. But if they lose weight by going on a diet, their insulin levels are adequate to cope.

Which brings us back to the question – can eating a lot of sugar cause diabetes? The answer is that it is not a direct cause. A meal of pounds and pounds of carbohydrate will not immediately give anybody high blood sugar levels that result in the symptoms of the illness. But such meals, taken often, can cause overweight, and overweight people may develop many of the symptoms of diabetes.

This tendency of a rich, high-calorie diet to increase diabetes was noticed dramatically in the inhabitants of the Yemen. When they lived sparse lives in considerable poverty, their diabetes rate was low, but when they emigrated to Israel and started to share the Israelis' richer diet, the Yemenites developed diabetes at the same rate as other Israelis.

So, eating less sugar is one way of keeping weight within control, and of avoiding late-onset diabetes.

Because diabetes is due to a shortage of insulin, the obvious treatment is to replace the missing hormone.

For many years that was impossible. Not only was the cause of the illness unknown to doctors – insulin simply was not available. But in 1921, two Canadian doctors, Banting and Best, isolated insulin, proved its absence to be involved in diabetes, and made it available to sufferers. Since then, regular injections of insulin have saved millions of lives, especially those of young people in whom the disease is more worrying and more severe.

But users of insulin have to follow a diet that contains measured amounts of carbohydrates and it can be extremely tedious for them not only to have to watch every bite they eat but also to have needles stuck in them once or twice a day. So a search for a simpler solution went on for some time.

It was found in 1954. Two German doctors discovered that one of the sulphonamides – an antibiotic drug given to combat bacterial infections – had a side effect of lowering blood sugar. These drugs, when given to sufferers from late-onset diabetes,

especially the marginal cases, provided some considerable benefit. Today, a great many older diabetics take tablets regularly, while younger ones use regular insulin injections. And quite a lot of the older diabetics can manage to control their problems with diet alone by just not eating too much, especially not too much carbohydrate.

The function of insulin

Insulin, made by the special cells in the pancreas, is essential to the body's use of sugar. Glucose is produced by the digestion of sugars and is carried around the body by the blood. Provided that the pancreas is producing adequate amounts of insulin, some glucose is taken up by the tissues for use when energy is required, while some is stored in the liver. But in a person suffering from diabetes, not enough insulin is made. The liver and tissues cannot take up the glucose, and the victim loses weight, lacks energy and becomes ill. The kidneys fail to absorb the excess glucose present in the blood and large quantities appear in the urine

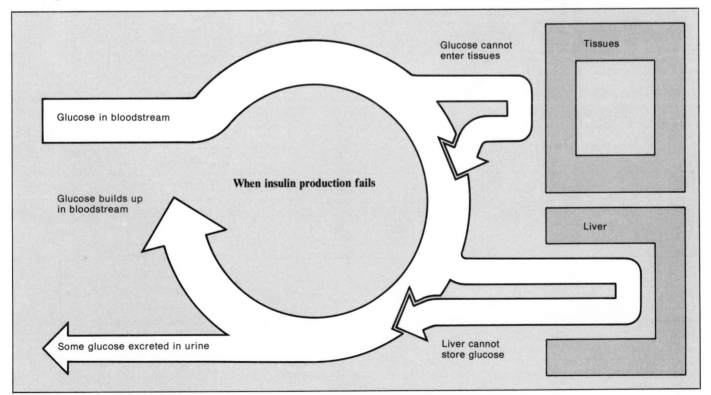

Glucose in bloodstream

Glucose cannot enter tissues

Tissues

When insulin production fails

Glucose builds up in bloodstream

Liver

Some glucose excreted in urine

Liver cannot store glucose

Glands and hormones

The thyroid gland
Growth is controlled by the dark red lobes of the thyroid gland, located in front of the windpipe (trachea) and just below the Adam's apple (the thyroid cartilage)

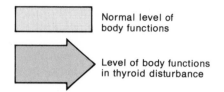

Normal level of body functions

Level of body functions in thyroid disturbance

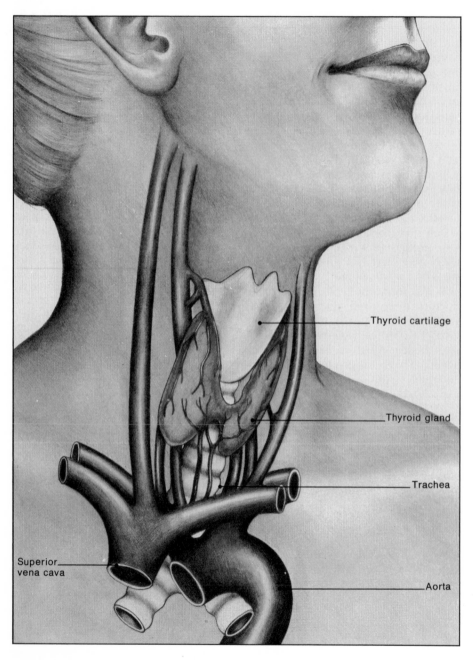

Thyroid cartilage

Thyroid gland

Trachea

Superior vena cava

Aorta

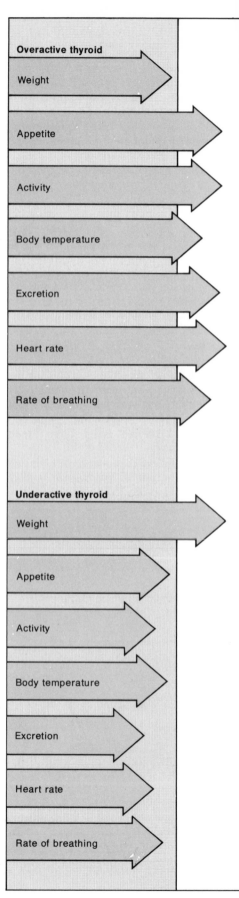

Overactive thyroid

Weight

Appetite

Activity

Body temperature

Excretion

Heart rate

Rate of breathing

Underactive thyroid

Weight

Appetite

Activity

Body temperature

Excretion

Heart rate

Rate of breathing

Disturbances of the thyroid gland have serious effects on the body (*right*). When too much thyroid hormone is produced, many body functions speed up and the weight decreases as energy stored in body fat is used up, even though the person may eat more. The sufferer often becomes irritable. When the thyroid gland is underactive, body functions slow down, the appetite decreases, yet the weight increases. The skin becomes puffy, the hair thins and the victim suffers more from the cold. Both disorders are relatively easily corrected by giving the patient doses of synthetic thyroid hormone or anti-thyroid medicines by mouth

Over-oxidation
(causing weight loss)

→ Thyroxine produced by thyroid gland

• Oxidation – burning up of body fuels

Under-oxidation
(causing weight increase)

→ Thyroxine produced by thyroid gland

• Oxidation – burning up of body fuels

Why do some people with a goitre get very thin, and some not?

A goitre is the swelling of an important gland called the thyroid which lies at the root of the neck. It looks rather like a couple of upside-down saddle-bags, connected by a narrow bridge which crosses in front of the larynx – the Adam's apple.

The thyroid has a complex job to do: it is concerned with regulating the rate at which the body burns its fuel. Like all the endocrine glands it operates in concert with the others, so disturbances of its function show in many different ways. For example, if the gland becomes overactive, the heart speeds up, there is breathlessness, restlessness and irritability. The appetite goes up – people with overactive thyroids seem to be always hungry – though the weight goes down and the sufferer may get positively gaunt. Menstruation is affected with periods becoming scanty or disappearing altogether, and there may be difficulty in starting a pregnancy. (It is women who suffer most from disorders of the thyroid.)

The disease caused by a non-active thyroid is called thyrotoxicosis or, sometimes, Graves' disease, after the Irish physician who first described it.

An underactive thyroid gland, on the other hand, causes generalized slowing down. The sufferer becomes heavy and slow, is always cold, eats little but stays bulky. The hair gets thin and coarse, there is a tendency to lose eyebrows, the skin becomes dry, the face dull and puffy and there is a hoarseness and deepening of the voice. This state is called myxedema. If a baby is born with an underactive thyroid, he becomes steadily more mentally handicapped and physically slow. This condition is called cretinism, and fortunately it is curable these days by giving the missing hormone as a regular medicine for the whole of the child's life.

However, a goitre does not always mean that there is disease in the thyroid gland. It can happen for a number of reasons and cause no symptoms at all.

For example, there is the physiological goitre. This happens in young girls at around the age of puberty, and sometimes in pregnant women, or those going through the menopause (the link between the thyroid and the ovarian hormones is obvious here). This sort of goitre causes no problems unless it gets really large (in which case a hormone called thyroxine can be given to reduce it) and indeed an enlarged goitre is regarded as a sign of beauty among some peoples. If you look at portraits of women painted during the Renaissance you will see that many of them have been shown with full, curving necks, due to this sort of goitre, and it was obviously a feature much admired.

Then there is also the simple goitre. This condition happens to both men and women, which makes it unlike other forms of thyroid swelling, and it happens because of a shortage of iodine in the diet. This substance is a vital part of the gland's function and is the main ingredient of the thyroid hormone, thyroxine. If there is not enough iodine available the gland grows larger, trying desperately to compensate and to make more hormone. The result can be an enormous swelling which presses on the windpipe, makes breathing difficult and, if it is an uneven swelling with one lobe bigger than the other, pushes the head sideways. Such goitres used to be common in certain parts of the world where there is inadequate iodine in the local soil or water, for example, in England's Derbyshire or Gloucestershire (the condition was popularly known as 'Derbyshire Neck') and in the American heartlands, a long way from the iodine-rich seashores. Nowadays, traces of iodine are added to table salt in most countries, so this sort of goitre is becoming rare.

So the only sort of goitre that makes people thin is the one due to an overactive thyroid gland, the toxic goitre. It can be treated sometimes by giving drugs such as thiouracil or imidazoles or potassium perchlorate, or by giving a radioactive isotype of iodine (I_{131}) which is eagerly taken up by the gland and has the effect of destroying some of the excess tissue. But the most effective treatment is still surgery, an operation to remove part of the goitre (not all of it, of course, because then the patient would be left with myxedema). Other kinds of goitre need no treatment at all, unless they get large enough to be unsightly or uncomfortable.

Glands and hormones

Why is cortisone used for so many different illnesses?

Actually, it isn't anymore. When the remarkable substances called steroids were first identified they were hailed as the 'wonder drugs of all time' and the answer to almost all the ills of mankind. But it was found in time that these powerful treatments could do harm as well as good.

Cortisone – properly called hydrocortisone – is one of more than 30 hormones produced by the outer shells of the adrenal glands, which perch over the kidneys in the small of the back. These hormones have a bewildering array of jobs to do; they shunt sugars, proteins and minerals about the body to do their work at cell level; they control salt and water metabolism; they are intimately involved with sex hormones and so with sexual appearance, behaviour and reproduction, and they also reduce inflammation and allergic and rheumatic reactions.

All of which sounds very useful indeed. Take, for example, the case of inflammation which, after all, is painful. It causes redness and heat and swelling and, above all, pain, and anyone who has ever suffered from, say, a skin condition due to inflammation (such as lots of boils) will pounce on a treatment that will relieve it.

But, and this is the important point, inflammation is useful. It is a vital part of the body's defences against disease and damage. It happens in response to any threat, notably bacteria and viruses, the organisms that cause disease, and is part of fighting off that threat.

Sometimes the threat that triggers the inflammatory response is a mild one, and the response is so exaggerated that it causes more trouble than the original threat. For example, in some people,

merely breathing in a few grains of pollen, or a few cat hairs, can lead to such swelling of the lining of the breathing tubes, and such an outpouring of mucus (the thin slippery material which the mucous membrane lining secretes) that the person can hardly breathe. In other people, it causes the fine muscles that form the walls of the breathing tubes to tighten into such a spasm that the sufferer has to fight for every gasp – the classic asthma attack.

This is called an allergic response, and many, many people suffer misery because of it. They may come out in great itchy lumps called hives whenever they eat a shrimp or a strawberry. Their faces may swell up and look like great puffballs whenever they go near a potted primula. They may almost choke as their noses clog and their chests fill up

The hormones of the adrenal glands
The adrenal glands, perched on the kidneys, are two of the busiest glands in the body. The hormones they produce control a range of body functions, of which some are shown here

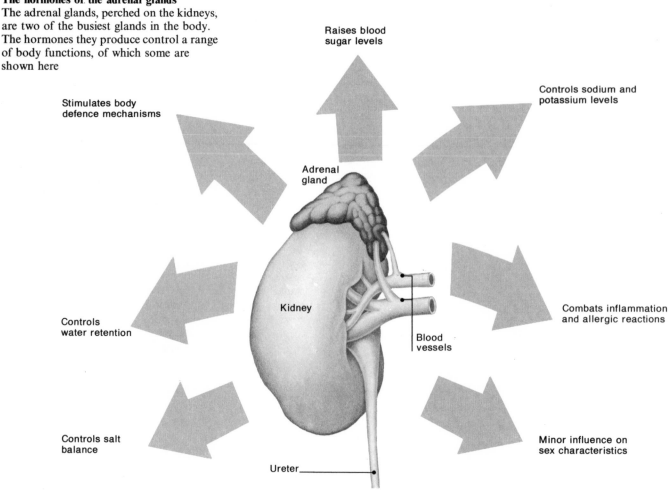

Raises blood sugar levels

Controls sodium and potassium levels

Stimulates body defence mechanisms

Adrenal gland

Combats inflammation and allergic reactions

Kidney

Blood vessels

Controls water retention

Controls salt balance

Minor influence on sex characteristics

Ureter

whenever they go near a rose. For them, the chance to use a hormone drug that will banish such hateful symptoms seems like heaven.

But, as the doctors found when they started using cortisone for reducing inflammation and fighting allergic symptoms, the kick-back effects were sometimes worse than the original problem. The drug is not selective: that is, you cannot tell it to 'go and stop the inflammation on that patch of skin, but do nothing else'. Cortisone affects the whole body, and if, as well as the inflamed skin, there is a bacteria or virus invasion elsewhere, the presence of the cortisone will damp down the disease-fighting mechanism in that area and allow it to flourish. In some cases, people who had been given cortisone for long periods to relieve the painful and unpleasant inflammation of severe acne

became ill with tuberculosis, which had been able to take hold because of the treatment.

Not only does cortisone control the body's fight against germ invasion and inflammation when given in doses large enough to have an effect on a disease, but it also slows down wound healing, causes weakening of the bones, thinning of the skin (which develops permanent reddish stretch marks), enlargement of the face, shoulders and belly and can also affect the mood and emotional state, as well as, in some cases, causing permanent damage to some of the endocrine glands. It is altogether an exceedingly powerful substance.

So, nowadays, cortisone is used sparingly and with great control. In some forms of rheumatism, which is a blanket term for a whole range of inflammatory conditions involving

joints, direct injections of cortisone into an afflicted joint can give considerable relief. In certain skin conditions, its short-term delicate use can be effective. In some allergic conditions, such as asthma, it can, if sparingly applied, control some of the more disagreeable symptoms.

In cases of acute shock – after a severe accident, say, or in a violent and life-threatening attack – it can be a life-saver, helping severely damaged patients to survive until their own body defences and repair mechanisms take over. And in people having transplant operations, where there is a risk that the body may reject its vital new organs, it can be of immense help.

But this drug, and the many others that are similar to it (and which are called steroids in medical shorthand), are not the answer to every illness.

Cortisone inhalers

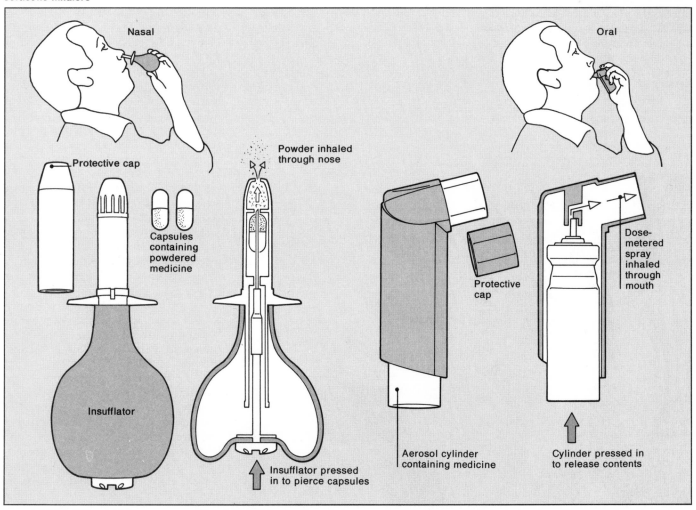

Nasal

Protective cap

Capsules containing powdered medicine

Insufflator

Powder inhaled through nose

Insufflator pressed in to pierce capsules

Oral

Protective cap

Aerosol cylinder containing medicine

Dose-metered spray inhaled through mouth

Cylinder pressed in to release contents

Glands and hormones

Why do some athletes take hormones?

Because some of the steroid hormone – the ones derived from the adrenal glands – have the job of shunting proteins about the body, they are intimately involved with muscle-building, since muscles are made almost entirely of protein.

When it was found, in the early days after the development of the first steroid drugs, that some of them actually had the effect of enlarging muscles, there was great excitement among athletes. Such a drug is useful if you want to be stronger or faster than other people. These steroids – they were called the anabolic hormones because they actually created new muscle substance – were therefore seized on by some Olympic performers and their trainers and were used to improve their physique. But then it was found that their side-effects were far too powerful; they can cause cancer of the liver because the liver is the place where excess hormones are broken down and disposed of; some changes in sexual function and a dangerous anti-inflammatory effect. No athlete who has any sense ever takes steroids now.

Why do some doctors say that hormone creams on the skin are dangerous when we all have hormones in our bodies anyway?

Because it is possible for substances to reach the bloodstream, and therefore the whole body, via the skin, any substance put on the skin can have a wide-reaching effect. For a hormone on the skin to be of any cosmetic use, it has to be given in large quantities for a long time, and when these are absorbed, as they usually are, all the unpleasant side-effects already described in the previous question can happen.

So, using a hormone cream on your skin to get rid of wrinkles on the face, or to enlarge the breasts, is potentially dangerous. In any event it is a waste of time. When the cream is stopped the original condition returns, and is usually worse than it was before.

Can taking hormones make a person feel more sexy?

That all depends on the person's hormone state to begin with. If someone is actually lacking in a vital sex hormone – for example, a man who has an abnormally low testosterone level, due to disorder of the testes – then his libido (the psychic drive or energy especially associated with the sex drive) will probably be absent. In his particular case, giving testosterone may well wake up his desires. However, if a man is going through a patch of impotence because he is worried, or not at his most healthy, or doesn't really fancy his partner anymore, then taking hormones will not help in the least. You can pump in testosterone interminably, but it cannot solve the business worries, or cure anaemia or influenza and it certainly will not make his wife seem more alluring. In fact, using sex hormones in this way can have a positively damaging effect on a person's sex drive. We all have a feedback loop built into our endocrine system. When the blood level of a hormone is what it should be, the pituitary switches off production of more hormone. So, giving sex hormones can actually reduce the hormone blood levels.

The same applies, of course, to the use of hormones for women. There was a widespread belief, largely disproved now, that women going through the menopause are deficient in estrogen and for that reason have a low sex drive. The theory accompanying that belief is that giving extra estrogen as Hormone Replacement Therapy (HRT) will restore sex drive like magic. But, of course, it cannot. The most common reason for loss of sex drive in menopausal women is not hormone deficiency, but self-esteem deficiency. The woman who feels aging and tired and bored cannot feel very sexy.

In fact, it is natural for many women to feel more sexy at the menopause, because of lower estrogen levels, rather than lose their drive. This is because estrogen is the natural opposer of androgen, the male-type hormone that both men and women have, although women usually have much less of it. But when estrogen falters at the menopause, androgen comes into fuller play and leads to an increase in sexual interest, provided, that is, that the woman likes herself, enjoys her life, and is loved by and loves her partner.

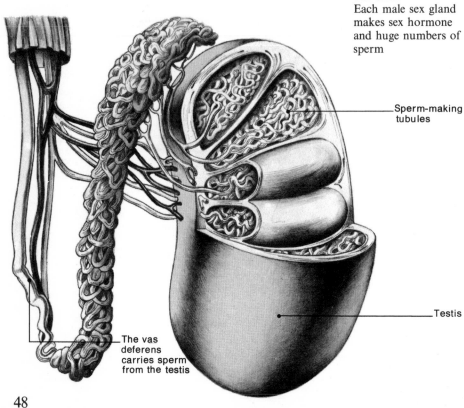

The testis
Each male sex gland makes sex hormone and huge numbers of sperm

Sperm-making tubules

Testis

The vas deferens carries sperm from the testis

Why do some women get hair on their faces and on their breasts and bodies? And why do some men never get any hair on their chests?

Although it is more common for men to have hair on their faces, chests and bellies than it is for women, it is by no means a universal rule. There are marked genetic differences around the world. For example, white people who originate in Central Europe tend to show abundant beard and body hair growth, while black people who originate from the Bushmen and Hottentot peoples tend to have no beard or body hair at all. Women of Mediterranean stock often have marked upper lip hair growth as well as strong growth on arms and legs, while some Northern European men, and also some Asian men, show little body hair but marked beard growth.

In addition to these genetic tendencies to grow hair on face or body (or not, as the case may be) there will be individual differences. There are women who are perfectly normal and healthy but who have a mild degree of hormone imbalance that results in heavier-than-usual hair growth on the face or around the nipples. And many women find, as they grow older, that hair starts to appear on their chins and upper lips, just as many men find that though they were smooth-chested in their teens and twenties they are quite door-matted between the nipples by the time they reach their thirties. This is due to slowly changing hormone patterns as the years go on, and is absolutely normal, if tiresome, for a woman who would rather be smooth than stubbly, or a man who dislikes his marble-like chest.

Only an unusually heavy and new growth of hair, or loss of hair, needs to be taken to a doctor for investigation. For the vast majority of us, it is a cosmetic problem to be dealt with as best we can, either with good depilatory creams or waxes or electrolysis for females' faces, or chest wigs for males' chests – if it matters that much.

Male and female body hair
Apart from the facial hair, the classic difference between the sexes is the female's pubic triangle and the male's diamond-shaped pubic hair

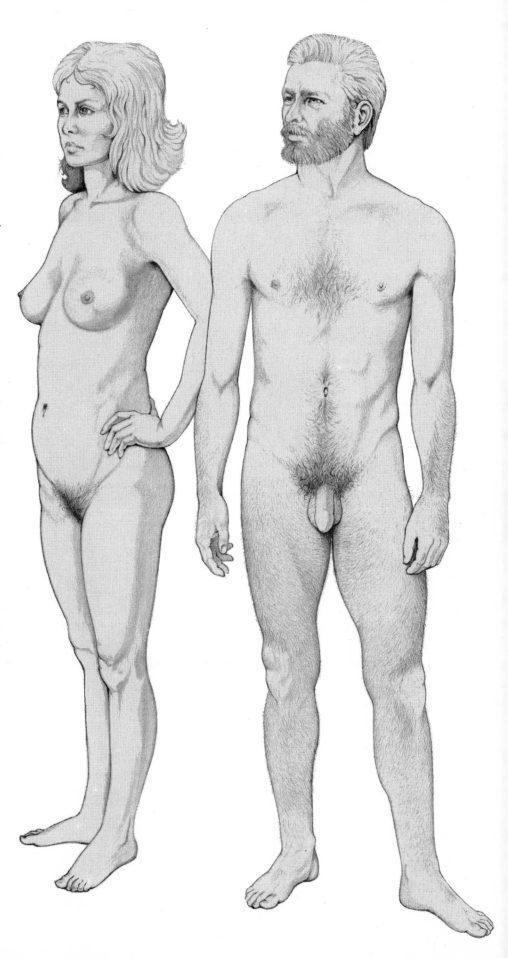

Skin and hair

The skin is the largest organ in the human body, and is also the only one which is totally unprotected on one side; every other body tissue is safely enclosed inside the body and is therefore less vulnerable. The skin is also the main organ of sexual arousal, since it is via the skin that we receive touch, and is also closely involved with sexual attraction, since it is skin which is the most obvious part of us. Hair is part of the skin and is another sexual characteristic on which we place great store. Hair loss, in both sexes, is always a distressing experience. All of which means that skin disorders cause a great deal of anxiety, and doctors who specialize in the treatment of such disorders are busy people. However, they are rarely called to their patients in the middle of the night or on Christmas Day which makes the speciality less exhausting for its practitioners than some other disciplines.

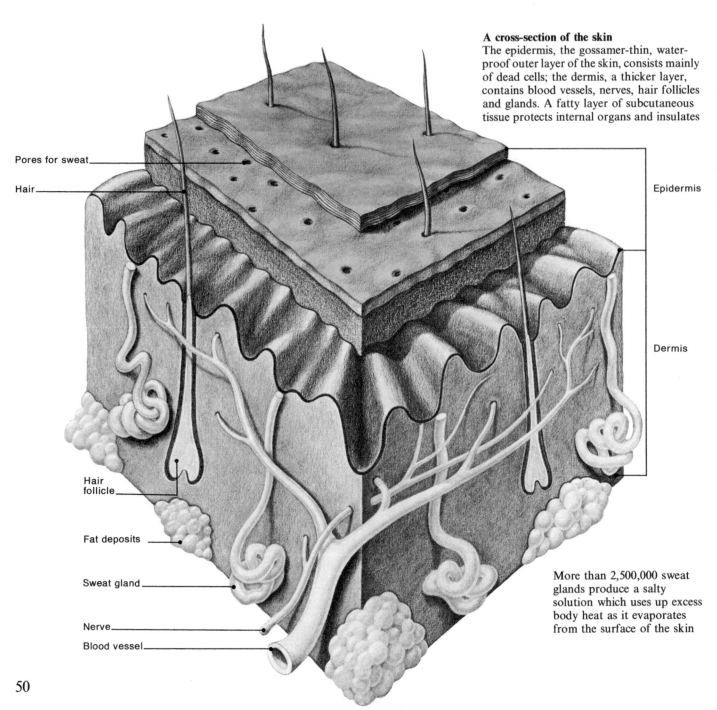

A cross-section of the skin
The epidermis, the gossamer-thin, waterproof outer layer of the skin, consists mainly of dead cells; the dermis, a thicker layer, contains blood vessels, nerves, hair follicles and glands. A fatty layer of subcutaneous tissue protects internal organs and insulates

Pores for sweat

Hair

Epidermis

Dermis

Hair follicle

Fat deposits

Sweat gland

Nerve

Blood vessel

More than 2,500,000 sweat glands produce a salty solution which uses up excess body heat as it evaporates from the surface of the skin

Why do fingertips wrinkle after being in water for a long time?

The skin is waterproof up to a point, but it can and does absorb a lot of water if it becomes sodden. When the hands spend long periods in water the cells take up a lot of it and the skin becomes stretched and collapses into folds. Slow drying out allows the skin to return to the normal size and the wrinkles then disappear. Wrinkling shows most on the fingertips because the area is particularly sensitive, but it would affect any skin eventually if it were soaked for long enough.

Why do old people get brown patches on their skins?

No one really knows. It does not happen to all old people, and those who experience it show no other special characteristics. Although these patches are often called 'liver spots' it is known that they have nothing to do with the liver.

Unless they darken, enlarge rapidly and start to bleed they are of no significance.

Why is sun tanning so healthy?

Sometimes it is and sometimes it isn't. The skin contains cells which, under the influence of the sun's rays, make Vitamin D, and as the vitamin is synthesized, the cells darken. That is the source of the sun tan. It is healthy if we are short of Vitamin D, and for many of the underfed peoples of the world the sun is indeed a vital source of this vitamin.

However, excess exposure to the sun may burn the skin, and that is far from healthy because it is painful and makes the skin vulnerable – the burned areas may be attacked by infecting organisms. A more worrying fact is that excess sun on pale skin can cause cancer. The highest skin cancer rates in the world are in California and Australia, where white-skinned people lie about in the sun.

Frequent tanning also accelerates the aging process of the skin. This is why the other main complaint from women in places like California and Australia is premature wrinkling.

How the skin wrinkles

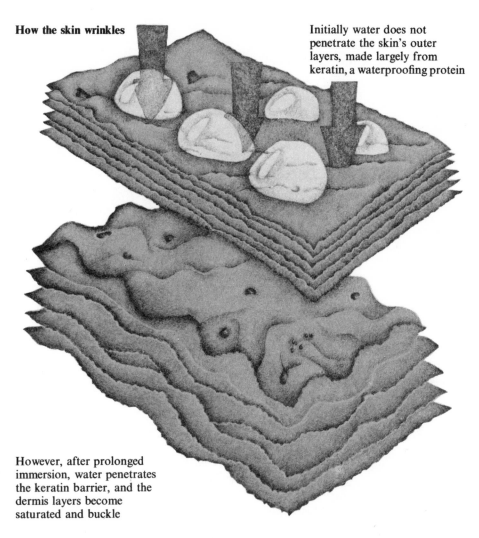

Initially water does not penetrate the skin's outer layers, made largely from keratin, a waterproofing protein

However, after prolonged immersion, water penetrates the keratin barrier, and the dermis layers become saturated and buckle

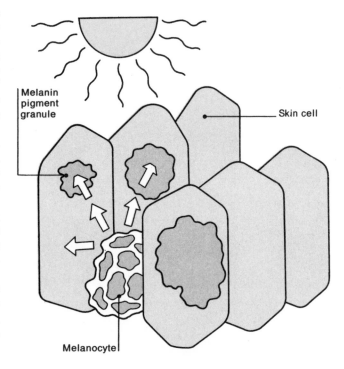

Melanin pigment granule

Skin cell

Melanocyte

What causes suntan
Stimulated by the sunshine, melanocyte cells in the lower layers of the epidermis produce extra pigment granules of melanin, a protein which protects the skin by absorbing the sun's harmful ultra-violet rays. The granules are injected into the surrounding cells; the extra pigment darkens the skin, causing suntan. Sunburn occurs when the melanin cannot absorb all the ultra-violet rays hitting the skin

Skin and hair

Is plastic surgery a good idea for sagging or damaged skin? Does it really work and does it last?

People have always sought the secret of perpetual youth and smooth unblemished skin for ever, and when cosmetic surgery developed, many believed they had found the secret. But it can only offer a certain amount of success and this, in the patient's eyes, depends entirely on his or her ability to recognize the limitations of the technique.

People who have developed very wrinkled skin early in life may benefit from an operation which consists of an incision round the hair line on each side, and a pulling back of the stretched skin to give it greater tautness. This is called a face-lift. Eyelids can have 'tucks' taken in them, and frown lines can be removed. But the face cannot ever be made to look as though it has never been stretched. Even the best of results on a 50-year-old cannot mimic the youthful skin of 17. People who expect such a degree of success are doomed to disappointment. But cheerful sensible people who have developed ugly lines may well be satisfied with an operation that in part removes them. The effect usually lasts up to 10 years, so the younger the patient when the first operation is done, the more likely is the need for a repeat. The limit for face-lifts is usually three.

Cosmetic surgery to the skin is like cosmetic surgery anywhere. A skin job, a nose job, and an ear job change only your skin, your nose and your ears. They cannot change you, nor can they change your life because that you can only do yourself.

The work of the cosmetic surgeon

Some surgeons specialize in improving on the looks that Nature has given to a person, or in repairing the wear and tear of the years. To a large extent, wrinkles can be smoothed, sagging skin and bags under the eyes removed, bustlines remoulded and noses reshaped. The sense of well-being such an operation can bring about in a patient is sometimes as great as that resulting from more conventional surgery directed at physical disease or injury

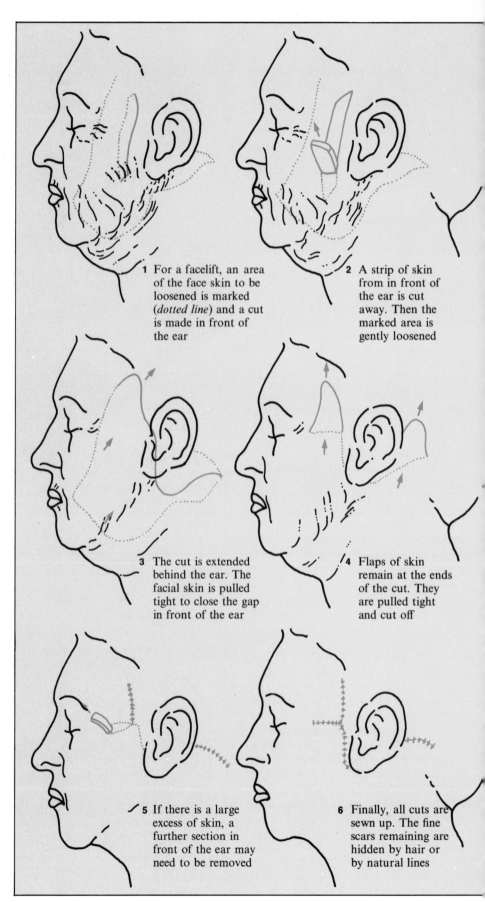

1 For a facelift, an area of the face skin to be loosened is marked (*dotted line*) and a cut is made in front of the ear

2 A strip of skin from in front of the ear is cut away. Then the marked area is gently loosened

3 The cut is extended behind the ear. The facial skin is pulled tight to close the gap in front of the ear

4 Flaps of skin remain at the ends of the cut. They are pulled tight and cut off

5 If there is a large excess of skin, a further section in front of the ear may need to be removed

6 Finally, all cuts are sewn up. The fine scars remaining are hidden by hair or by natural lines

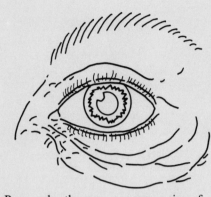

1 Bags under the eyes, a common sign of middle age, can be dealt with surgically

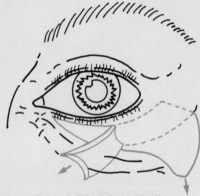

2 A flap of skin is lifted from the lid and pulled downward, and fat is removed

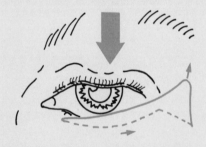

3 The surgeon gently pushes down the eyeball and stretches the lower eyelid to estimate how much of its skin must be removed

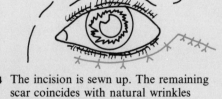

4 The incision is sewn up. The remaining scar coincides with natural wrinkles

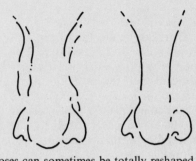

1 Noses can sometimes be totally reshaped. Here, a lumpy shape has been improved

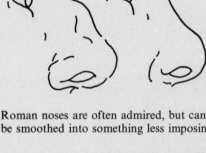

2 Roman noses are often admired, but can be smoothed into something less imposing

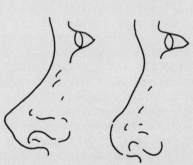

3 It may be possible to straighten a nose that originally was severely twisted

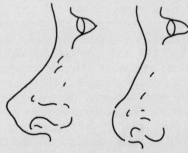

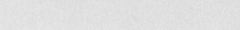

4 A small alteration has completely changed the appearance of this nose

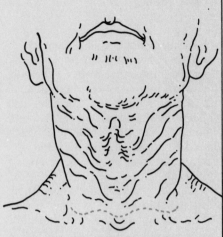

1 An operation to improve a 'turkey skin' neck begins with the cut shown

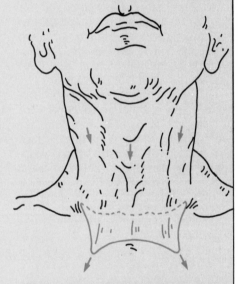

2 A broad flap of skin is pulled away and down from the neck and then removed

3 The skin of the neck is pulled down and made taut to close the cut before sewing

Skin and hair

How can you tell what sort of rash is significant? So often spots come up and then go before you can see the doctor.

If spots go that quickly then they cannot be all that significant. It is those which linger, or which are accompanied by other symptoms, that matter. (The only time when this is not entirely true is in the case of syphilis – a transient rash which appears after sexual contact with a possibly infected person and which should be discussed with a doctor.)

Many of the infectious fevers of childhood – measles, chicken-pox, rubella – are generalized illnesses which affect the skin as well as other tissues and cause eruptions there. Treatment of the disease deals with them. The rashes themselves are not important, unless they are of the sort that if scratched and teased leave scars. Chicken-pox is like that, and a child with it needs help to prevent long-term scarring (medicines to relieve the itching, gloved hands to prevent the scratching, entertainment to distract the mind from the spots).

The spots that appear in adolescence – acne – afflict up to 90 per cent of teenagers, many of them mildly, but others quite severely, with the face and neck and the back showing widespread pustules, blackheads and scars. A happy outgoing child can become a morose, withdrawn and very unhappy adolescent because of acne.

The cause is not fully known. Some people seem to have skins which produce great quantities of sebum (skin lubricant) and this clogs the pores and leads to the lesions. Certainly there is a genetic component: a child with parents who had acne is more likely to have the same problem than one whose parents did not.

Many treatments have been tried, ranging from savage dietary controls to any number of medicines. The most effective treatments seem to be sunlight (many patients report relief of symptoms in the summer months), antibiotics, to control secondary infection of the spots and, for girls, hormone therapy using the Pill. There seems to be a connection with hormone balance and the skin's production of sebum.

More hopeful now is the development of a new treatment with retinoic acid, a cousin of Vitamin A. Promising results are reported from recent trials and this may be the answer of the future. For people already severely scarred by acne, dermabrasion, in which the upper layers of the skin are surgically rubbed away, thus making the scars less noticeable, is a possible answer.

Every winter I get chaps and chilblains. Are these avoidable?

Winter conditions with chilling drying winds can attack vulnerable exposed skin and cause either drying out and flaking, chapping (cracks) or red, doughy, itching swellings (chilblains or coldburns). Severe chapping can lead to deep and painful cracks in the skin, especially around the heels and the hands.

Prevention is the best answer. A film of oil over exposed areas will prevent the drying effect which is the cause of the problem, and protection of other parts, for example, the hands, with warm, dry loose covering is essential. Once chapping has happened, patient application of emollient creams is the only answer.

Chilblains are similar to chapping, in that they are due to cold injury but blood vessels as well as the skin are affected. There seems to be a constitutional component; in some people the tiniest blood vessels (the capillaries) seem more easily constricted and so prevent the passage of blood to the extremities. In a way, chilblains are like frostbite and some people are more likely to experience that in bad weather conditions than others.

Here again the only solution is prevention, with ample warm clothing over threatened areas. It may help to use vasodilating medicines which dilate skin vessels and adjust body temperature.

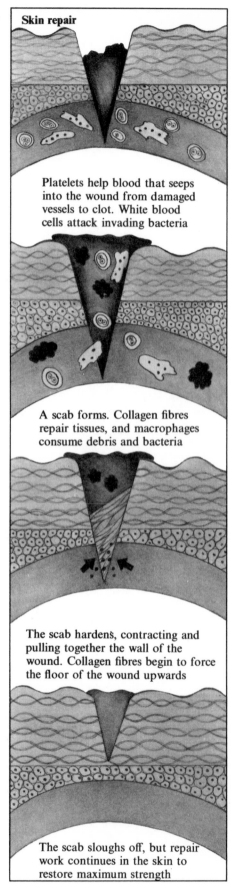

Skin repair

Platelets help blood that seeps into the wound from damaged vessels to clot. White blood cells attack invading bacteria

A scab forms. Collagen fibres repair tissues, and macrophages consume debris and bacteria

The scab hardens, contracting and pulling together the wall of the wound. Collagen fibres begin to force the floor of the wound upwards

The scab sloughs off, but repair work continues in the skin to restore maximum strength

Why do old people get wrinkled faces when the skin on their bodies doesn't seem to change all that much?

Skin, as well as being the largest organ in the human body, and a very tough and effective one, being thick, self-regenerating, waterproof and elastic, is vulnerable. It is particularly vulnerable to the environment – the drying effect of wind and sun and air, the soaking effect of humidity. In our young years, the skin is elastic and brisk in its responses to the need for self-repair. Its cells are plump with moisture and the sebaceous (oil) glands produce plenty of lubricating material. So, tanning by the sun and drying out by the wind or soaking by humidity will not matter.

But, as time goes on, the skin, like every other organ, becomes less effective, less swift at self-repair and above all, less resilient. The pull of underlying muscles shows more and more on the surface and lines created by expression become 'set'. The result is the wrinkling of exposed skin that we all eventually recognize.

On unexposed skin, under which there are fewer individual muscles – the belly doesn't need nearly as many muscles as the face which has to do a great deal more work – lines are less easily produced and, of course, the skin is protected from wear and tear by clothing. So the skin stays smooth much longer. However, it does slowly get thinner, and in extreme old age the skin of the body seems papery and fine and may become as wrinkled as that of the hands and face.

I have a red birthmark on my arm which I hate. Doctors refuse to remove it. Why? And will my children inherit this from me?

It may be that it is too big to be removed without leaving a scar which you would hate even more. 'Port wine stains', which are the dark red birthmarks some babies have, can be large and distressing, but removing them is a problem because of their size. This is probably the situation in your case. Smaller ones are much more easily dealt with.

As for children inheriting birthmarks – no, they do not inherit one exactly like the one which a parent has or had. But there is a range of birthmarks which are very common, so it is all too easy for several members of a family to have them without actually getting them from each other.

Small 'strawberry' marks are very common indeed, and usually fade before the child starts full-time school, though they may seem to grow larger for a while before they break up and disappear. Small red marks on the eyelids and forehead are common, and are charmingly called 'stork bites'. They, too, usually fade early in life. Pigmented moles, sometimes with hair growing on them, may appear and can be surgically removed if they are unsightly. 'Port wine' stains are, fortunately, much the least common and many cosmetic firms have developed cover-up makeups which men can use as discreetly and effectively as women.

My doctor advised me always to keep an eye on the moles I have, and to report any changes. Why?

A mole is a collection of pigmented cells in the skin. The pigment they contain is melanin (from the Greek word for black; the popular name Melanie means 'the black one'). Most of these marks are harmless. They may be present at birth, or develop slowly over the years or be put down during pregnancy (a time when extra moles often appear, especially in dark-haired women) or after frequent sunbathing. Usually they are harmless but in a few cases they undergo a malignant change. The cells enlarge and there may be bleeding. This sort of malignancy – it is called a melanoma – is particularly powerful and needs prompt treatment if it is not to lead to a severe and dangerous widespread disease. That is the kind of change that your doctor wishes to know about.

I keep getting warts. I have tried everything to get rid of them, but they keep coming back. Is there any permanent cure?

Warts are due to another virus, called a papovavirus, deep in the skin, and afflict between seven and 10 per cent of the population. They keep reappearing because the virus is not eradicated when individual warts are treated. Like herpes simplex, they can affect the genitals and be sexually transmitted.

Treatment is varied and not always effective. Unsightly warts can be removed by electric or chemical cautery, being 'burned' off. Some dermatologists freeze them off, using a cryoprobe. Others leave them alone, because up to three-quarters of them will disappear by themselves anyway.

Oddly enough, they seem to be susceptible to all sorts of 'magical' treatments. There are many authenticated reports of people being cured of their warts by the use of spells being said over them, sympathetic magic, in which the warts are rubbed with meat which is then fed to a dog (the idea is that the warts will then afflict the animal instead – a shade unkind, but reasonable to a wart sufferer) or the use of a somewhat repellent range of plant and animal materials, including sheep and rabbit dung and the slime from a toad's back.

These may well be just as effective as scientific treatments, with their rather disappointing cure rate.

Skin and hair

What causes cold sores? Is it just having colds in your head? And why doesn't it happen to everyone?

Cold sores are due to a virus called herpes simplex. It can be enduring and lives, dormant, in the skin for long periods. When resistance is lowered because of an infection such as a cold the virus is activated and the result is painful, slow-healing watery blisters which break out on lips and nose. In severe cases they can spread widely and make the sufferer feel really ill and in need of hospitalization.

Many treatments have been tried but none yet have shown much success. Chilling of the sores, with cubes of ice applied continuously for an hour at a time, is the latest treatment thought to be of some use.

A form of herpes simplex can affect the genital organs and become a sexually transmitted disease. This again is hard to treat, but a venereologist can do a good deal to give relief. It is always worth seeking help for such an infection.

A cousin of the herpes simplex virus is herpes zoster. This is the causative organism of chicken-pox and also of shingles, in which the path of a nerve is covered by painful watery blisters.

Why does hair go grey when you get older?

No one really knows why hairs lose their pigment with time. It is a widespread phenomenon, although it does not happen to everyone. There have been authenticated cases of people over 70 years old who are as black-haired as ever they were. The tendency to early or late loss of hair colour runs in families.

In fact, hair does not go grey at all. Some hairs lose their pigment and become white. Then the mixture of white hairs and dark hairs give the overall pepper-and-salt effect we call greyness. The greyness gradually lifts as more and more hairs turn white until the whole head seems snowy.

My small son has fair hair, as I did when I was his age. My hair is now brown; will my son's hair change colour?

Almost certainly it will change. Hair goes through three stages as a child grows. First there is lanugo which is finely soft and usually pale in colour. In most cases it is present only before birth, which is why small premature babies have a hairy look. Some full-term babies still have it, however.

This gradually gives way to vellus. This is a little coarser, and slowly becomes more pigmented, and longer in length, though rarely longer than an inch or so.

As time goes on vellus gives way to terminal hair which is coarser, longer and darker. Nearly all children have hair that is lighter than its final colour will be, unless they are particularly dark, in which case the pigment will be settled early on.

I am 22 and my hair seems to be receding fast. What can be done to prevent baldness? My father was bald before he was 30, and I don't want to be like him.

Male-pattern baldness is ineluctable. You can worry and fret, pour on vast quantities of expensive lotions and potions, and nothing will halt it. It is an inherited trait, and a man whose father and other male relations were bald has a high likelihood of being the same. Unfortunately, few men are willing to believe this, and they spend large sums of money making barbers rich and doing themselves no good at all. A man with male-pattern baldness just cannot grow hair.

The basic reason for the loss is the amount of testosterone (male sex hormone) in the man's body Eunuchs, who have had their testicles removed and so have low levels of testosterone, do not go bald. So, a balding man is in a sense displaying his virility – although in fact he has no higher levels than his better thatched friends. It is not true that a rich head of hair points to a low sex hormone level, but it is true that baldness indicates a normal one.

Why do some people have curly hair and some straight?

For the same reason that some have blue eyes and some have brown. It is a trait that has developed during the aeons of evolution, possibly as a mutation that was associated with a useful adaptation – for example, more heavily pigmented skin which would protect its owners in high sunshine areas of the world – and which has been passed down the generations. There is nothing anyone can do to make essentially straight hair grow curly, or vice versa.

Sometimes children have curly hair and become adults with straight hair. This is because the finer hair of childhood finds it easier to curl and later on the thicker, heavier terminal hair pulls against the springing tendency.

What causes dandruff? And what can be done to cure it?

True dandruff is not a disease, but a hurrying up of a normal physiological process. The skin of the scalp regularly sheds little flakes of itself, as does all skin, but in people with true dandruff this seems to happen more quickly and more lavishly. It seems to be most common in late adolescence, and may be associated with acne, but not always. The incidence tends to decline in middle age and is rare in the old.

Some older people have a condition of seborrhoeic dermatitis which also causes the shedding of skin flakes; other people, of all ages, may have psoriasis, another skin disease which results in flake-shedding.

The treatment depends on the basic cause. For true dandruff, most doctors recommend the use of special shampoos containing either selenium sulphide, or zinc pyridinethione. These can be prescribed by the doctor, or bought in most pharmacies. A number of commercial anti-dandruff shampoos are marketed and reading of the small print on the label will tell you whether either of these ingredients is present.

There is one comfort: true dandruff declines in late spring, and is least prevalent in summer. And in winter you can wear a hat for part of the time.

How does hair go white overnight?

It doesn't. It cannot do so, even though there have been so many tales told of it happening (Sir Thomas More's hair was said to have whitened the night before his execution, and General Gordon's during the siege of Khartoum). But, despite all the stories, it is just not possible for it to happen as quickly as has been claimed. A fully grown hair, even though it is held in the follicle which gave it birth, is actually dead tissue and not accessible to change. It can only fall out, in time, leaving the follicle to grow a new hair. We all normally lose about 75 hairs a day, and always have new hairs growing. If you brush your finger tips gently over your scalp, inside the long hair, you will probably feel the bristly new growth.

Why, then, the stories? What can and, perhaps, does happen, is a fairly heavy loss of hair – more than the usual 75 a day – following illness, severe emotional shock, even pregnancy. It happens three months or so after the experience because it takes that long for the hairs to be detached from their follicles. For a not yet fully understood reason, white hairs seem to have a firmer hold on the scalp than pigmented ones, so a heavy loss will usually remove far more dark hairs than white ones. The result of such a loss can leave the remaining hair looking a great deal lighter than it used to.

There is a condition called alopecia areata in which there is sudden heavy hair loss; this can happen very quickly indeed – perhaps within a week or so. Again, the white hairs are spared, so a person with this condition who had only five to 10 per cent of white hair, and so looked quite dark, could be left with a thin thatch of totally white hair fairly quickly. But this metamorphosis would still not happen overnight.

Hair

Hair is found on all skin surfaces except the palms and soles – the scalp alone has about 100,000 hairs. Each hair consists of a shaft (the visible hair), composed of dead tissue, and a follicle which contains the roots and live tissue (growing about 1 inch every 2–3 months). The papilla feeds the follicle with nourishment from the bloodstream

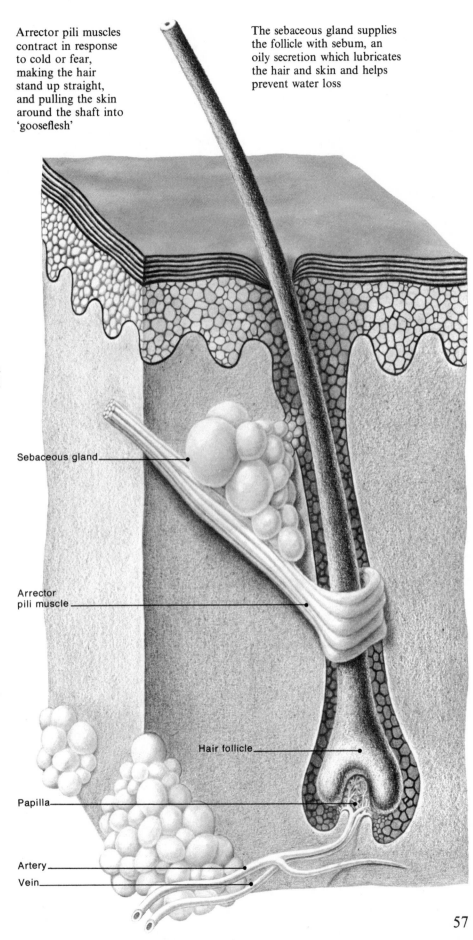

Arrector pili muscles contract in response to cold or fear, making the hair stand up straight, and pulling the skin around the shaft into 'gooseflesh'

The sebaceous gland supplies the follicle with sebum, an oily secretion which lubricates the hair and skin and helps prevent water loss

Sebaceous gland

Arrector pili muscle

Hair follicle

Papilla

Artery

Vein

Bones and muscles

Orthopaedic specialists are great engineers. They need a deep understanding of all the structural stresses and strains to which human bones, joints and muscles are exposed, as well as the detailed understanding of the basic human anatomy and physiology that every doctor has. They tend to be considerable innovators, too. The invention of complex systems for splinting or straightening damaged or misshapen bones and joints has always been a vital part of the orthopaedic craft. Finally, orthopaedic specialists are often very strong physically. Operating on other people's bones and joints demands a great deal of surgical muscle as well as manual delicacy.

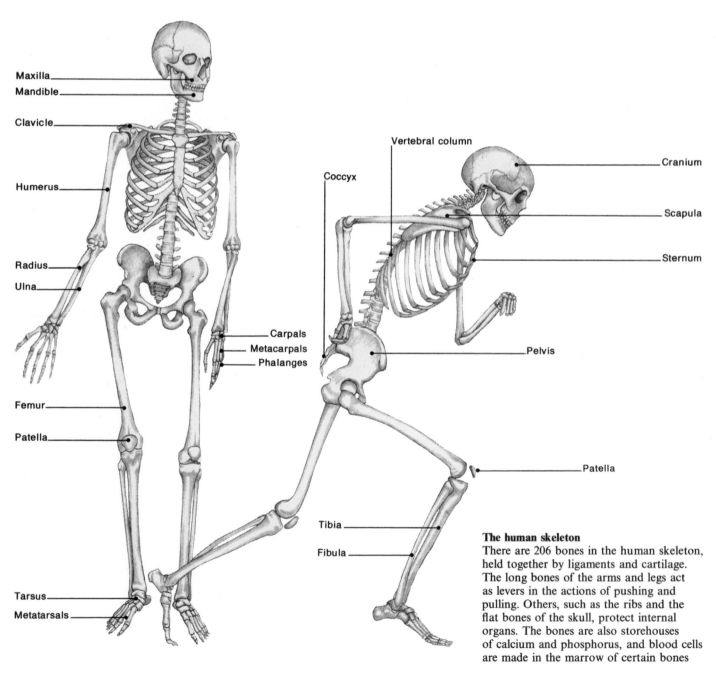

Maxilla
Mandible
Clavicle
Humerus
Radius
Ulna
Carpals
Metacarpals
Phalanges
Femur
Patella
Tarsus
Metatarsals

Vertebral column
Coccyx
Cranium
Scapula
Sternum
Pelvis
Patella
Tibia
Fibula

The human skeleton
There are 206 bones in the human skeleton, held together by ligaments and cartilage. The long bones of the arms and legs act as levers in the actions of pushing and pulling. Others, such as the ribs and the flat bones of the skull, protect internal organs. The bones are also storehouses of calcium and phosphorus, and blood cells are made in the marrow of certain bones

What is the difference between a fracture and a break?

None. The word fracture means break. But a 'fractured tibia' sounds more interesting and important than a 'broken shin', which is probably why people prefer the fancier expression.

Types of fracture
1 Simple – single break. 2 Compound – associated wound. 3 Comminuted – more than two fragments. 4 Complicated – involving another structure, e.g. a blood vessel. 5 Greenstick – partly fractured and bent.

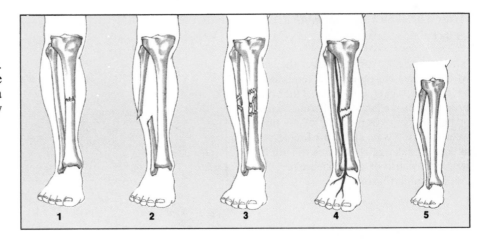

Why did I have to lie in bed in hospital and have my leg pulled by weights when I broke it? Why couldn't I just have it in a plaster cast and carry on at school the way my brother did when he broke his leg?

Because you broke different bones, in different ways. When a bone breaks, the muscles which run alongside it, and which are very powerful, don't just go limp. They go into spasm, bunching up tightly, and this has the effect of bringing the broken edges together. If they stayed that way, held neatly together, that would be ideal. They would then heal easily and safely. But where the muscles are particularly powerful, what usually happens is over-riding of the broken ends so that the limb actually shortens. When this occurs, the bone ends have to be pulled apart, and then fitted together so that they are able to heal correctly.

When the broken bone is one of those in the lower leg (the tibia or fibula) it is usually possible for the ends to be held together by first pulling them apart (under an anaesthetic of course!) and then holding them in place by splinting. A plaster cast is put on, fitted exactly to the leg's contours, very often immobilizing the knee as well as the ankle so that the break is held firmly in place. Once the plaster has set hard, and is fitted with a reinforced heel, the patient can walk about on the leg because the cast is taking the strain.

However, if the bone in the upper leg (the femur) is broken, then it is much harder to immobilize the injury in a cast. First of all the thigh muscles are much more powerful than those of the lower leg, and second, it is much harder to immobilize the joints at either side of the break.

Often the only way to do this is to put the patient to bed with traction applied to the break. This means that weights (often passed over a beam) are hung on to the leg, and these pull all the time on the lower section of the injured bone, ensuring that it stays firmly against its other fragment. The patient usually has a cast on the leg as well, to give extra splinting, although sometimes the traction is applied by passing a metal rod through the leg, below the knee, and applying the traction to that.

Whichever method is used, the aim is the same; to keep the broken ends of bone against each other so that they can heal, and restore the limb to its former strength.

Plaster cast equipment

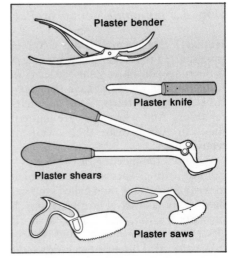

Traction for a thighbone fracture
The leg is supported by weight **A**, while weight **B** pulls the thigh by means of a cord attached to a pin through the shinbone

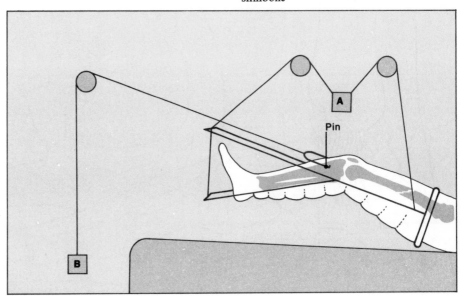

Bones and muscles

After a broken bone has healed, is it weaker?

Not because of the break. In fact, the area where healing has taken place tends to be harder and thicker. Of course, if the bone originally broke because of some illness or because of extreme age, it may be a weak bone anyway, and more fragile and likely to break again. But this will not be weaker because of the first break – for just the same reason.

Structure of bone

Fracture

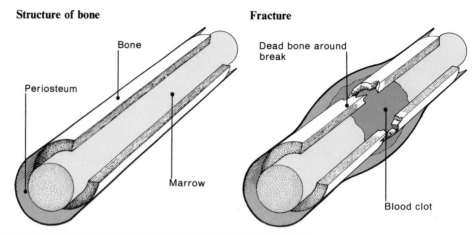

Why did my ankle get so swollen when I twisted it?

Human joints are marvellous pieces of precision engineering. They provide a wide range of movement yet remain stable themselves, they have their own lubricating systems, and are self-repairing. And when they are injured, they can even provide their own protective splint.

A joint – the meeting of two bones – is lined with a special capsule which makes a fairly thick fluid called synovial fluid. This acts as a lubricant, which prevents friction, and acts as a shock absorber. The amount of fluid is carefully controlled because too little would allow the bone ends to grate together and cause limited movement, pain and damage to the moving parts, while too much would cause swelling of the joint and, again, limited movement and pain.

When there is damage to a joint, of the sort that happens when the ankle is violently twisted into a movement outside its normal range, there may be actual tearing of the capsule and of the tough ligaments which bind the bone ends together to give stability. This is a dislocation, because the joint goes out of true. If there is no actual tearing, but still severe stress, then the membrane lining the capsule may be damaged, and will pour out more of its fluid as a result. This is a sprain.

The swelling of the joint is caused by the extra fluid together with the rush of blood to the soft tissues around the joint, the muscles and skin, and supportive tissue.

The rush of blood happens because it is part of the body's natural defence mechanism. Extra blood, and with it food and oxygen supplies, are rushed in, just as a general sends reinforcements and munitions to the part of the battlefield where the enemy attacks.

All this has the effect of immobilizing the joint. It hurts when you move it because of the pressure exerted by the swollen tissues, so you don't move it. And that ensures that the joint rests, and so has time to repair itself.

Twisted ankle

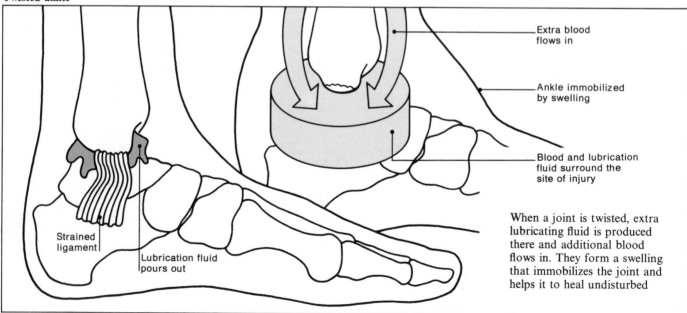

When a joint is twisted, extra lubricating fluid is produced there and additional blood flows in. They form a swelling that immobilizes the joint and helps it to heal undisturbed

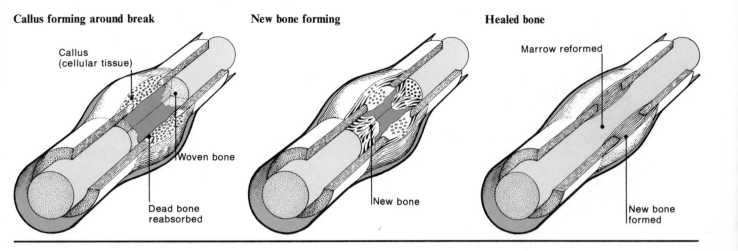

Callus forming around break

Callus
(cellular tissue)

Dead bone
reabsorbed

Woven bone

New bone forming

New bone

Healed bone

Marrow reformed

New bone
formed

Why do old people break their bones so easily?

As time goes on, our bones become more brittle as the tissues of the body shrink and lose their suppleness. It is not only skin and muscles that shrivel and lose elasticity in time. So young bones have a degree of 'bounce' in them, while older bones are inevitably more fragile. Also, older people may be less stable on their feet. They may lose balance more easily, be less able to see hazards and be less likely to hear oncoming danger. All of this adds up to greater likelihood of accident, and with it a greater likelihood of bone injury.

Incidentally, some people think that the breaking of the femur (the thigh bone) in old age is a cause of death. It is not, in itself, but it is true that a very old person may die after such an injury. (George Bernard Shaw is a case in point: he was 94 when he fractured his hip and then he died.)

The reason for this is a combination

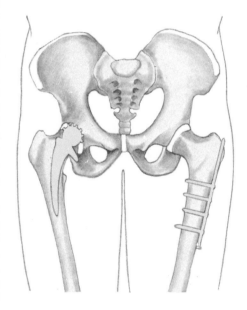

of things. First, there is the shock of the experience which, in a frail old person, is very damaging, and then there is the enforced idleness of bedrest which may be used for treatment. The old person is all too likely to become bedfast, develop pneumonia because of shallow, poor breathing, and will die from that cause.

That is why nowadays every effort is made to get an old person with a broken limb back on to his or her feet as soon as possible. Pinning or plating of a broken hip – the upper part of the femur – is often done on really old people for this reason. Then they have every hope of living for several more enjoyable and mobile years.

Surgery of pelvis and femur
Far left: A ball-and-socket artificial hip joint. *Near left:* A thighbone is held by a pin after surgery

Why don't little children, who fall over such a lot, break their bones?

In small children, the bones are not yet fully formed. At each end of the long bones there are areas of cartilage – thick, tough, jelly-like material – called epiphyses. It is from these special areas that the new bone develops as the child grows. (Bony growth usually ends by the age of about 25 or so.) This means that small children have far more separate bony areas than older children

and adults, so they are less likely to break their bones because there is always an adjoining soft area that can take the shock of a fall.

In addition, babies' bones are far more flexible than older bones – just as green young wood on a tree is much more flexible than fully grown wood. But, in fact, small children do sometimes break their bones in what is called

a 'greenstick fracture'. Only one side breaks, while the other holds firm, just as green wood does when you try to break it.

There is also another reason why small children are much less likely than adults to break bones. They are smaller and lighter so that when they tumble they have less far to go, and they land much less heavily.

Bones and muscles

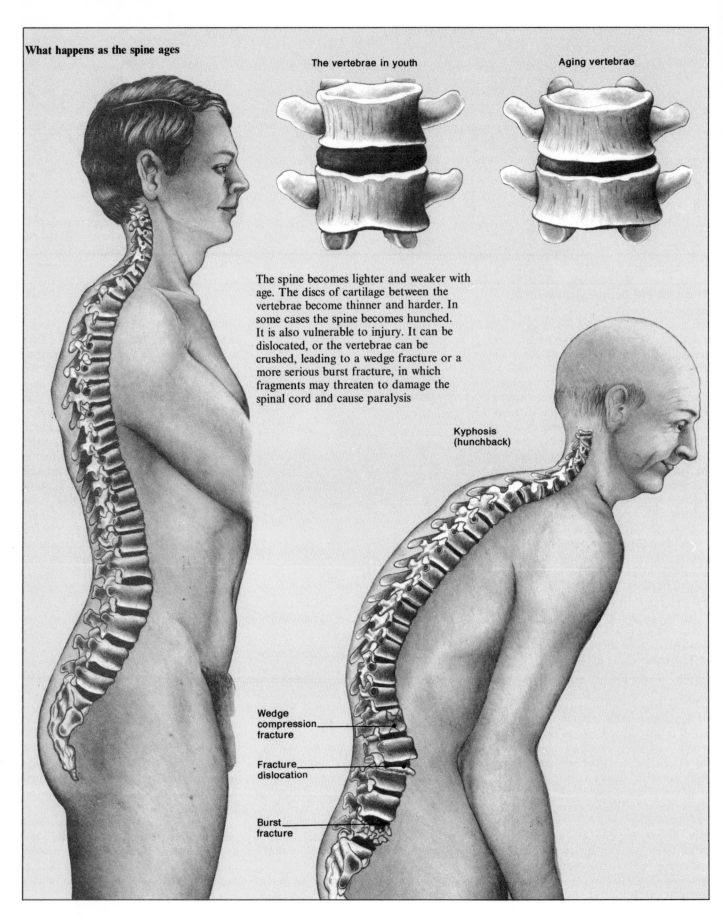

What happens as the spine ages

The vertebrae in youth

Aging vertebrae

The spine becomes lighter and weaker with age. The discs of cartilage between the vertebrae become thinner and harder. In some cases the spine becomes hunched. It is also vulnerable to injury. It can be dislocated, or the vertebrae can be crushed, leading to a wedge fracture or a more serious burst fracture, in which fragments may threaten to damage the spinal cord and cause paralysis

Kyphosis (hunchback)

Wedge compression fracture

Fracture dislocation

Burst fracture

Why do old people grow shorter as they grow older?

When bone ages it not only becomes more brittle and fragile, it actually loses some of its substance. It 'thins' and there may be some shortening as well. This is called osteoporosis, and it is absolutely normal. Everyone loses about 15 per cent of the skeleton in the course of aging. This process starts at around the menopause in women and goes on at the rate of about 0.5 per cent each year. Men, always the more physically favoured of the sexes, start their bones loss about 10 years later, and it goes on more slowly in them.

One effect of this bone loss in older people may be the actual collapse of one or more of the small bones that make up the spine – the vertebrae. They are squashed, and the effect, in addition to a nasty backache, is bending and shortening of the spine.

In addition to the effect of age on bone, there is also the effect of age on cartilage. Between each of the bones of the spine there is a soft fat cushion of this firm jelly-like material – it's the same as the gristle you find in a joint of butcher's meat – which in the young is resilient and bouncy as well as tough. But in older people the cartilage, like all other body tissue, gets thinner and harder – and the result is loss of height. All of which explains why there are so many little bent old men and women about.

Some of this loss is avoidable; not all the bent backs and backaches of the old are due to squashed vertebrae and thin cartilage. Often it is the result of years of sloppy posture.

If you spend all your young years flopping over and letting your shoulders sag, there is no way that you can expect to be upright in your eighties. Learning to walk tall while you are young can do wonders for you when you are old. And a healthy, well-balanced diet, rich in fresh fruits, vegetables, wholemeal grains and whole milk, will provide the necessary raw materials, including calcium, which will keep bones young as long as possible.

Slipped disc presses on spinal cord
When the cartilage between two of the lower vertebrae bulges, it may press on the spinal cord and cause pain along the sciatic nerve

What causes lumbago and sciatica?

These are two words that are often used very inaccurately, together with another term – 'slipped disc' (the technical term is intervertebral disc) – that a lot of people bandy about.

In simple terms, lumbago is pain involving the lower part of the back. Sciatica, which may accompany it, is pain which goes from the lower back, down the buttock and back of the thigh into the back of the calf and foot. It gets its name from the sciatic nerve, which is the biggest nerve in the body and which runs from the lumbar region of the spine (the bottom five vertebrae, just above the solid part called the sacrum and the little 'tail' called the coccyx) down each leg to the foot. If there is pressure on the sciatic nerve it results in the pain and sometimes in tingling and 'pins and needles'.

Why does it happen? The commonest cause is a bulging of the disc of cartilage that lies between each of the small back bones. This bulge puts pressure on the nerves, especially the sciatic nerve, which run through, and emerge from, the spinal column. This is indeed a major problem, and the sufferer may need to spend some time in bed, on a very hard base, to allow the bulge to return to place and relieve the pressure. In severe cases the answer has to be surgery – removal of the offending bulge.

Unfortunately, the idea of a 'slipped disc' has become so popular that people who have backache for other reasons *(see the next question)* will say importantly that they have this condition when they have nothing of the sort. Even some doctors use the label as a lazy way of dealing with a patient with persistent backache and pain in the legs. Sciatica, and certainly lumbago, are not always due to this. They can be caused by the nerve being pinched farther down, perhaps at the point where the nerve leaves the spine, if there has been collapse of the bone of the sort that happens in some old people. Or it can occur where the nerve goes round the fibula, the small bone in the lower leg, on its way to the foot. Severe sciatica is a more likely indicator of 'slipped disc' than lumbago, however.

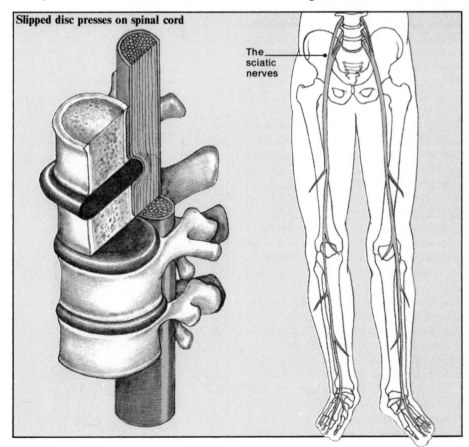

Slipped disc presses on spinal cord

The sciatic nerves

Bones and muscles

Why do I get so much backache?

Backache is one of the most tiresome disorders of modern times. Every year millions of working days are lost because people with bad backs have to stay at home, which is an expensive waste of time as well as being misery for the people with the pain.

Perhaps it is not too surprising that backs cause so many problems. A back is a very complicated creation, made up of nearly three dozen oddly shaped little bones, all surrounded by a cats-cradle of ligaments and muscles, carrying in its centre the most vital communication structures in the body. All too often the muscles and ligaments are strained, even torn, and the bones, especially in older people, become squashed, or the cartilages which cushion them bulge or harden – all of which can lead to back pain.

Only about five to seven per cent of people with backache have disc problems. Most of them suffer as they do for a host of other reasons.

Maybe they are overweight: carrying a lot of excess baggage about in the form of fat puts a great strain on the back.

Perhaps they move and stand and sit badly. Lazy posture, as well as looking dismal, stretches and strains the back painfully. High-heeled shoes can contribute to this; they put an unnatural forward strain on the body.

Some people don't know the best way to lift things. Bending down with straight knees to lift a heavy weight such as a shopping basket, or a two-year-old who wants to be carried, puts extra pressure on the back at its curves which are its weakest points. Crouching down with bent knees is much safer, and enables you to lift heavier weights, too.

People often expose their backs to needless strain by not studying their working conditions. Women in particular suffer this way because their kitchen surfaces are the wrong height for them. Far too many kitchens are designed for the under-five-foot-five, so-called average person – and the thousands of women who are around five-foot-seven or more and who have to use these kitchens feel the result in their backs.

Some people sleep on soggy beds that give no more support than a string hammock. Hours spent on such a surface strains back muscles and ligaments quite severely. A firm bed surface is much healthier.

And some people get backache not because there is anything wrong with their backs, but because they are unhappy. Why the back should carry the load of misery in people who are depressed, frustrated in their jobs or marriages, or unhappy about their life styles and future prospects, no one quite knows. But the fact is that over and over again, doctors find that there is no apparent cause for a person's backache, but that they are undoubtedly suffering from emotional stress. Dealing with the emotional stress – marriage guidance or sex counselling, a new job, a changed life style – can and does lead to miraculous cures in such cases.

Wrong posture   **Correct posture**

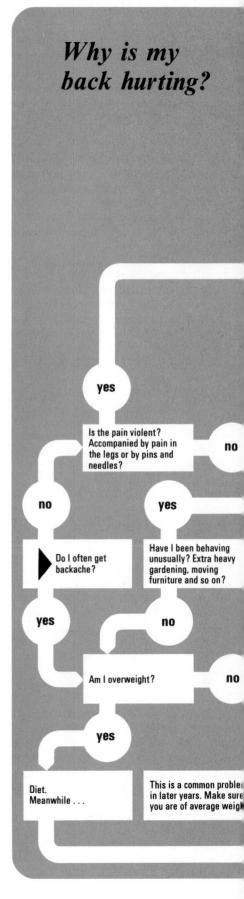

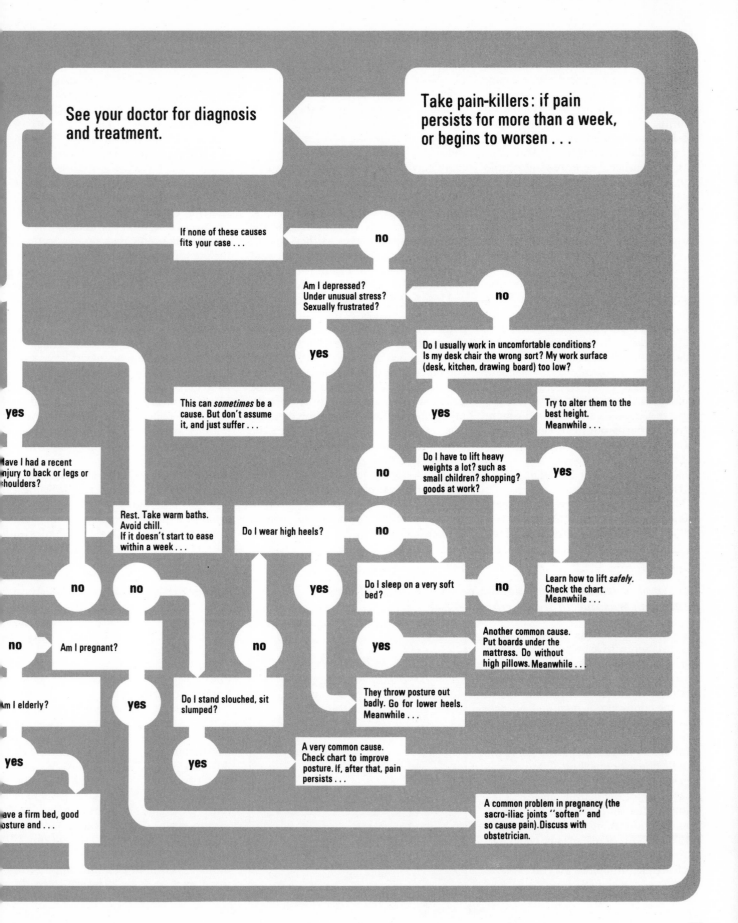

See your doctor for diagnosis and treatment.

Take pain-killers: if pain persists for more than a week, or begins to worsen . . .

If none of these causes fits your case . . .

no

Am I depressed? Under unusual stress? Sexually frustrated?

no

Do I usually work in uncomfortable conditions? Is my desk chair the wrong sort? My work surface (desk, kitchen, drawing board) too low?

yes

This can *sometimes* be a cause. But don't assume it, and just suffer . . .

yes

Try to alter them to the best height. Meanwhile . . .

yes

Have I had a recent injury to back or legs or shoulders?

no

Do I have to lift heavy weights a lot? such as small children? shopping? goods at work?

yes

Rest. Take warm baths. Avoid chill. If it doesn't start to ease within a week . . .

Do I wear high heels?

no

Learn how to lift *safely*. Check the chart. Meanwhile . . .

no

no

yes

Do I sleep on a very soft bed?

no

Another common cause. Put boards under the mattress. Do without high pillows. Meanwhile . . .

no

Am I pregnant?

no

yes

They throw posture out badly. Go for lower heels. Meanwhile . . .

Am I elderly?

yes

Do I stand slouched, sit slumped?

A very common cause. Check chart to improve posture. If, after that, pain persists . . .

yes

yes

Have a firm bed, good posture and . . .

A common problem in pregnancy (the sacro-iliac joints "soften" and so cause pain). Discuss with obstetrician.

Bones and muscles

What causes rheumatism, because I've had it for years?

There are about fifty different conditions that can be called rheumatism. Some of them are severe illnesses such as Still's disease, which is a rheumatoid arthritis affecting children, and some are little more than vague aches and twinges that come and go, often linked with the weather. There are some people who reckon that they can tell when it's going to rain or snow, because they get an 'attack of the screws'.

Fibrositis is a label given to the muscular aches and pains many people complain of, and for which no other reason can be found.

There is no osteoarthrosis – the degenerative condition in which joints become stiff and less mobile as the cartilage in them thins and hardens, and bony overgrowths appear. There is no inflammatory disease such as rheumatoid arthritis, a potentially severe illness in which there is fever and general ill-health as well as pain and stiffness in the joints of the hands and feet, and which, before it 'burns out', can cause severe deformities of the joints.

There is no disc lesion, that is, the spine shows no signs of bulging discs between the small bones.

There is no sign of error of the body defence mechanisms – auto-immunity – that is now believed to cause some of the rheumatic illnesses. There is just this ill-defined aching.

Fibrositis got its name because the problem was thought to be one of inflammation of the fibres of the muscles, but nowadays few doctors think this actually happens. They say there may be localized muscle spasms – a form of minor cramp, or weak spots in the tough covering of the muscles which allow fibres to bulge through and be pinched, or minor irregularities in the spine which nip nerves as they emerge from the central spinal column, and cause pain in the muscles to which those nerves send their messages.

Most sufferers find out for themselves what triggers their attacks of pain. In some people it is bad posture – sitting slumped for long hours in one position. Their muscles get stiff and sore and take a long time to recover. In other people, it is getting chilled; these are the people who are sensitive to weather. In others it is caused by emotional stress. There is nothing like a fight with the boss to bring on an aching shoulder.

Once you recognize what causes the pain it obviously helps if you avoid the cause whenever that is possible. And using enough simple pain-killers early in an attack, before the pain really builds up, helps as well.

I never play tennis, yet my doctor said the pain I suffered in my arm was due to tennis elbow. Why?

The condition could as easily have been labelled 'screwdriver elbow' because it can be caused by heavy use of this tool by a person who is not used to it, just as it can be caused by excessive tennis playing. In fact the condition of pain and stiffness involving the elbow can be caused by any sustained and unusual activity of the joint. It may be due to a partial tear of the muscle fibres, or pinching of the nerve as it passes through the muscles at the elbow or swelling of the capsule enclosing the joint – bursitis. Treatment may be by manipulation or injection of cortisone into the elbow, or rest may be enough to cure it. The condition usually resolves itself in time, although it may take several months.

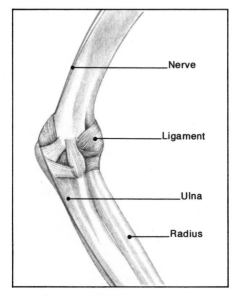

Nerve

Ligament

Ulna

Radius

Why does cramp come on at any time, even when I'm asleep?

Cramp is a painful hard spasm of a muscle that feels as though someone has tied a knot in it and is pulling cruelly on both ends at once. There are lots of causes of cramp and most doctors admit that they just don't know all of them.

Sometimes cramp is due to known disease. Narrowed arteries which are caused by atheroma (deposits of fatty material on the walls of blood vessels) or arteriosclerosis (hardening of the vessel walls) can cause angina pectoris, the chest pain due to a heart starved of an adequate blood supply, or intermittent claudication, cramp in the legs brought on by walking. Treatment of the underlying illness relieves the cramps.

Salt hunger is a possible cause of cramp in healthy people. Those who have been playing a fast game of squash or a hard round of golf, or sitting in blazing sunshine, lose so much salt as the sweat pours out of them that their muscles are starved of salt because the blood levels fall. It can also happen to people who work in sweaty, hard jobs, such as mining and stoking. The remedy is to replace the salt, and the pleasantest way is to take a glass of fresh orange or grapefruit juice topped up with soda water, sweetened with glucose and with a hearty pinch of salt added. Take this once an hour during such heavy exercise. It is also useful to eat salty food if you live in a hot climate, or regularly do sweaty work – there's a good health reason for all those salty anchovies and olives which are so important a part of the Mediterranean diet.

Swimmer's cramp is thought to be due to the blood being diverted from the limbs to the stomach to digest food – which is why people should not swim within an hour or two of eating a meal. Writer's cramp is probably more emotional than physical. So many different muscles are involved in holding a pen and moving it over paper that true cramp which affects all of them at once is highly unlikely, unless the person really doesn't want to do the writing any more. Pregnancy cramp is sometimes due to the baby's use of the mother's salt and calcium supplies, or there may be some pressure from the enlarged and heavy uterus on the vessels supplying blood to the legs so that they are starved of essential blood (and salt, of course). And no one has yet come up with a satisfactory answer to the agonizing attacks of cramp which wake perfectly healthy people and make them scream with pain in the middle of the night.

The best way to deal with sudden cramp is to try, gently, to stretch the afflicted muscle. Rubbing the painful area only makes it hurt more. If the calf is affected – and it's the likeliest area – pushing the heel down on to the ground and pulling the toes up towards the knee usually ends the pain dramatically.

There is one other kind of extremely embarassing and painful cramp from which some people suffer and which is rather more difficult to deal with. This is cramp of the levator ani muscle – a thin sheet of tissue which is in the pelvis and which when it goes into cramp causes excruciating pain in the anus, the exit of the bowels. The only way to stretch the muscle here is to gently and evenly push open the anus – not an easy task, especially if you are a bit squeamish about handling this part of your body. A useful gadget for such stretching is one of those large alabaster eggs that are sold in so many gift shops. It must be large enough to avoid the risk of pushing it in too far and losing it, and the blunt end should preferably be used. Keeping the pressure on for a few minutes should relieve the pain.

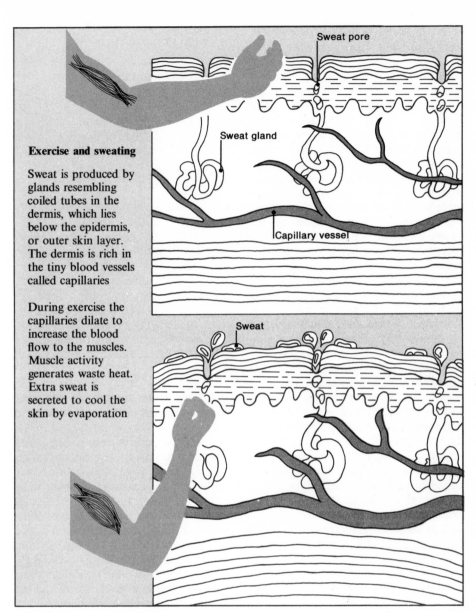

Exercise and sweating

Sweat is produced by glands resembling coiled tubes in the dermis, which lies below the epidermis, or outer skin layer. The dermis is rich in the tiny blood vessels called capillaries

During exercise the capillaries dilate to increase the blood flow to the muscles. Muscle activity generates waste heat. Extra sweat is secreted to cool the skin by evaporation

Cramp after exercise

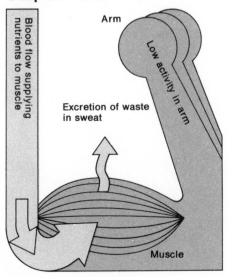

Blood flow supplying nutrients to muscle

Arm

Low activity in arm

Excretion of waste in sweat

Muscle

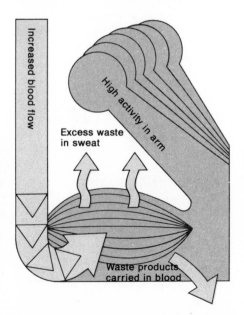

Increased blood flow

High activity in arm

Excess waste in sweat

Waste products carried in blood

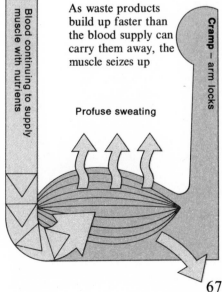

Blood continuing to supply muscle with nutrients

As waste products build up faster than the blood supply can carry them away, the muscle seizes up

Cramp – arm locks

Profuse sweating

Bones and muscles

Why do some people get knobbly joints on their hands as they get older?

It is not only the cartilage between the small bones of the back that thins and hardens as time goes on; so does the cartilage between all the joints, including those in the hands where there are at least 15. This thinning causes painful rubbing inside the joints, and the linings try to reduce the friction by pouring out more lubricating fluid, which, in turn, causes swelling and stiffness of the joints. But there is more going on than that; there is a tendency for little extra bits of rough bone to grow, and these can push the joint out of line.

As well as all this, some people suffer from gout, an illness in which showers of crystals of uric acid (a by-product of the digestion of protein foods, especially meat such as liver and kidney, and vegetables such as peas and beans) are deposited as painful lumps in the joints, often in the feet, but also in the hands and elsewhere. It is not true, by the way, that gout is always due to rich living and the drinking of too much port and brandy and sherry. It is usually an inherited tendency, and however careful you are with your diet, if you are a member of an affected family, you are a candidate for gout.

Add all this together, and the result is the knobbly stiff hands with which some old people are afflicted. But it isn't all bad news. These days surgery can eliminate many of the problems.

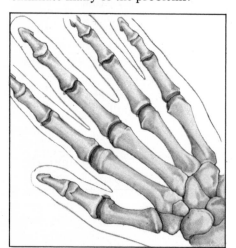

Where arthritis strikes
Arthritis of the finger joints in old age is due to degeneration of the cartilage between them

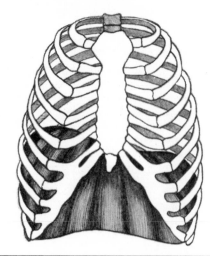

The position of the diaphragm in relation to the rib cage

Why do I get a stitch when I run?

A stitch is a cramp of the diaphragm, the great sheet of muscle that lies between the chest and belly, or of the muscles between the ribs, the intercostals. Bending over and reaching for the toes usually stretches the cramp enough to relieve it.

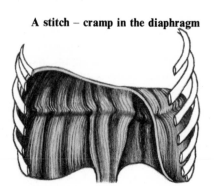

A stitch – cramp in the diaphragm

Why are some people double jointed? My sister can do the splits but I can't.

No one has double joints, but some people have very mobile ones; that is, their joints are capable of a somewhat greater range of movement than other people's. This can be an inherited tendency; some black people have greater joint mobility than some white people, which could account for the development of such dances as the West Indian 'Limbo' in which people have to bend backwards from the knees and get under a low bar. The Limbo can be done by white people, of course, but most of them find it very difficult.

Also, some people are more willing than others to try unusual movements. Maybe both you and your sister have hip joints of equal mobility but you don't want to risk the possible pain of stretching the joints as far as she does.

However, you may be wiser than she is, if a bit less adventurous, because over-stretching of ligaments in joints can lead to long-term damage. Dancers who regularly punish their joints and muscles as part of their performances often suffer from osteoarthrosis (creaking, painful joints) at a younger age than other people. Athletes, such as gymnasts, carry the same risk.

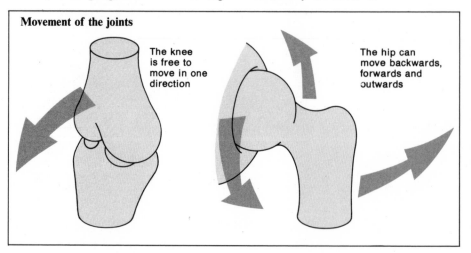

Movement of the joints

The knee is free to move in one direction

The hip can move backwards, forwards and outwards

Why have I got corns and bunions on both feet, while my husband has none? Are women more liable to these?

Corns are areas of hardened skin over the knuckles of the toes, and at the side of the small toe. Sometimes soft corns appear between the toes.

Bunions are enlargements of the big toe joints. Sometimes they consist of swelling due to excess fluid in a little sac covering the joint (this condition is called bursitis) and sometimes they are due to actual bony enlargement and displacement of the joint.

Often, where there are corns and bunions, there are also callouses. These are areas of hardened skin on the sole of the foot, around the heel, and on the back of the heel.

The cause of all these things is much the same, namely pressure. It is a rule in nature that constant pressure causes atrophy, that is, withering away and dying of the part under pressure, while intermittent pressure causes hypertrophy, that is, extra growth of the area under pressure. If a person were constantly to wear shoes so tight that the toes were crushed together and couldn't move, then in quite a short time the toes would lose all their blood supply and die; they would develop gangrene. But because we don't go to bed in the tight shoes that so many of us insist on wearing during the day, we develop corns instead – the skin grows thick pads in an attempt to protect itself from the constriction of the shoes. The hard skin builds up and up until it causes pressure on the deeper structure of the toe, and it causes pain that continues after the shoe that started the corn in the first place is taken off. If the corns are between the toes, they tend to be soft, as the sweat works on them, but they are still painful.

Bunions are caused in the same way. The big toe is forced across its neighbours by being scrunched up in a pointed toe, and the small toes often fold upwards to create hammer toes which get corns on their knuckles because of their pressure against the uppers of the shoes. The swelling happens when the little sac of fluid appears to try to protect the underlying joint.

Some people are more likely to suffer bunions than others. They have an inherited tendency to the bony change in the big toe joint (doctors call it hallux valgus) because they are born with a bony structure that is particularly vulnerable to such development.

Men suffer corns and bunions less often than women because at present the fashion in men's shoes is a sensible one – wide toe sections, giving room for movement of the toes and good supporting insteps which prevent the foot from sliding down and being crushed up against the end of the shoe. Women still tend to go for shoes with small, pointed toes and high heels with open fronts which push the feet down into trouble. But if the fashion for men changes to the 'winkle-pickers' of the nineteen-fifties, they will suffer the same foot troubles as women do now and which they did then.

People who regularly go barefoot do not entirely escape these problems, however. They get callouses on the soles of their feet and around the edges of their heels.

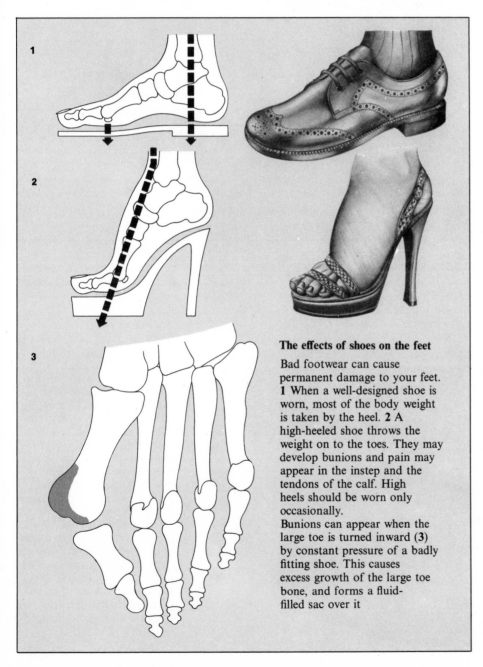

The effects of shoes on the feet

Bad footwear can cause permanent damage to your feet. **1** When a well-designed shoe is worn, most of the body weight is taken by the heel. **2** A high-heeled shoe throws the weight on to the toes. They may develop bunions and pain may appear in the instep and the tendons of the calf. High heels should be worn only occasionally.
Bunions can appear when the large toe is turned inward (**3**) by constant pressure of a badly fitting shoe. This causes excess growth of the large toe bone, and forms a fluid-filled sac over it

Eyes

The eyes are actually part of the brain; the only part of it that is in contact with the outside world. The remainder of the nervous system is enclosed safely inside the body. This means that the eyes are not only the organs of sight, but are also a source of information about what is happening inside the brain. Ophthalmologists therefore deal with the disorders of the eyes that interfere with satisfactory vision, and also with eye diseases which may involve the brain. Working with ophthalmologists are opticians who are experts on the provision of lenses to improve the eyes' ability to collect visual images. Although opticians do not treat eye diseases, they are often well able to make early diagnoses of them and advise people to seek the further help of an ophthalmologist.

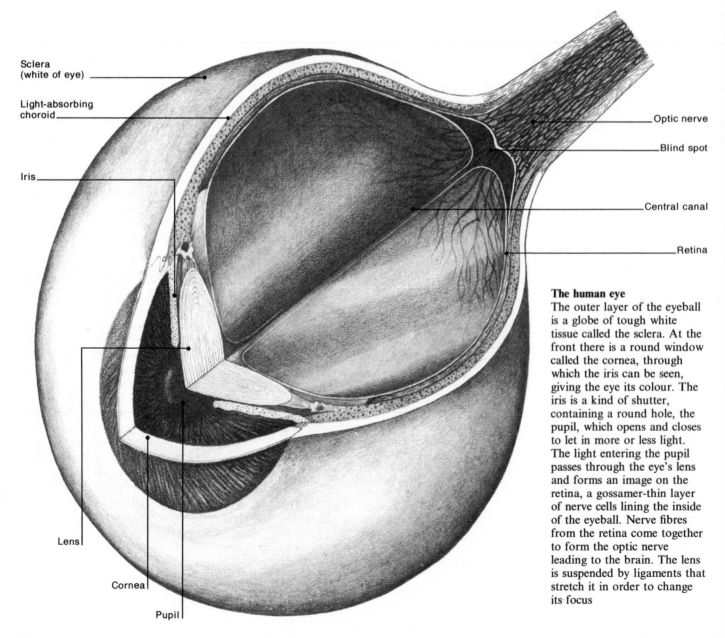

Sclera
(white of eye)

Light-absorbing
choroid

Iris

Lens

Cornea

Pupil

Optic nerve

Blind spot

Central canal

Retina

The human eye
The outer layer of the eyeball is a globe of tough white tissue called the sclera. At the front there is a round window called the cornea, through which the iris can be seen, giving the eye its colour. The iris is a kind of shutter, containing a round hole, the pupil, which opens and closes to let in more or less light. The light entering the pupil passes through the eye's lens and forms an image on the retina, a gossamer-thin layer of nerve cells lining the inside of the eyeball. Nerve fibres from the retina come together to form the optic nerve leading to the brain. The lens is suspended by ligaments that stretch it in order to change its focus

Why is it that some old people need glasses and some never do?

Clear vision demands that the rays of light coming from the object at which you are looking should reach the back of the eye (where they are collected to be transmitted to the vision centre in the brain) exactly together (*see the illustration*). The rays are bent (refracted) on the way in by the lens at the front of the eye. The lens is a tiny transparent body which is capable of changing its shape to produce the necessary degree of bending.

In many people the shape of the eyeball (which varies greatly, shape being inherited from both parents) does not allow the bent rays to meet at the right point. Sometimes the rays meet just in front of the retina. This leads to short sight, or myopia. If objects are brought close to the eye, then the rays meet at the right spot on the retina, and can be clearly seen. This is why myopic people hold things that they want to see close to their eyes. (And a charming story is told of Mary Norton, the children's writer. She was severely myopic in childhood and no one realized it. When she went for walks in the countryside near her home she had to peer very closely into hedges and grass

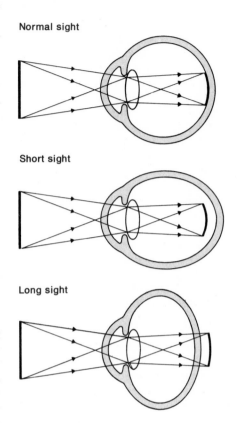

Normal sight

Short sight

Long sight

to see anything; and when she grew up she wrote 'The Borrowers' – a story about tiny people inhabiting a world full of huge structures.)

Long sight, hypermetropia, happens when the light rays meet at a point beyond the retina. It is something that tends to happen to all of us as we get older, because the lens loses its suppleness and hardens and is not as good as it was at bending the rays. This is why people who have always had good eyesight tend, after the age of 45 or so, to hold things which they want to see clearly away from them – the long-arm posture. The proper name for this is presbyopia.

People who were short-sighted when they were young come into their own as presbyopia develops (as it does in all of us sooner or later) and makes the short-sighted eye more long-sighted. They are the ones who can go on happily without spectacles for much longer than the rest of us.

However, even short-sighted people, as the years go on and the lens hardens more, are likely to find that they eventually have to resort to glasses.

Is it true that reading a lot or doing a lot of close, fine work can weaken your eyesight?

Absolutely not. Vision does not come in limited quantities, like packs of sugar. As long as the eye is healthy it will pick up visual signals and transmit them to the brain to be interpreted and will go on doing it all the time and never get fatigued.

However, the eye muscles which control eye movement, and therefore the amount of visual signals that can be picked up, can tire, and long periods of

concentrated reading or sewing or painting may weary them so much that they just cannot go on responding to the demands put on them. The result is reddening of the eye (*see the earlier question*) and tiredness of the lids which makes them want to close; indeed they insist on closing. But the vision under the closed lids is as lively as ever.

The sad thing about the widespread myth that vision can be 'worn out' is the

way in which some older people, or people with eye disorders, limit their pleasure in reading or watching television for fear of losing their remaining eyesight. They need not. Using whatever vision you have never causes it to deteriorate.

To avoid glare, direct lamps on to your work or reading, not into your eyes, and have some lights on when you watch TV

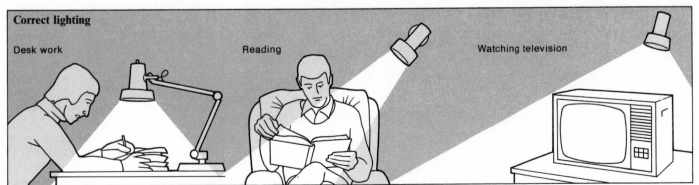

Correct lighting

Desk work

Reading

Watching television

Eyes

Why do I keep on blinking? And why can some people prevent themselves from blinking, as actors sometimes do?

The eye is the only part of the brain that is in direct contact with the outside world – and as well as being a complex structure it is a delicate one.

It is covered on its outer surface with a transparent, supple membrane (called the conjunctiva) which folds back on itself at the top and bottom to line the eyelids. The membrane is needed to keep the eye surface moist and slippery so that the eye can move about constantly.

Even when you think you are staring at something unwaveringly, your eyes are actually making tiny flickering movements. This is necessary for really sharp vision; when the eye picks up the image the small movements 'spread' it over a larger area of the seeing part inside the eye (the retina) and so sharpen the picture.

Obviously, this frequent movement would be difficult if the eye were dry; there would be rubbing and friction. So with the aid of tears (a salty liquid produced in special glands beneath the upper lids) the eyelids keep the globes of the eyeballs at the ideal level of moistness by sweeping tears regularly over the conjunctivae and pushing the tears into the corners of the eyes.

Blinking is something that happens by itself as a reflex action – you don't have to think about it – even though the eyelids are under conscious control. You can close them and open them when you want to, blink as often as you want to, and stop blinking when you want to – though that does take rather more effort. This is because the drying out of the conjunctivae triggers the reflex blink that is needed for remoistening. Whether asleep or awake, the stimulation of the eyelashes causes blinking.

With practice, the reflex can be inhibited for quite long periods, but even the most gifted of actors would find it difficult to maintain a non-blinking pose for more than a minute or so at a time. It would be a dangerous thing to do, anyway; if the conjunctivae do dry out the result is pain and possibly damage to the delicate structures. However, it is possible to prevent yourself blinking for up to five minutes if you are under water, because the water keeps the eyes wet. But even in these circumstances blinking is unavoidable for any longer.

Lubrication of the eyeball and eyelid

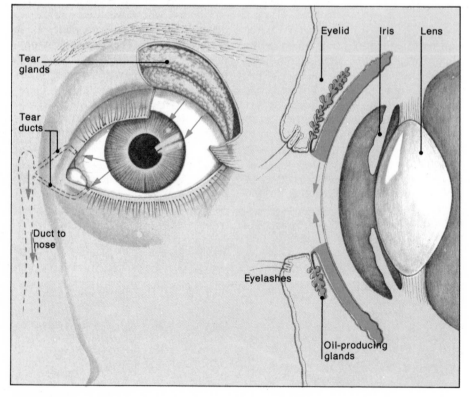

Tear glands

Tear ducts

Duct to nose

Eyelid   Iris   Lens

Eyelashes

Oil-producing glands

Why do my eyes sometimes feel gritty, especially when I'm tired?

Irritation or dryness of the conjunctivae causes a pain message to be sent to the brain, where it is registered as a feeling of grittiness. It is common, and often normal. When a person is tired and needs sleep, for example, fatigue is signalled as grittiness. This has led to the rather charming notion that a sandman comes and throws sand in the eyes of children at the end of the day to tell them that it's bedtime.

Persistent gritty pain plus redness and stickiness probably means conjunctivitis, which needs treatment.

Why do I get spots in front of my eyes?

The most likely reason is 'floaters'. About 80 per cent of the population complain about these at some time or another. They are flecks that look like tadpoles or motes of dust and they are much easier to see when you are looking at a blank white surface. They are due to tiny specks of dead tissue – a few cells – which come away from the lining of the eyeball and bob about in the fluid with which it is filled. People who are nervous, worried, depressed or tired tend to complain about floaters more than relaxed, unworried people, not because they have more of them, but because they are more aware of them.

Generally speaking they are of no significance at all, though tiresome. But if they increase greatly in amount over a short period of time, get a medical check. They may be a sign of inflammation at the back of the eye, or just possibly a threatened detachment of the retina. This is an alarming experience which results in sudden partial blindness but modern techniques have made it much more easy to treat successfully.

Other causes of seeing spots may be fainting: when someone feels shaky and groggy and is about to pass out they may get a sort of dazzling of the vision which looks like fast-moving spots. Excess alcohol can cause it, as can some medicines. In a few cases, people with high blood pressure get this sort of visual disturbance as well. If in any doubt, seek expert advice.

Why do the pupils of my eyes change size from time to time?

Vision depends on the amount of light that gets into the eye. The pupil controls the amount of light that can enter. It really is as simple as that. When light is bright the pupil contracts, allowing in only enough light to see, and not enough to damage the delicate retina (as, of course, excess light can – staring at the sun can cause blindness). When light is limited, the pupil widens to allow in as much light as it can.

But there are other reasons for pupil activity. Drugs affect the size of the aperture. For example, the opiates – morphine, heroin and so on – cause it to contract to a very tiny space; hence the pin-point pupil of the drug user. Atropine, on the other hand, causes it to enlarge hugely.

Which brings up a rather interesting point. Another reason for enlarging of the pupils is interest or excitement – people watching a dramatic football game have enlarged pupils, and a man or woman seeing a handsome member of the opposite sex also has wide pupils.

Atropine is also known as belladonna or 'beautiful lady'. Renaissance women used it to enlarge their pupils and so make their eyes look as though they were in a perpetual state of sexual excitement, because nothing excites a man's sexual interest more than seeing a woman who appears to be sexually interested in him. And vice versa, of course. This is why so many fictional heroes are described as having 'big eyes' or 'dark eyes' or 'deep eyes.,

Pupil wide open –
more light enters the eye

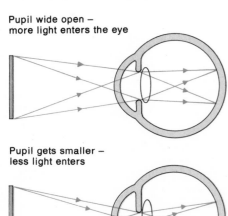

Pupil gets smaller –
less light enters

How the eye lens focuses

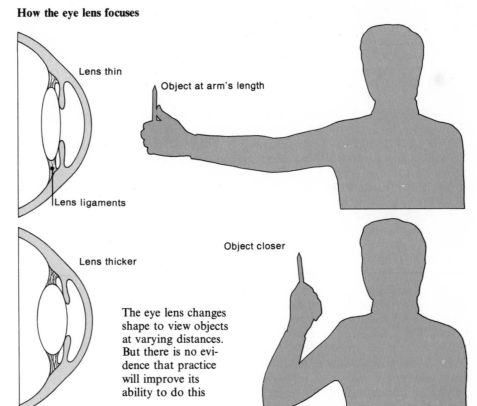

Lens thin

Object at arm's length

Lens ligaments

Lens thicker

Object closer

The eye lens changes shape to view objects at varying distances. But there is no evidence that practice will improve its ability to do this

Can sight be improved by exercises? And isn't it better to do without glasses for as long as you possibly can? Using them too soon must weaken your vision.

There are some people who think that frequent practising of eye movements – such as focusing first on a distant object and then on a close one – will improve the lenses' ability to accommodate and so improve sharpness of vision. There is no evidence whatsoever that this is true. All the exercises cause is frustration and fatigue which limits comfortable vision.

However, there are some people who, after illness or any other tiring experience, find that their vision becomes blurred for close work. They are suffering from a tendency to lose control of their eyes muscles, not failure of the lenses to accommodate. The eyes drift outwards when they try to look at close objects.

For them there is a simple exercise which they can try. They should take a pencil, hold it at arm's length and then slowly bring it in towards the nose, focusing on the tip of the pencil, and go on until it actually hurts to continue. That is about when the pencil is four inches away. If they do this once a day for a month, they may be able to correct the tendency to outwards drift.

The time when a person needs glasses depends as much on personality as on visual sharpness. There are some happy-go-lucky souls who can move through the world in a blissful blur and not really mind that everything looks muzzy. There are others who are so impatient and quick that they cannot tolerate any loss of sharp definition, and clamour for glasses at the first hint of fuzziness.

It is certainly not true that glasses hasten the loss of the ability to see clearly; but people do become lazy and come to depend on their glasses more and more once they start using them. Fatigue comes into it, too. There are many of us who can read the paper without glasses in the morning but not in the evening. Also, light matters greatly. Low diffused light is pretty in a living room, but it can make seeing difficult for someone with presbyopia. If you provide a bright clear light for close work, it can help you to do without glasses for quite a while.

Eyes

Why do some people squint?

The eyes are controlled by three pairs of muscles apiece, which together can create a remarkable array of movements. They can make the eyes swivel in their sockets in Eddie Cantor style; they can roll the eyes upwards, downwards and sideways, boxing the compass.

This great range of movement is needed to give us our full stereoscopic vision. Each eye collects a different image and adjusts it by fine movements of the eye muscles, and of the lens. These two images are then 'married' in the brain to give us the final complete picture.

In a new baby, focusing ability is limited, if present at all (no one can be quite sure about how clearly new babies see, since they can't tell us) and the eyes tend to swivel around all over the place. This is why a tiny baby will sometimes produce the most ferocious squint (the medical name incidentally is strabismus). As long as this is a temporary thing it is not important. As the baby develops he will gradually learn to move his two eyes in harmony with each other. It is only if there is a constant squint that treatment may be needed, so a new baby with a squint that persists should be seen by a doctor.

If the occasional squinting of the young persists after the age of six months or so, again, medical assessment is needed, especially if there is a family history of squinting, because this tendency can be inherited.

The problem can be treated either by the use of special glasses and exercises which teach the child to use his eye muscles in harmony, or, in some cases, by surgery which corrects the error in the muscles. The eye itself is not operated on – only its muscles.

In older people the appearance of a new squint should be medically assessed; it may indicate some disorder of the nervous system or brain as well as of the eye. However, again, an occasional squint is less important. Many adults will squint when they are tired, or relaxed by a few drinks. It is a new, constant squint that needs attention.

Incidentally, in some parts of the world a degree of squint is regarded as exceedingly beautiful. A wall-eyed lady in a yashmak can be very desirable in some Middle Eastern countries. And even here in the West we don't find it all that disagreeable.

Why can I make both of my eyes turn inwards, but not outwards?

The ability to make the eyes converge is needed in order to see small objects close to us. It is possible to bring the eyes inwards so far that vision actually blurs, as the eyes 'cross' and look in opposite directions from usual. The muscles are used to moving in this way.

However, we do not need to turn our eyes outwards simultaneously. Rabbits do – their eyes are at the sides of their heads, and this means that they can see in front of them when they make their eyes converge, and behind them when they diverge. If we did this, we would get a very distorted view of our world; the different pictures we get because of the inch or so that our eyes are apart makes it difficult enough for us to get clear vision. It would be much more difficult if the eyes could stare out to the sides at the same time. So, the muscles which pull the eyes sideways and outwards are incapable of acting together.

Movements of the left eye

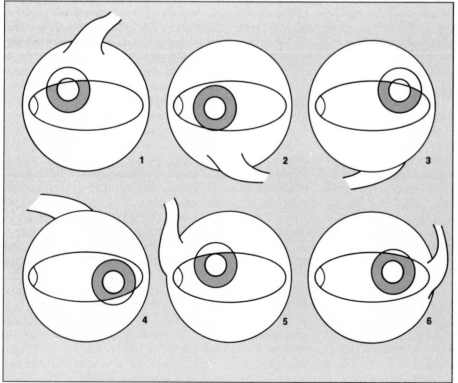

Trochlea

5 Medial rectus

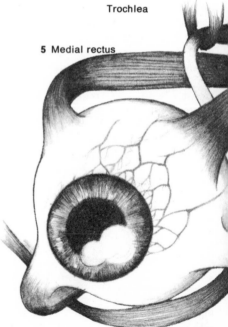

3 Inferior oblique

Six muscles move each eyeball. The diagram at the left shows the effect of each muscle of the left eye when it acts alone. The numbers correspond to the numbering of the muscles in the picture above. In most eye movements, several muscles act together

Eyes

Can make-up or eye lotions damage your eyes?

Generally speaking, any make-up which is comfortable to wear is harmless. But some people suffer allergic responses to some brands which cause reddening of the eyes, excess tear production and swollen lids. When that happens, they stop using it since it was meant to make them look more beautiful, and allergic responses are not a pretty sight. They can then try a hypoallergic brand.

The use of branded eye lotions or baths is different. They really are not necessary unless you work in a particularly dusty or dirty atmosphere (in which case you ought to wear protective goggles anyway) when eye bathing may be comforting. However, there is no need to invest in heavily advertised brands of lotion. Make your own with a teaspoon of salt dissolved in a pint of boiled water with a pinch of bicarbonate added (to prevent it from stinging). Never use eye ointments without a doctor's recommendation.

What is a stye? Why does it happen?

A stye is simply an infected eyelash root, or sometimes an infected sebaceous gland. These tiny glands are all over the skin and produce a skin-lubricating and soothing material called sebum. We collect the sebum made by sheep (it is called lanolin) for many uses.

Germs get into the tiny opening of the follicles or the gland, start to multiply, and the local blood supply immediately increases as the body's defence systems are mobilized. The result is redness, pain and swelling. Later, when the build-up of pus in the area causes the stye to burst, the pus discharges (pus consists of the dead germs and the white cells which had rushed to the site to destroy them, together with broken-down tissue from the inflammation).

An occasional stye can happen to any of us. But if they are frequent and multiple and stubbornly resist healing you may have an underlying disorder which needs medical treatment.

A stye

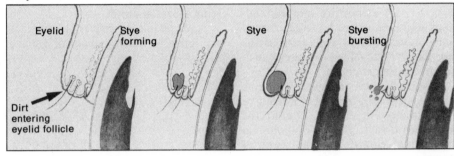

Eyelid • Stye forming • Stye • Stye bursting • Dirt entering eyelid follicle

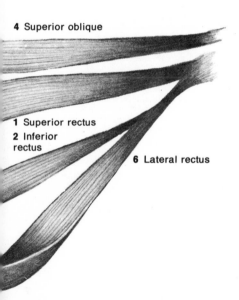

4 Superior oblique
1 Superior rectus
2 Inferior rectus
6 Lateral rectus

Why do my eyes sometimes go bloodshot?

Together with every other part of the body the eyes are plentifully supplied with blood to provide fuel – food and oxygen – for the work of their cells. The eyeballs have their blood vessels, and so do the conjunctivae. Usually you do not see the ones supplying the conjunctivae –

although if you look in a mirror and gently lift your upper lid and pull down the lower lid you will see the delicate tracery of some of the tiny vessels glowing redly because the blood inside shows through. There are even smaller vessels, usually invisible, on the rest of the conjunctivae.

Sometimes the blood supply to the area is greatly increased, and the blood vessels swell up with their greater quantity of blood inside, and so do the very small, usually invisible, ones. The result is the engorged redness called bloodshot eyes.

The reasons it happens are many. Local irritation can do it – dust flying in, tobacco smoke, or small foreign bodies. The tear glands respond by making more tears to wash out the invaders, and they call up more blood to help them to do the extra work.

Sometimes the cause is irritation to nearby structures rather than to the eyes themselves. Irritation of the nose, for example, can result in red eyes, as anyone who has ever had hay fever or a really bad cold knows. In this case, the nerve supply to the nose is stimulated and some of the stimulation is passed on to the eyes' nerve supply.

Fatigue can cause bloodshot eyes, too. When any muscle anywhere gets tired, it demands more blood to supply it with its needs, and the eye muscles, of which there are 12 – six to each eye – are no different. And again, more blood supply shows as red streaks.

These causes are relatively unimportant – removal of the irritation or resting will get rid of the redness. But if the cause is infection and inflammation of the conjunctivae (a condition called conjunctivitis) it is different. When this happens the result is not only redness but pain and often the production of a sticky discharge which can almost glue the lids together. There may also be swelling of the eyelids. The condition – popularly called 'redeye' – is highly infectious and can spread around a family like wildfire if its members share towels and wash flannels with each other. A doctor can treat conjunctivitis with antibiotics. Strict hygiene for the afflicted individual protects the family.

In a few cases, red eyes may indicate the illness of glaucoma, a potentially severe condition, so always check persistent red eyes with your doctor.

Eyes

What are the causes of blindness?

Blindness may be caused by conditions that interfere with the entry of light into the eyes; conditions which impair the eye's ability to react to light; interruptions in the delivery of messages to the seeing part of the brain; and conditions which damage the brain's ability to handle light messages.

For example, inflammation of the outer tough coating of the eyeball, the cornea, may result in scarring. The scar tissue is not transparent, as the cornea should be, so light cannot get in. This can be the result of direct injury to the eye, especially with corrosive poisons. In the past, babies born of mothers with untreated gonorrhea suffered corneal scarring and loss of sight because the gonococcus organism causes such severe inflammation.

People who lack adequate Vitamin A or B may develop drying and scarring of the cornea, but this is rare in the Western world. It is tragically common in underdeveloped tropical countries however, as is trachoma, an infection of the eye which is the world's most important cause of blindness, leading to millions of cases a year.

Another cause of blindness may be an increase in the pressure of the fluid inside the eye. This fluid is a vital part of the eye's structure, and in the illness of glaucoma the amount builds up and cannot drain away as it should. Untreated glaucoma leads to severe pain and blindness as the nerve at the back of the eye is constricted. Fortunately, nowadays, it can be treated successfully, as long as it is diagnosed before any permanent nerve damage is done.

In some cases there is hardening and blurring of the lens, the part of the eye that 'bends' light rays to provide focused vision. This blurring, which is called cataract, prevents the passage of light. Luckily, this condition can also be treated surgically with a considerable degree of success.

If the retina, the part of the eye that receives light messages and transmits them onwards, is damaged, vision is altered. In some cases, there may be detachment of the retina, which also can be treated by modern techniques – including laser beams – with considerable success.

Other diseases of the retina include blockage of its central blood vessels, a complication of the condition of hardening of the arteries. Once the damage has happened, it cannot be reversed, so prevention is important. Treatment for hardening of the arteries is therefore protective treatment for the eyes.

Another form of blood vessel disorder affecting the retina is linked with diabetes. Again, careful treatment of the diabetes reduces the risk.

There may also be blood vessel disease linked with high blood pressure, and once more, treatment of the underlying illness is protective.

Some people suffer from a disease of the retina in which patches of pigment are laid down and interfere with vision. This is called retinitis pigmentosa and at present it remains difficult to treat.

Afflictions of the optic nerve, which carries vital messages to the brain, may include damage caused by heavy alcohol drinking (especially methylated spirit drinking), heavy tobacco use, and lead poisoning. They may also occur in some of the neurological diseases including multiple sclerosis, though this is usually a late development in the course of the disease.

Damage to the brain, perhaps following fracture of the skull, may also result in blindness if the visual cortex – the section which is involved with seeing – is affected.

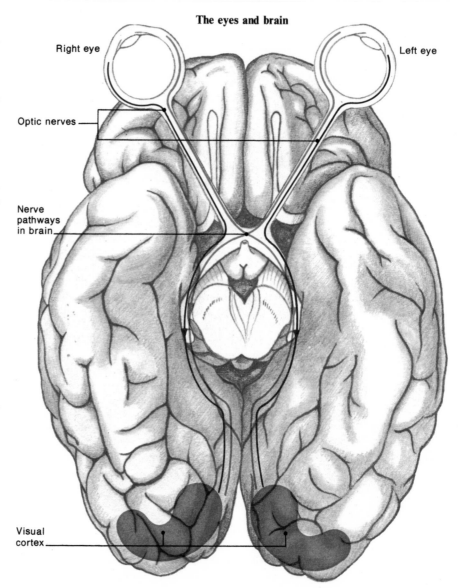

The eyes and brain

Right eye

Left eye

Optic nerves

Nerve pathways in brain

Visual cortex

Why are people's eyes different colours?

Eye colour is carried from generation to generation by the genes – the tiny shreds of material carried in our cells which instruct our bodies in the way that they will grow and develop and behave.

The basic eye colours are blue and brown. There are some variations, with blue eyes perhaps showing as grey, or greenish and brown eyes as hazel or amber, or almost black.

Brown eyes are called a dominant trait, while blue eyes are a recessive trait. That is brown eyes are 'stronger' than blue. It means that two brown-eyed people may marry and produce a blue-eyed child, because they carry blue eye genes, which are masked by their own brown eyes. Blue-eyed parents, however, are much less likely to produce brown-eyed offspring.

But the shuffle of the genetic pack can produce all sorts of surprises; there are people who have one blue eye and one brown, for example. When you consider that we each inherit half our genes from parents who inherited theirs from their parents, who inherited theirs from their parents, you will see just how many different traits we each have the chance to end up with.

Why do babies' eyes change colour as they grow older?

All white-skinned babies are born with apparently blue eyes, though in fact they are not at all. They have very little pigment in their eyes because it is laid down shortly after birth. Their eyes look blue because light is reflected from the deeper layers of the iris – the part that is coloured – and appears blue, much as blood vessels shining through pale skin look blue. Babies with black skins are a little different; they tend to have more pigment in general, so their eyes even at birth look dark. But their irises, too, will darken more as they grow older. Final eye colour is usually established by the age of six months or so, though it may take rather longer in some babies.

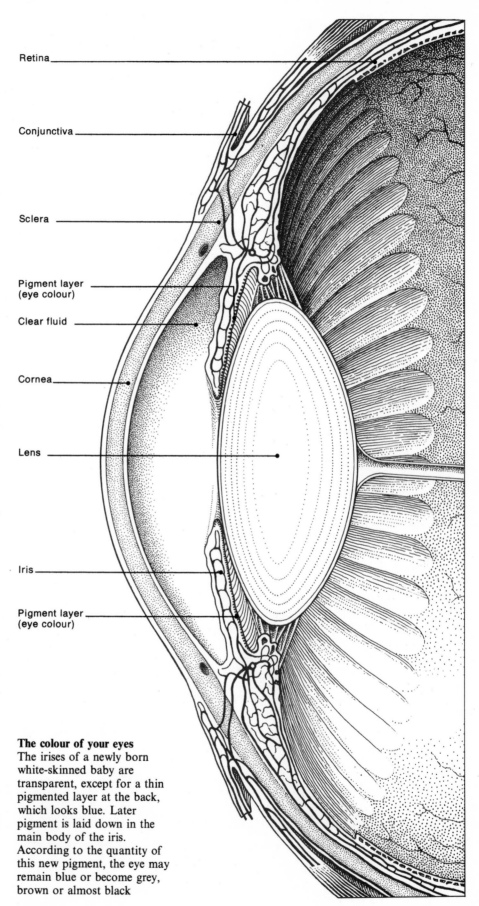

Retina

Conjunctiva

Sclera

Pigment layer (eye colour)

Clear fluid

Cornea

Lens

Iris

Pigment layer (eye colour)

The colour of your eyes
The irises of a newly born white-skinned baby are transparent, except for a thin pigmented layer at the back, which looks blue. Later pigment is laid down in the main body of the iris. According to the quantity of this new pigment, the eye may remain blue or become grey, brown or almost black

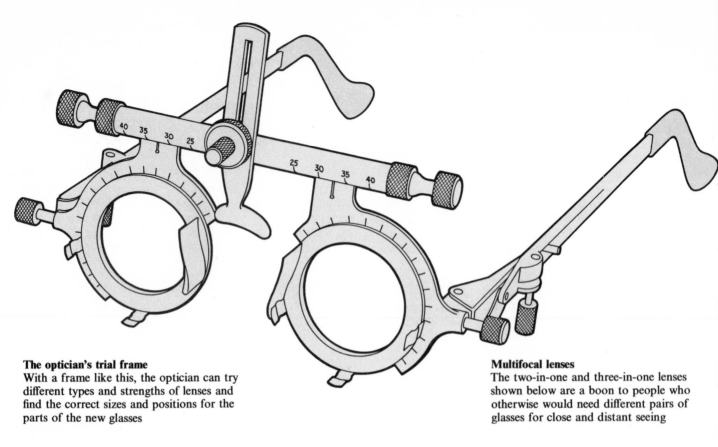

The optician's trial frame
With a frame like this, the optician can try different types and strengths of lenses and find the correct sizes and positions for the parts of the new glasses

Multifocal lenses
The two-in-one and three-in-one lenses shown below are a boon to people who otherwise would need different pairs of glasses for close and distant seeing

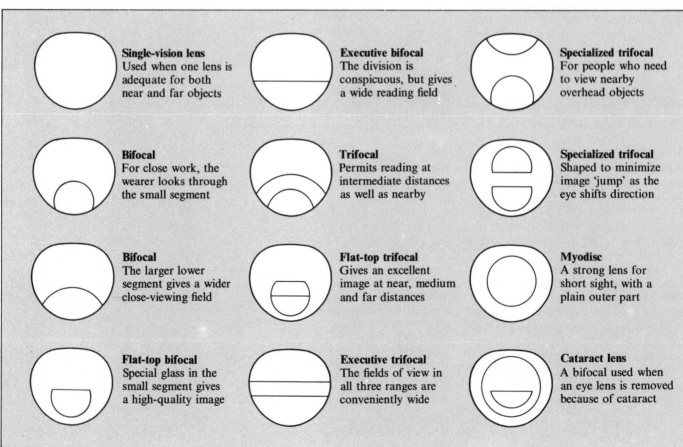

Single-vision lens
Used when one lens is adequate for both near and far objects

Executive bifocal
The division is conspicuous, but gives a wide reading field

Specialized trifocal
For people who need to view nearby overhead objects

Bifocal
For close work, the wearer looks through the small segment

Trifocal
Permits reading at intermediate distances as well as nearby

Specialized trifocal
Shaped to minimize image 'jump' as the eye shifts direction

Bifocal
The larger lower segment gives a wider close-viewing field

Flat-top trifocal
Gives an excellent image at near, medium and far distances

Myodisc
A strong lens for short sight, with a plain outer part

Flat-top bifocal
Special glass in the small segment gives a high-quality image

Executive trifocal
The fields of view in all three ranges are conveniently wide

Cataract lens
A bifocal used when an eye lens is removed because of cataract

What is colour-blindness? How do you avoid it?

You can't avoid it, and you can't 'catch' it. It is an inherited trait – or rather an inherited disability. In fact, colour-blind people are neither blind nor colour-unconscious. They simply have trouble seeing certain colours. Some are unable to identify red, others green. A few rare cases have difficulty in seeing blue.

The fault lies in the cones of the retina; each colour has its own special sensitive cones, and in people who inherit this problem the cones are missing or in short supply. The tendency is sex-linked: that is, it is usually suffered by men, but passed on to the next generation by women. So a man who is colour-blind and who has a daughter and son may find that his son is colour-blind while his daughter is not, but her son is colour-blind, though the son's daughter is not.

Colour-blindness is only a handicap in certain activities. For example, car drivers who need to see red lights and green lights may have trouble, though they can usually identify instructions by the position of the light in the traffic-light line-up. Pilots need perfect colour vision, however, as do electricians. Painters, designers and interior decorators can cope well enough as long as they know of their defect. It is said by some that the painter, Constable, was colour-blind and that this accounts for the subtle shading of his landscapes.

Why do I see green or red for a while after I come in from bright sunshine, or after someone has flashed a bright light, such as a camera flash, at me?

The retina, at the back of the eye, picks up images in structures called rods and cones. The rods contain a substance called 'visual purple' (its proper name is rhodopsin) which breaks down in dim light into two different chemicals, and it is these which trigger the message to the brain. The 'visual purple' takes up to half an hour to be replaced in the rods after it has been used. Usually we are not aware of this happening because only a few of the rods have lost their 'visual purple'. Also, much of the replacement happens at night, in the dark, when the body uses Vitamin A, derived from the diet, to replace the 'visual purple'.

However, when a great deal of white light is thrown on to the retina, there is a bleaching effect because the 'visual purple' breaks down quickly, and a great many rods are affected. Once back in the dimmer light, you become aware of the shortage of 'visual purple' by seeing dimly with an overlay of red and/or green, because now the colour-collecting cones are dominant. It does no harm to the eyes or to the vision, unless, of course, there has been enough bright light to do actual damage. It's as well to remember that staring at the sun or any violently bright scene can destroy areas of the retina.

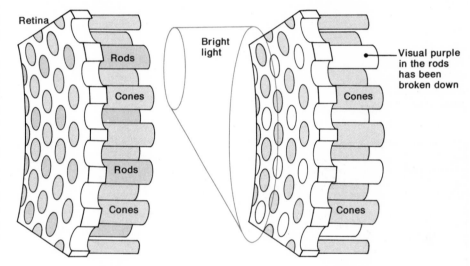

I had severe bronchitis which caused me to cough a great deal and several times a red mark appeared in my eye, and wouldn't go away for a long time. The doctor said it was a burst blood vessel and was not dangerous, but surely burst blood vessels must be a severe problem?

The tiny vessels which feed the membrane that protects the eye – the conjunctiva – can enlarge and contract a great deal and so usually cope well with a sharp rise in pressure. However, sometimes the pressure rise is so great, as during a severe bout of coughing (it happens in children with whooping cough, as well as in adults with bronchitis) that a vessel cannot cope and the wall breaks down and releases its contents. The result is the rather large red patch you can see on the white of the eye. But there is no need to worry because the burst is a form of fail-safe mechanism. When it happens it releases the pressure and so protects the rest of the eye. It need cause no problems to the person who has it, as it is painless and does not interfere with vision.

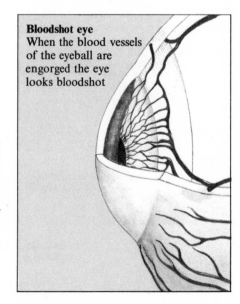

Bloodshot eye
When the blood vessels of the eyeball are engorged the eye looks bloodshot

Ear, nose and throat

It is obvious to all of us that the nose and throat are closely related to each other. Air that enters the nose continues its journey to the lungs by way of the throat. But why should the ears be bracketed with these other structures? The ears are for hearing, and apparently have nothing whatsoever to do with breathing, after all.

But the ears are connected to the nose and throat, and ills that afflict them may affect the nose and throat and vice versa. A narrow tube runs from each ear to the back of the nose; these two tubes are called the Eustachian tubes, and have the function of allowing the air pressure between the middle ear and the outer atmosphere to be kept in balance. But they also allow infection to travel from the nose and throat into the ear, which is why doctors who specialize in the care of one of these structures also need to be knowledgeable about the others.

The nose and throat in relation to the ear

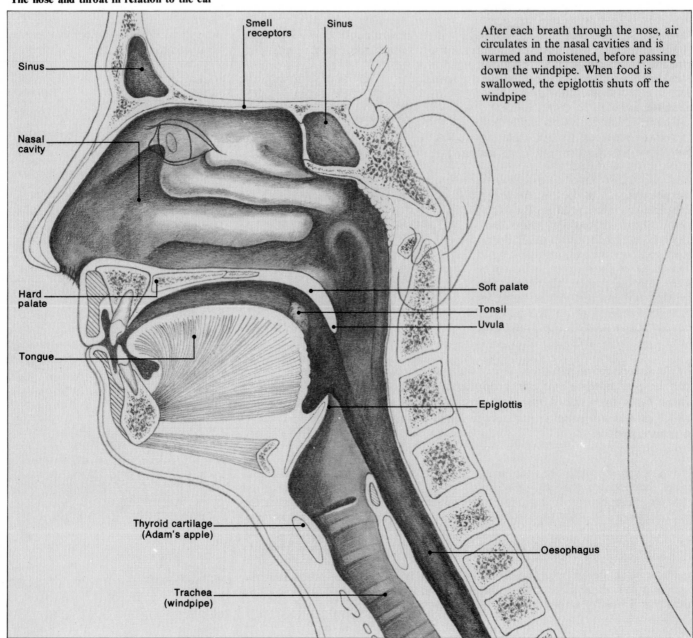

Smell receptors

Sinus

Sinus

Nasal cavity

After each breath through the nose, air circulates in the nasal cavities and is warmed and moistened, before passing down the windpipe. When food is swallowed, the epiglottis shuts off the windpipe

Hard palate

Soft palate

Tonsil

Uvula

Tongue

Epiglottis

Thyroid cartilage (Adam's apple)

Oesophagus

Trachea (windpipe)

Why do noses bleed? And what's the best way to deal with them?

Once again, there can be lots of reasons. Direct injury is the obvious one – being bashed on the nose with a baseball can make the nose spurt like a fountain. Injury elsewhere in the head can do it, too – a crack on the head that fractures the skull can cause bleeding from the nose (and the ears) and this is a symptom that must be treated at once by a doctor because it shows that a severe injury is present.

Some noses bleed because the small blood vessels just inside the nostrils – and the nose is richly supplied with these blood vessels – are damaged. They contract and expand busily in response to a great many stimuli, for example, cold outer air, or hot air, or damp or dry outer air, or sharply increased exercise such as running about or climbing hills; and these blood vessels are rather more vulnerable than other, less active, ones.

There are some blood vessels on the septum (the resilient cartilage which separates the nostrils) which are part of a section called Little's area which is particularly vulnerable, and some people have frequent and copious nose bleeding from this source.

The best treatment is first to pinch the nose hard between thumb and forefinger, because pressure always stops blood flow, and then to close up the vessels. The simplest way is by using a chemical which will cauterize the vessels and block them off for good, and any doctor can do this.

It is not true that the best way to stop nose bleeds is to put a cold key down the back of the neck or that the afflicted person is more comfortable with his head held back. The key is useless, and the head-back posture is extremely uncomfortable and actually encourages the blood to go down the back of the nose into the throat, which is sickening. Sitting up with the head poked forward so that the blood can be caught in a cloth or a bowl is much better – though accurate pinching should prevent any dripping.

Less common causes of nose bleed include infections such as colds which affect the nose. They can affect the blood vessels and cause bleeding as, too, can forceful blowing of the nose. Picking with sharp fingernails, of course, can cause blood-letting damage.

Some people suffer nose bleeds because of a general disorder affecting the whole body, rather than just the nose. For example, in people with hardening of the arteries and associated high blood pressure a marked increase in the pressure can cause the blood vessels in the nostrils to open. This can work as a safety-valve effect: the blood loss brings the pressure down a little and prevents bleeding in a more dangerous place such as the brain.

Also, certain forms of blood disorder in which the clotting mechanism is not as effective as it should be can result in nose bleeds, and these can be difficult to control.

Some people get nose bleeds as a result of great mental effort, which seems to lead to a rise in blood pressure and in intra-cranial pressure. This occasionally happens to students who are taking examinations, to musicians playing in concerts and to tense, stressed people trying to deal with anxiety.

Whatever the cause, the best way to deal with it is first to stop the bleeding with the pinch method, and then to get a doctor's diagnosis, and with it removal of the cause.

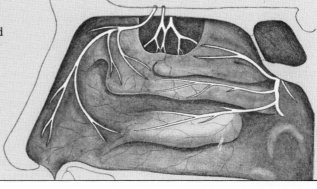

Blood supply to the nose
The walls of the nasal cavities are rich in blood vessels which warm incoming air and moisten it – water vapour passes out of the blood vessels through their lining. Air inhaled through the mouth is less moist and tends to dry the air passages

Stopping a nose bleed

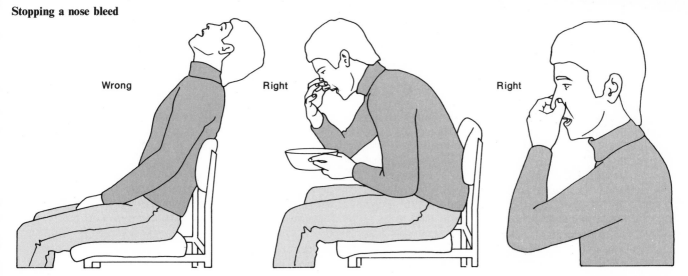

Wrong

Right

Right

Ear, nose and throat

Whenever I drink wine I start to sneeze. Why?

You could be allergic to wine or to some component in it. Since you mention wine in particular rather than alcohol in general, the trigger substance in your case may be one of the natural chemicals that give wine its flavour or bouquet.

Most people think that the reason for allergic responses such as wheezing, coughing, eye-watering, nose-running and sneezing has to be an allergen that is breathed in, such as grass pollens or animal hair. But you can get just the same responses from swallowing a substance if you are sensitive to it.

What is the cause of sinusitis? What can be done about it?

The skull is full of air pockets, especially around the nose and the forehead.

They lighten the weight of the bony skull and also act as resonators for the voice. When sound vibrations are applied to solid bone the result is dull and heavy; when it travels through the air it is clear and slightly echoing – resonant. Many singers possibly owe their success more to the holes in their heads than to their vocal cords.

These air spaces are linked with the nose via narrow channels each of which, like the sinuses themselves, are lined with mucous membrane. And when infection swells the mucous membrane in the nose, and causes an outpouring of sticky mucus, it can have just the same effect on the sinuses as the infection travels into them.

The answer is the same as it is for other upper respiratory infections. Wait patiently until nature puts an end to the process (as it will, in time, as your body defences win the battle) or, if it becomes chronic, painful and constant, attack it with medicines that destroy the germs (antibiotics) shrink the membrane (decongestants) and limit the discomfort (analgesics).

In some cases the infection gets so firm a hold that the condition goes on and on, with pain, dripping of pus down the back of the nose and general misery. Then surgery may be advised to wash out the offending material and to give the mucous membrane a chance to heal.

What are the sticky black blobs we get in our noses?

The nose has almost the most active area of mucuous membrane of the whole respiratory tract. It pours out a great deal of mucus and has very active cilia. It needs all the mucus and cilia because it is the point of entry for most of our air and it takes in, unavoidably, a great deal of dust, bacteria and other particles. These could cause considerable irritation and possible disease if they reached the lungs, so the nose has the task not only of getting air in, but also of filtering it of detritus. And, incidentally, warming it too, because that is what the many blood vessels are for – they heat the air that passes over them.

The hairs inside the nose trap the dust particles and bacteria, and hold them in sticky mucus. If this is not cleared by sneezing, then it builds up into the 'bogeys' that are so familiar.

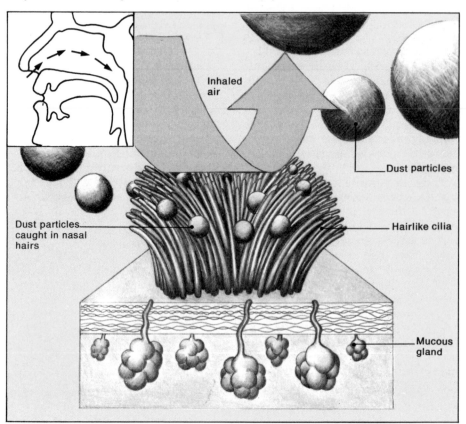

Inhaled air

Dust particles

Dust particles caught in nasal hairs

Hairlike cilia

Mucous gland

What causes sneezing anyway?

A sneeze is a reflex, that is, you cannot control it, nor can you consciously initiate it. It happens in response to irritation somewhere in the upper air passages (the nose and pharynx), and a complex series of actions rapidly occurs. A large amount of air is gulped in – up to two-and-a-half litres – and the breathing muscles make an explosive and forceful movement which pushes a great deal of air out through the nose and mouth at great speed. This has the effect of clearing the passages and is designed to remove the cause of the initial irritation.

If sneezing doesn't work first time, then it may be repeated several times, which is what tends to happen when there is an allergen such as pollen present, or the debris of a cold in the nose.

Apart from allergens and organisms that cause colds, anything that is irritating causes sneezing. Cigarette smoke, snuff, a sharp change in air temperature or humidity, even bright light or shrill noises in the case of very sensitive individuals.

What is the little dangling bit at the back of my throat for? What does it do?

To be perfectly honest, no one can be quite sure. It is part of the soft palate and is called the uvula and it may just possibly ensure a good seal when the air passages have to be shut off from the gullet, during swallowing. If there was not a good seal there, we would breathe in our food and choke to death. But people who, for any reason, have had their uvula removed are not in the least incapacitated by its loss.

One thing is sure: despite the way it tends to be shown in cartoon characters to be wobbling in a frenzy when they shout or sing, it has no connection whatsoever with the voice.

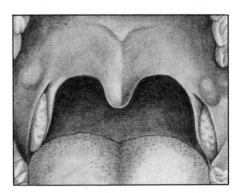

When the mouth is wide open, the uvula can be seen hanging down above the throat

Whenever I see a slice of lemon on my plate, the sides of my face hurt. Why?

At each side of your face and under your tongue are the salivary glands. They produce the slippery, watery saliva which is needed to make food chewable and to start the digestive process.

They are very swift glands – they react fast to a stimulus, and they tend to react extra fast to acids, because the saliva itself is mainly alkaline, and one of its jobs is to neutralize acid foods.

A sour substance will always call up a fast supply of saliva, so fast in some cases that the gland actually hurts as it swells a little and goes into production.

Occasionally, a small blockage may appear in the tube that leads from the gland to the inner cheek, and this can cause 'kick-back' into the gland and cause pain and obvious swelling. If this happens to you a lot, see your doctor. He may be able to diagnose and remove the pain.

Interestingly, it is not necessary for you to see a sour fruit like a lemon or some other tasty food for the gland to operate. Thinking about it can be enough of a trigger; the chances are that just reading this has made your mouth water.

This fact is used by some doctors as a little diagnostic trick. Mumps – infective parotitis (the salivary glands in the cheeks are called the parotids) – causes swelling and pain in the gland. When the swelling is well established it is easy to diagnose the illness but in the early stages it isn't so obvious. So, a doctor who suspects that the face pain of which his patient complains is mumps will ask him to close his eyes and imagine that he is sucking a lemon. If the patient claps his hands to his face and yells with pain, it's mumps.

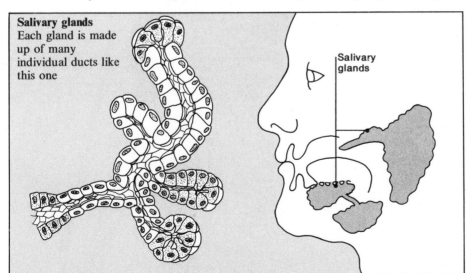

Salivary glands
Each gland is made up of many individual ducts like this one

Salivary glands

When I was continually getting sore throats my doctor sent me for a blood test. Why?

Sore throats can be due to any one of a number of causes: inflammation of the mucous membrane of the sort that happens with a cold (which is a virus infection) or an illness such as scarlet fever (which is a bacterial infection), or irritation (say, from breathing heavily dust- or smoke-laden air) or allergy (from breathing or swallowing something to which you are sensitive, say, grass pollens), or muscular strain (which can happen to people who have to use their voices a lot, such as teachers or singers) or direct injury (swallowing something too sharp or too hot). The diagnosis can only be made in an individual patient by a doctor who can take into account other signs and symptoms.

In your case it could be that your doctor suspects that you might have infectious mononucleosis – glandular fever. This is a tiresome illness caused by a particular virus which was first identified by Epstein and Barr in 1964. It causes a considerable range of symptoms, including a sore throat with swollen glands in the neck, fever, occasionally jaundice and a swollen liver and spleen, sometimes a fine, German measles-type rash – and it can go on for some time with repeated attacks.

The diagnosis is made by means of blood testing which shows increase in some white blood cells and, more importantly, an increase in antibodies – the body's special way of fighting off the infection. The test for this is called a Paul-Bunnell, again after its devisers, (or Mono-spot in the US).

Ear, nose and throat

Why does getting a cold in my nose make me lose my voice?

One of the effects of a cold, which is a virus infection attacking the upper breathing passages, is the swelling of the mucous membrane which lines all of them – the mouth, the nose, the throat, the larynx (voice box) and the lungs. It does this as part of the defence system because the swollen membrane produces more mucus to wash out the invading organisms.

Unfortunately, it can also happen that the cilia, the tiny hairs which line the membrane and which normally wave about and so sweep excess mucus and dust particles on their way to the exit, are knocked out by the infection. They cannot work properly, the mucus builds up, thickens and gets sticky. This is the disagreeable 'catarrh' that is so much a feature of a heavy cold.

When the larynx is also affected by swelling and thick mucus, the movement of the two flaps of membrane, which are the vocal cords, is impeded and the result is hoarseness and possibly loss of sound altogether at the top end of the sound register. And when the cords seize up altogether there is total voice loss.

It is important when this happens to try not to talk. Forcing the cords to move when they are swollen and clogged increases the pressure on them, enlarges the swelling and prolongs the problem. Even whispering, by the way, involves movement of the cords, so real silence is needed.

Why does my nose get blocked when I have colds?

For the same reason that the larynx does – swollen membrane, paralyzed cilia and thick mucus.

Why can't I taste food properly when I have a cold?

Taste depends not only on taste buds picking up flavours, but on the nose picking up smells. When the nose is blocked with mucus, scents cannot reach the endings of the olfactory nerves in the nostrils, smell sensation cannot reach the brain, and taste loses its subtlety.

Whenever I get a cold I get sores round my lips which take ages to clear up. Why does this only happen to some people?

This is a condition called herpes simplex. The sores are caused by a tiny virus which, it appears, lies dormant in some people until such time that they are in less than perfect health. Then it can flourish, since the body's defence systems are occupied elsewhere.

There is no point in putting anything by way of ointment on them – they just won't respond. Nor will the use of drying agents such as surgical spirit do much more than make them sting. One new treatment being recommended is to chill them.

If a cube of ice is wrapped in a piece of gauze and applied to the sore, and held there continuously for 45 to 60 minutes (replacing the cube as it melts, of course) it is said that the sore will disappear within 12 to 24 hours. It works for some people, apparently, and if you have the patience to do it, it can do no harm, and may help.

How a cold spoils taste
When the membranes lining the nose, throat and mouth produce large quantities of mucus, smells are prevented from reaching the olfactory nerve endings which contribute strongly to the sense of taste

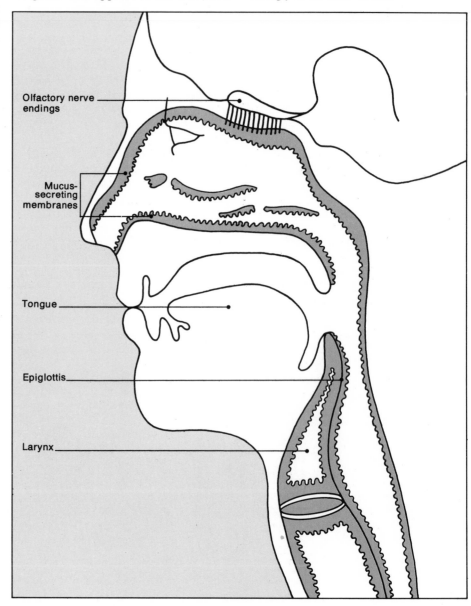

Olfactory nerve endings

Mucus-secreting membranes

Tongue

Epiglottis

Larynx

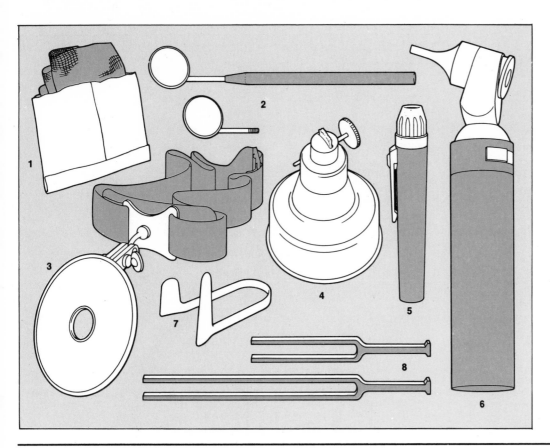

Some of the instruments used in a routine examination of the ear, nose and throat

1 Swabs for cleaning and taking samples of mucus or saliva. **2** Hand mirror for inspection of the throat – also magnifying mirror for use on the same handle. **3** Mirror worn on the surgeon's head to reflect light on to the area he is examining. **4** Spirit lamp to warm hand mirrors and so prevent steaming before they are used in the throat. **5** Pen torch. **6** Otoscope, containing a built-in light and used for examining the ear. **7** Nasal speculum, which holds the patient's nostril open. **8** Tuning forks. The doctor may test hearing with them, or find out whether passages in the head are blocked by listening to the sound obtained when the foot of the vibrating fork is held against one of the bones of the head

Why do so many children have to have their tonsils and adenoids removed?

Fashion has a lot to do with the operations that people have. Tonsillectomy and adenoidectomy are classic cases.

The tonsils and adenoids have a function: they are part of the body's defence system, and when micro-organisms invade the mouth, nose or throat, they go into action, and show the classic inflammation response – swelling, redness, pain and heat. Tonsils and adenoids also help in the production of antibodies to fight the invaders more effectively.

Sometimes, but by no means all the time, repeated attacks of infections in the upper respiratory tract cause permanent enlargement and thickening of the tissue, and this results in a degree of blockage. The child with permanently enlarged and scarred tonsils and, more particularly, adenoids, tends to breathe through his mouth (creating the classic 'adenoid face') and to speak with a marked nasal twang because the air passages which usually give the voice resonance are blocked. He may also breathe noisily, snore heavily, and

become droopy because breathing really is quite a chore for him. He is a dismal, underactive and unhappy child – and if there is a chronic infection in the tissues as well, then he is even more wretched.

The obvious answer for such a child is to remove the offending structures. They are doing him no good and he

The position of the tonsils and adenoids

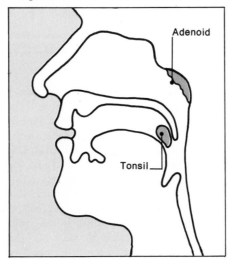

Adenoid

Tonsil

will be better off without them. And for many years this was precisely what surgeons did for any child who had recurrent sore throats. They didn't wait to see if he developed all the signs of chronic tonsil and adenoid enlargement.

Then, some more conservative surgeons, encouraged by parents who were unhappy about exposing their children to surgery, tried a wait-and-see policy. They used antibiotics to control the attacks of infection, which helped a great deal, and they found that a large number of these children who were at first thought to need surgery never developed the full-blown adenoidal look, were perfectly fit and well between their bouts of sore throat and tonsillitis, which they admittedly had a couple of times a year, and, most importantly of all, lost their tonsils naturally in late childhood. They just shrivelled up and virtually disappeared.

So, although between the two World Wars children in large numbers had painful surgical assaults on their throats, today it is an operation that is far less commonly done.

Ear, nose and throat

What causes deafness?

Hearing depends on a combination of several things. The first is a healthy brain, with its area which receives and interprets messages to do with sound, intact and in full working order.

The second is a healthy and fully functioning nerve running from the brain to the ear.

The third is a healthy and fully functioning sound-collecting apparatus to transmit sound from the outside world to the nerve to take it to the brain.

The two most important of these are the brain and nerve supply; the collecting apparatus is the least.

So let's start with the collecting apparatus. First, there is a passageway along which sound waves can travel (sound makes the air vibrate and it is the vibrations that have to be collected). Then, there is a drum which vibrates when it is hit by the air vibrations. After this there is a series of little bones (charmingly named the hammer, anvil and stirrup – the Latin versions are *malleus*, *incus* and *stapes* – because of their shape) which carry the vibrations from the drum across the space of the middle ear to the inner ear, where the auditory nerve has little fibres poised ready to pick them up and take them the rest of the way to the brain.

There can be failure of the collecting apparatus anywhere along that line. A firm block in the outer passage – wax or a foreign body – holds the vibrations back.

A damaged drum that does not vibrate stops them getting through.

Blocking of the middle ear space with fluid or pus stops the little bones from vibrating and sending messages on.

Blockage of the tiny window at the point where the small bones connect to the inner ear also holds the sound back.

However, lack of all of this need not mean total deafness as long as the nerve fibres are there at the inner ear, and are in good order, and the relevant brain area is ready to accept messages. The nerve fibres can still pick up the vibrations that sound creates through the bony tissue which surrounds the inner ear – the skull.

But if the nerve is damaged or the brain-receiving centre is damaged, then even the clearest and most receptive of collecting apparatus will be useless. The result will be deafness.

There can be damage to the auditory nerve, of course. Severe infection of the area where the nerve fibres pass used to be common and caused much deafness. This was the condition called mastoiditis – it is named after the part of the skull it affects – but since the advent of antibiotics this infection is much less common. It used to happen as infection ascended from the mouth or nose through the Eustachian tube to the middle ear and on to the inner ear.

Some people have an inherited tendency to failure of the auditory nerve. So far, we know of no way to reverse or prevent this.

Age also diminishes the auditory nerve's effectiveness.

Some people are born with profound damage to the nerve. Babies whose mothers had German measles in the first three months of the pregnancy that produced them may suffer this sad affliction. In others, the cause cannot always be identified.

The ear

Skull · Auditory nerve · Cochlea · Eustachian tube · Outer ear · Middle ear · Inner ear

How sound passes through the ear

Eardrum · Oval window · Cochlea · Outer ear · Middle ear · Inner ear · Fibres of auditory nerve

The vibrations of the eardrum are passed through the bones of the middle ear to the oval window, travel through the fluid of the cochlea, and then trigger nerve signals

How do hearing aids work?

By amplifying the vibrations that cause sound. People with a poorly functioning auditory nerve may cope well as long as the sound is loud enough, so a simple amplifier is all they need. This can be put into the outer ear, and works by picking up sound in its collection apparatus – often a small box or gadget worn on the clothing – which amplifies the sound and sends it on its way.

Other people need help in picking up sound without using their outer ears – maybe it is not possible to ensure that vibrations will make the complete journey as they should because of damage to some part of the transmitting system. Then the same apparatus is used, but instead of an ear piece there is a behind-the-ear piece. These are less obtrusive, and have become popular in recent years.

New developments in hearing aids are promised as research into tiny, transistorized gadgets is developed.

One type of hearing aid

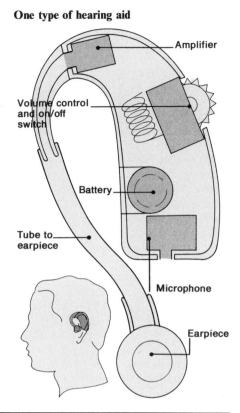

Amplifier

Volume control and on/off switch

Battery

Tube to earpiece

Microphone

Earpiece

Why do I sometimes get ringing in my ears?

Just as muscles, even when they are at rest, are always a little tensed and ready for action, so also the hearing nerve is always firing off little sound messages, even when it is not picking up any of the air vibrations that create sound. So, in really quiet conditions, we can all hear a faint ringing.

In some people, however, it is more than faint and is a really tiresome sound that interferes with daily life. Over and above speech and radio and television and traffic there's that noise, going on and on. It is called tinnitus, and severe cases can drive sufferers to distraction.

The cause in these cases is disorder of the hearing (auditory) nerve. It may be associated with other disturbances such as deafness and loss of balance. Unfortunately, there is not a great deal that can be done about it because treatment of the nerve which would result in loss of the sound would also result in loss of hearing. Counter-irritation helps some sufferers – always having a radio on or a loudly ticking clock – because at least that provides a little distraction.

Why do my ears pop when I am in an aircraft taking off?

Your middle ear contains air at a stable pressure and when the pressure of the atmosphere outside – the one we live and move around in – changes, then the pressure inside is matched to the one outside via the Eustachian tube, a tiny structure that runs between the inner and outer worlds.

If the air pressure changes sharply, as it does in a vehicle that is moving rapidly up or down (air pressure is lower the higher you go, and vice versa), then the passage of air along the tube will be felt as a 'pop'. If it doesn't change there will be a sense of dullness in sound and the Eustachian tube may need help. The simplest help is first to swallow and, if that doesn't work, to close the nostrils with thumb and forefinger and blow gently into the nose against the block. This forces air into the tube, makes the 'pop' and ends the problem.

Why can some people hear fine differences in pitch – musicians can – when others are, like me, tone deaf?

This has nothing to do with the ear itself – or probably not – but with the brain. The way sound is interpreted by different people is variable, and depends on individual personality, cultural differences, intelligence levels and so on.

So, what is music to one person is cacophony to another. What is an obvious sound difference to one person is imperceptible to another. Someone trained from childhood to respond to fine subtleties in music is better at recognizing differences in pitch than someone in whom this sense has never been specially encouraged. It is no accident that musical achievement runs in families; although there may be a tendency to inherit a particularly active and healthy auditory nerve and brain structure, the most important factor is the environment and the teaching.

You say that you are tone deaf – which almost certainly means that you have never been taught to recognize tone differences, not that you really cannot hear them. If you had to learn, the chances are that you could become as high-fidelity conscious as Menuhin or Heifetz.

This is not to say that these great musicians do not have a special ability in music; they do clearly find it easier to perceive sounds and translate what they perceive into music than others. But there is no magic about it. Anyone could learn to recognize tone differences in time, given normal auditory nerves and normal intelligence.

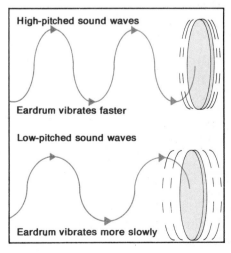

High-pitched sound waves

Eardrum vibrates faster

Low-pitched sound waves

Eardrum vibrates more slowly

Ear, nose and throat

Why does having things done to my ears make me feel sick and giddy? And why did my mother have to see an ear specialist when she got attacks of dizziness?

Ears are not only for hearing: they are for balance, too. There are shell-shaped structures in the inner ears which tell us where we are in space – upright or upside down, leaning sideways or forwards – and they work by responding to different fluid levels inside them. When you turn your head sharply sideways the fluid moves, the new position is transmitted to the brain, and the brain registers 'head sideways'.

If the changes in posture are rapid then the messages don't get through properly: by the time one arrives there is another contradictory one right behind it, and another and another. The result is giddiness – 'not knowing whether you're on your head or your heels'. We get it from twirling rapidly in a dance routine, or rolling down a hill – something children love doing for the pleasure they find in the giddy feeling.

Incidentally, have you ever noticed how ballet dancers, twirling like tee-totums, snap their heads round at each turn? They do it to ensure that the fluid levels shift once, sharply, instead of constantly, and the messages get through to the brain at an acceptable speed. The result is no giddiness.

But there can be abnormal giddiness. One form is travel sickness – the constant up-and-down and side-to-side movement of a ship or car or plane confuses the fluid levels and causes prolonged giddiness. This, in turn, leads to nausea and vomiting, although why this should affect the nerve connecting to the stomach is not as yet fully understood.

There is an interesting link between eye movements and balance disorder in travel sickness: people who try to read in a moving vehicle, that is, fix their eyes in one direction while their heads are moving in another, suffer a more rapid onset of nausea. Similarly, looking out at the shifting horizon from a heaving ship speeds up the heaving of the stomach.

Disorders of the auditory nerve and the labyrinth (a section of the inner ear) can also cause giddiness. The most common is Ménière's disease, in which there are attacks of recurrent deafness and tinnitus, plus giddiness. It is a very unpleasant illness, but many of its symptoms can be controlled with medicines, and even those which cannot eventually get better on their own.

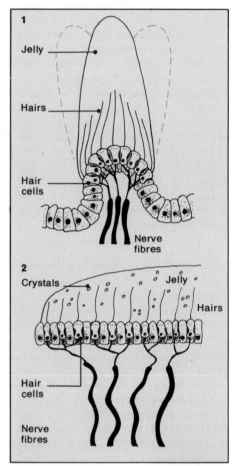

Why do I have wax in my ears?

Once again this is part of the protective system of the body. Wax is there to trap dirt particles, or even larger objects such as tiny insects which may get into so large an aperture as the ear. Usually the wax removes itself, as the cilia on the skin lining the passage of the ear sweep it to the opening, where it is removed when you wash your ears. Even if you did not wash, it would still get out – it would itch, and then when you scratched the wax would come away on your fingers.

Sometimes the wax does not get out easily, however, and a chunk of it builds up and leads to dullness in sound transmission, and possible giddiness if the wax is thick enough to press against the ear drums and the pressure is transmitted to the inner ear. This is rare but it does happen.

The answer then is to have it washed out by an expert. One famous ENT specialist used to warn his patients, 'Never put anything smaller than your elbow in your ears'. A wise warning, because much damage is done by people poking about with little sticks or hairpins, or those swabs on sticks which are recommended for the purpose by some misguided pharmaceutical firms. In particular, these should never be used on babies. If you cannot remove what you can see at the opening of the ear passage and wipe it easily, leave it alone. You will only push whatever it is farther in and hurt the ear drum, although there is a little natural protection against such meddling; the ear passage bends slightly, so the drum is tucked in at an angle.

If the wax really gets tiresome, and you don't want to ask a doctor to wash it out, you can get special dissolving drops to put in, which will melt the wax and let it trickle away. The drops smell unpleasant but are effective.

Sensing the body's movement and posture
When the head turns, the fluid in each semicircular canal swirls and disturbs a tiny blob of jelly (1, above), triggering nerve signals. In similar structures nearby (2), embedded crystals make a mass of jelly flow into different shapes according to the head's position, and stimulate nerves

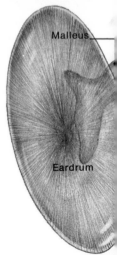

I always thought the ear drum was vital to hearing, yet I can hear perfectly well though one of my drums had to be perforated when I was a child, to release an infection.

Middle ear infection, in which the space fills up with pus, often results in a break in the drum, either naturally (it bursts by itself to let the hard-pressing pus out) or by surgical intervention. But it heals again, and usually hearing is restored. And remember, of course, that you also pick up sound through your bony skull. You can manage without a drum altogether.

The inner ear
The semicircular canals and the cochlea are the main parts of the inner ear. Vibrations from the eardrum pass through the oval window, spiral along the cochlea and return, and leave by the round window. The spiral organ of hearing, lying along the centre-line of the cochlea, converts the vibrations into nerve signals

My son has what is called a 'glue ear' and the doctor says he needs grommets. What on earth are they?

Some children develop a condition in which the middle ear fills with a thick, sticky germ-free material very like glue. It can happen as a result of an ear infection treated with antibiotics in which the treatment was not given for a long enough period. Sometimes mothers, and some doctors, don't bother to finish a course of antibiotics once the symptoms have subsided. This is not a good idea at all. It leads to this particular ear problem as well as to a species of super germs which thrive on antibiotics because they develop a resistance to them.

Sometimes Eustachian tube obstruction is present. This can happen as a result of infection, or after damage because of sudden changes in air pressure.

An allergy seems to be present in some of the children who develop glue ear, and it seems to be common in children who have cleft palates.

Whatever the cause, it leads to dulling of hearing and can considerably impede a child's education and progress. Treatment to remove the glue is needed. Sometimes treatment of the underlying cause, once it is identified, can resolve the problem. Sometimes surgery is needed, with an operation to drain the middle ear (myringotomy), and the insertion of a tiny tube called a grommet. This allows the liquid to escape to the outer ear and be drained harmlessly away.

Sometimes, there are problems with the use of grommets. They tend to push their way out in time, and so stop functioning, and it is also important to prevent water getting into the outer ear while they are in position. This is misery for a would-be swimmer. But grommets help a lot of children: long-term trials have shown that grommet treatment has resulted in superior hearing improvement for those for whom they remained in place.

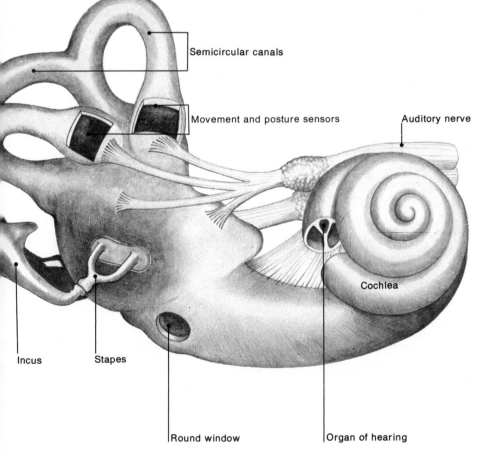

Semicircular canals

Movement and posture sensors

Auditory nerve

Cochlea

Incus

Stapes

Round window

Organ of hearing

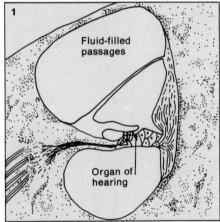

Fluid-filled passages

Organ of hearing

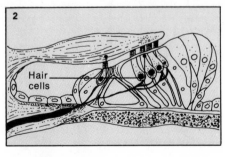

Hair cells

The organ of hearing
A cross-section (**1**) shows the cochlea's passages. Vibrations in the fluid stimulate the hair cells of the organ of hearing (**2**)

Lungs

Chest physicians were once the busiest of men who spent the bulk of their time and effort in fighting the tubercle bacillus. When pulmonary tuberculosis – TB infection of the lungs, also known as consumption, or phthisis, or the 'white plague' – was endemic all over the world, the disease killed hundreds of thousands, and the chest physicians were the people who had to find ways to combat that appalling death rate. Today TB has lost much of its sting although there are still parts of the world where it flourishes. However, this does not mean chest physicians are a disappearing breed. They are not. Today, they are as busy as ever they were dealing with another plague – smaller in proportion but no less significant – lung disease due to tobacco smoking. The incidence of lung cancer among people who smoke cigarettes is rising steadily and gives chest physicians much work they would obviously rather not have to do. They also work with cardiologists, helping patients suffering from various forms of heart disease, and for most chest physicians this is infinitely more satisfying.

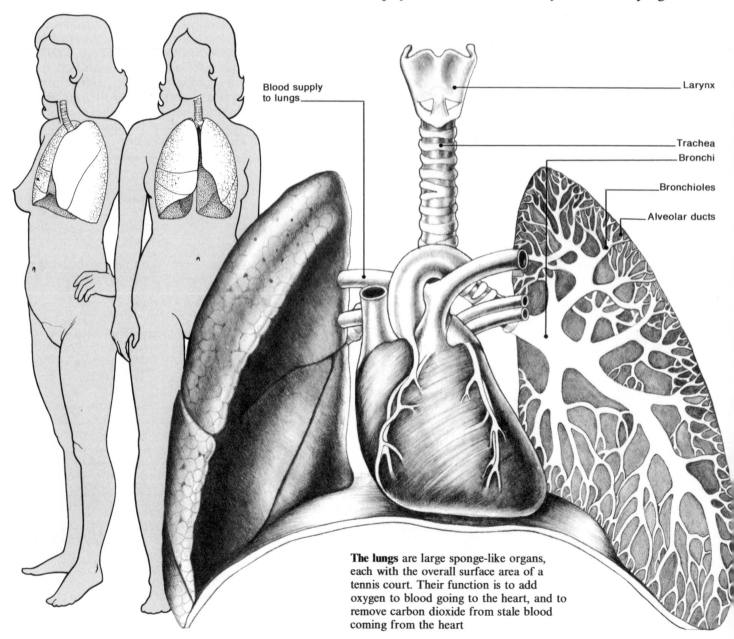

Blood supply to lungs

Larynx

Trachea

Bronchi

Bronchioles

Alveolar ducts

The lungs are large sponge-like organs, each with the overall surface area of a tennis court. Their function is to add oxygen to blood going to the heart, and to remove carbon dioxide from stale blood coming from the heart

The bronchial tree

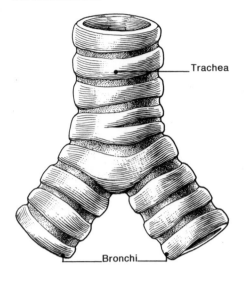

Trachea

Bronchi

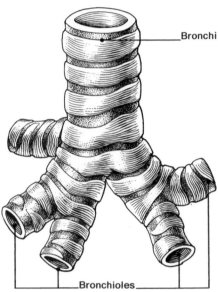

Bronchi

Bronchioles

Alveolar duct

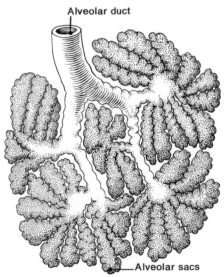

Alveolar sacs

What does the doctor listen for when he listens to my chest with a stethoscope? And what does the stethoscope do?

A stethoscope is merely a simple amplifier. The first stethoscope was a tube of rolled paper, one end of which was applied to the patient's chest, and the other to the doctor's ear.

The stethoscope makes the many sounds which can be heard in the chest both louder and more easy to identify. First, there are the heart sounds, and these reveal to an experienced listener what the heart is doing as it goes through its pulse-rest-pulse-rest cycle. The movement of the valves can be discerned, and the suck and gurgle of the blood in the aorta and the big veins. Although more accurate diagnoses can now be made by studying electrocardiograms which make tracings of the heart's electrical action, a trained ear can pick out a great deal of vital information through a stethoscope.

The other group of sounds are those connected with breathing. The doctor can estimate the state of the small air sacs in the lungs just by listening to air flowing in and out. He can tell whether the bronchi – the tubes that branch into ever smaller twiglets and carry air in and out of the lungs – are in good condition. He can listen for crepitations – harsh crackling bursts of sound which identify such illnesses as pneumonia, or he may hear rhonchi, continuous high- or low-pitched sounds occurring when the patient is breathing in and out, and which may be due to asthma. However, if the patient coughs and the sounds disappear, then they are due only to a little mucus in the larger bronchi. Another type of sound is râles and these are harsher discontinuous noises which may mean bronchitis or edema (waterlogging) of the lungs. Sometimes there is a friction rub, a crackling noise which is possibly due to pleurisy.

The stethoscope is sometimes used for other parts of the body as well as the chest. For example, it is useful to listen to the abdomen after a person has had an operation there, to ensure that the gut is still as active as it should be. And, of course, it is necessary to listen to the heartbeat of a baby in the uterus, although often a differently shaped, funnel type of stethoscope is used. The instrument is also used to listen to the arteries in the arm when measuring blood pressure.

The listening examination is called auscultation, and doctors take much personal pride in developing their skills in interpreting what they hear.

Why does my doctor tap my chest with two fingers when he examines me?

This is called, unsurprisingly, percussion, and is a search for areas of dullness and resonance. Dullness shows areas where the underlying tissue is more solid – the consolidation of pneumonia perhaps, or the presence of fluid in an area where it should not be (effusion of the sort that happens with pleurisy, for example). Excess resonance may show that there is air where there should not be. For example, there may be resonance over a section of the pleural cavity which has filled with air, and which has pushed the adjacent lung flat – this can happen after accidents where a broken rib pierces a section of lung. Sometimes the lungs may be deliberately flattened by the introduction of air into the pleural cavity. This is done to rest a section of tuberculous tissue so that it can heal. Resonance may also indicate the condition of emphysema, where the little air sacs in the lungs instead of being normal size are over-extended and blown up like little balloons.

Percussion can also demonstrate the size and position of the heart because the chest wall over the heart gives out a dull note. In a few cases it can also show enlargement of the liver, if it is displaced upwards beyond its normal limits into the chest.

The bronchial tree
The air passages within the lungs are similar to the trunk, branch, and leaf system of a tree. The trachea divides into two bronchi which in turn branch into bronchioles leading to the alveolar ducts and sacs, where the blood-gas exchange occurs

Lungs

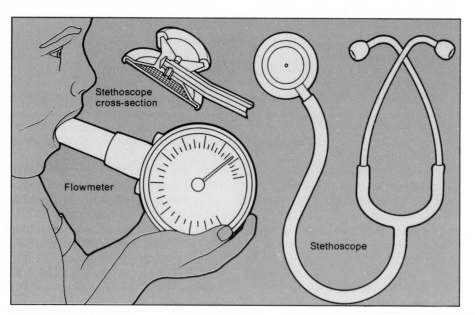

Stethoscope cross-section

Flowmeter

Stethoscope

Diagnostic apparatus
A flowmeter indicates the condition of the airways by measuring the rate of air-flow. A stethoscope amplifies sounds, enabling the doctor to listen to the body working. Its broader, lower side is used for listening to large areas; the narrower, upper half can pinpoint sounds more closely

Why does the doctor tell me to say 99?

This is a search for vocal resonance. If there is consolidation of a section of the lung, the sound of the voice will be more resonant through the stethoscope. If there is an effusion – the presence of fluid – resonance disappears altogether.

Sometimes the doctor asks the patient to whisper 99; this is used to show areas of underlying consolidation or cavitation, where the lung tissue has actually broken down and left a hole. In the days when TB was a severe and widespread illness doctors could map the lungs by listening to the pattern made by 99 resonance. Nowadays, fortunately, it is a skill which few doctors need.

What is it the doctor sees when he looks at a chest X-ray?

The ribs, mostly, and of course the breastbone (the sternum) and the collarbones (the clavicles). But there is also a good deal to see of the soft tissues – the heart and the position it holds in the chest; the lungs and the dome of the diaphragm that separates the chest from the belly.

Experienced X-ray viewers can identify a good deal of what is going on in the lungs by studying the shadows that are there. There may be areas of lung which are consolidated, with the little air sacs filled with mucus and fluid; there may be cavities, where disease has destroyed sections of tissue (this is seen on the X-ray of a tuberculous chest) or there may be new growths.

No patient should ever try to imagine he can see anything useful on a chest X-ray. The reading of these films is a specialist skill, and many doctors themselves prefer to send them for specialized analysis.

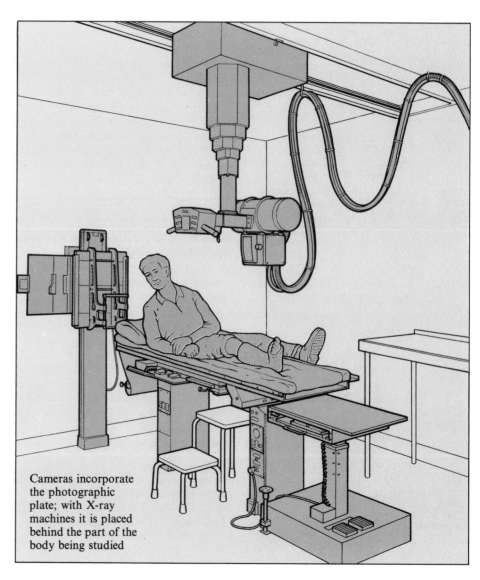

Cameras incorporate the photographic plate; with X-ray machines it is placed behind the part of the body being studied

While she was in hospital after breaking a leg, my grandmother caught pneumonia and died of it. Does this mean that they didn't take enough care to keep her warm?

There are two false assumptions in this question. Firstly, that pneumonia is always an infection which people catch, and secondly, that infections can be caught from being cold.

The first assumption is wrong because although it is possible to have a bacterial pneumonia, or a viral pneumonia, both of which are caused by inhaled organisms, there is also a form of pneumonia which owes nothing to them. When a person lies still for long periods, and does not breathe as deeply as she or he should, areas of the lung become unused and slowly fill with fluid. This sort of pneumonia is common in the old, especially after injury or surgery, and may be unavoidable even though good doctors always insist on vigorous physiotherapy, which encourages deep breathing exercises and adequate movement to keep the chest working as it should.

This sort of pneumonia has been called the 'old man's friend' since it may lead to a quiet and peaceful death for someone who is afflicted with an incurable illness. It is possible that despite attempts by her doctors to keep her lungs working well, your grandmother lost her interest in living after she broke her leg and so quietly succumbed to her pneumonia.

The second assumption – that chilling causes chest diseases – is also wrong. No one ever caught a cold from being cold, or pneumonia from being chilled. A cold is caused by a virus, and unless you inhale it, you cannot get the cold. An infective pneumonia also demands the presence of the causative organism.

All that chilling may do is to make a person less willing to be active and make some of his body responses less brisk. This may have the effect of lowering general resistance to infection, and it could account for the noticeable tendency for people to develop infections after they have been chilled. But plenty of other people do not get ill after being cold although most of us tend not to notice this fact.

All four of my grandparents died of TB. I'm told it runs in the family. Does this mean I am sure to get it? How can I be protected?

You have no need to protect yourself because TB is not an inherited disease. It is an infection, caused by the tubercle bacillus, and is passed from one individual to another, either as droplets in the breath, or as coughed out sputum or via the milk supply – cows can have TB, and their milk is laden with the bacilli if it is not treated. If humans drink untreated milk they may get TB of the bones, as calcium from the milk is carried to them.

The high incidence of hunch-backed people in the so-called Good Old Days was due to TB which destroyed vertebrae, made them collapse and so curved the spine. TB of other organs of the body, including the kidney and uterus, is also possible.

The most common form, by far, however, has always been pulmonary TB, also called phthisis, or consumption, or the White Plague. In the past it spread rapidly throughout the world and as many people were killed by it as they were by cancer. It is not surprising that all your grandparents had it: they were in the same family circle, caught it from each other, and were probably as ill-equipped to fight it off as most people then were because poor feeding, overworking and often poverty were the lot of the vast majority.

The development of such drugs as streptomycin, PAS and INAH, together with the strict control of the hygiene of milk production virtually brought an end to this disease. Today, it is rare in developed countries, although it remains a problem in the Third World which is still bedevilled by hunger and poverty, both of which are enthusiastic allies of infectious diseases such as tuberculosis.

Why do I get wheezy when I eat shellfish? I can understand people who wheeze because they are allergic to grass pollens or animal fur, but I don't inhale shellfish.

The allergic response – the way the body reacts when it meets a substance it regards as inimical – is variable.

In some people there is a skin reaction. Whatever the foreign substance which is objected to, be it a food which is swallowed, a substance which is inhaled, a material which is touched – the skin is the reactor. There may be a fine, widespread, red rash (nettle-rash) or there may be large, intensely itchy, red and white bumps (hives). Alternatively, there may be huge areas of swelling (angio-neurotic edema) usually found around the eyes or lips.

In other people, the response is centred on the gastro-intestinal tract and takes the form of nausea, vomiting and diarrhoea. This response is less common than the response which is centred on the mucous membranes of the upper respiratory tract and which involves the swelling of the membranes leading to blockage of the tubes (wheezing and breathlessness) and an outpouring of mucus (which leads to a running nose and a bubbly cough).

Clearly, you respond with the last type. That is why whelks make you wheeze and prawns make you puff.

Why do some people have weak chests and keep getting attacks of wheezing?

There are some people who are strongly sensitive to foreign substances and show an allergic response to several different ones. They do not have weak chests at all, but they do have strong immune responses.

Unfortunately, it can happen that repeated attacks of wheezing due to allergy can cause permanent damage to some of the lung structures, and then it can be said that the person is left with a weakness. But control of the allergy, using antihistamine medicines, should avoid this problem.

Lungs

I'm told that the X-ray of my chest showed 'calcification'. What does that mean?

Some time in the past, probably as a child, you had a tubercular infection which got better by itself, as your body's defence systems fought off the invader. But the section of lung – or adjacent glands – which was affected, hardened and filled with calcium salts as it slowly healed.

There is no need for you to worry about this at all. Indeed, you should be grateful for it. It means that you have a good resistance to tuberculosis and in the highly unlikely event of your being exposed to the disease again, you will not catch it. Modern children who rarely, if ever, are exposed to TB, and so do not build a natural resistance, have to have an immunizing injection (BCG – bacille Calmette-Guérin – named after the Frenchmen who developed it in 1906) to protect them.

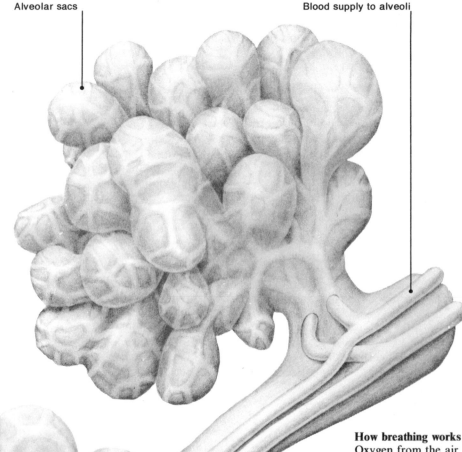

Alveolar sacs

Blood supply to alveoli

Carbon dioxide

Oxygen

Airflow

Capillaries

How breathing works
Oxygen from the air in the lungs is taken into the bloodstream and exchanged for carbon dioxide via the alveoli

I went to my doctor because I was breathless and he sent me for blood tests and didn't worry about my lungs at all. Why was that?

Breathlessness does not necessarily mean that there is anything wrong in the lungs. It can in fact show that they are working well and responding to a demand for extra oxygen with great efficiency.

One of the causes of breathlessness, and it is quite a common one, is anaemia. The blood is less efficient than it should be at carrying the breathed-in oxygen from the lungs around the body. It sounds as though your doctor suspects that this is your problem and that is why he wants blood tests. Once he knows the sort of anaemia you have, he can treat it, and that will cure your breathlessness.

What difference does it make whether you breathe through your mouth or your nose?

The nose does a most useful job, it warms the incoming air, filters it of large dust and other particles, and helps to deal with the inevitable load of bacteria present in every indrawn breath. Not to use your valuable nose if you can does seem extremely wasteful.

Why do some people only breathe through their mouths?

This is frequently caused by a bad habit. People who commonly sit with their lower jaws lax and their mouths drooping open because they have never learned to sit up and maintain a good posture of the whole body, including the face and jaw, will breathe through their mouths because they know no better.

In others, it is due to blockage of the nostrils – perhaps by a deviated nasal septum (*see the next question*) or because of adenoids.

Why do some people breathe so noisily?

Again it is just a bad habit. Tense people may tighten the muscles around the nose so that they narrow the air entry space and this makes the intake of air sound loud. In other people it is due to the actual narrowing of the space, perhaps by swelling of the mucous membrane because of allergic response or infection, or the nose may have a displacement of the central dividing wall (the septum). This creates one narrow and one wide nostril and the air makes a noise as it enters the narrow one. The condition is called DNS (deviated nasal septum).

Some people have asthma, a difficulty in breathing out, and this causes noisiness; others have bronchitis, inflammation and narrowing of the air intake tubes, and this causes noisiness when they breath in.

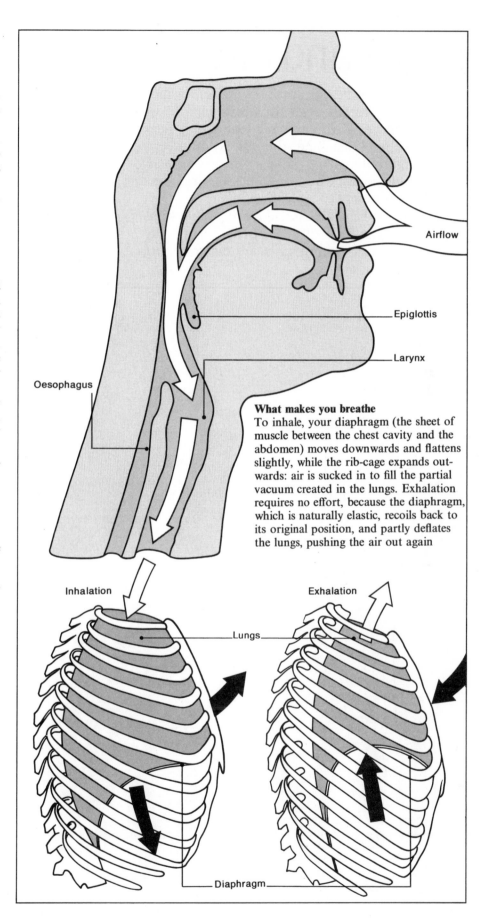

Airflow

Epiglottis

Larynx

Oesophagus

What makes you breathe
To inhale, your diaphragm (the sheet of muscle between the chest cavity and the abdomen) moves downwards and flattens slightly, while the rib-cage expands outwards: air is sucked in to fill the partial vacuum created in the lungs. Exhalation requires no effort, because the diaphragm, which is naturally elastic, recoils back to its original position, and partly deflates the lungs, pushing the air out again

Inhalation

Exhalation

Lungs

Diaphragm

Heart and circulation

The heart is indeed the heart of the matter for most of us. There are few who do not regard illness involving the heart with awe and fear, seeing heart disease as the 'worst kind' there is. Many people believe that a diagnosis of heart disorder means imminent death at worst or a life of prolonged invalidism at best.

Yet, in fact, heart disease, like many other kinds of bodily ill, can be controlled, treated and sometimes cured. And cardiologists are the specialists who have the task of providing that sort of care. Much of their work is involved with the precise identifying of disorder, and the use of the right drugs to correct it. But they may also offer surgical remedies. Today, new valves can replace damaged ones inside the heart, new sections can be inserted into damaged arteries, and hearts have even been transplanted. The work of today's cardiologists includes some of the most remarkable technical expertise of our times.

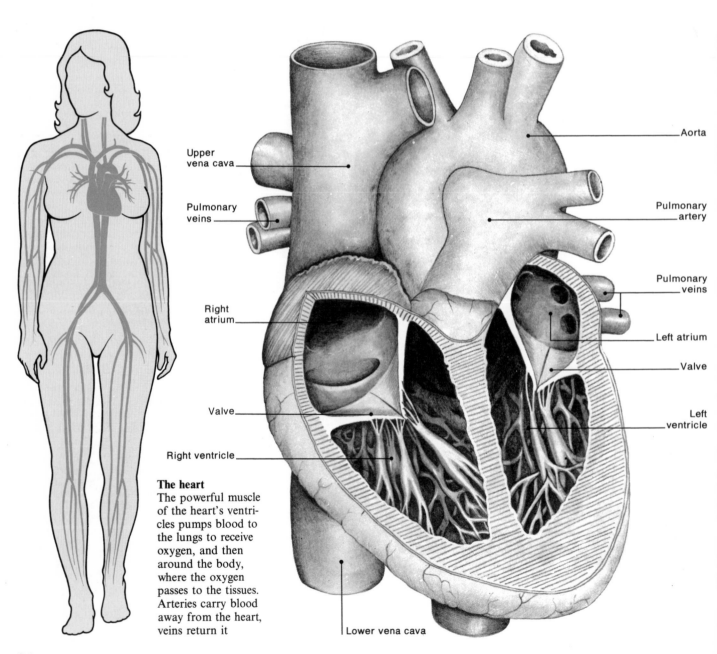

Upper vena cava

Pulmonary veins

Right atrium

Valve

Right ventricle

Aorta

Pulmonary artery

Pulmonary veins

Left atrium

Valve

Left ventricle

Lower vena cava

The heart
The powerful muscle of the heart's ventricles pumps blood to the lungs to receive oxygen, and then around the body, where the oxygen passes to the tissues. Arteries carry blood away from the heart, veins return it

Why does my heart sometimes miss a beat? Lots of doctors have said my heart is normal, but it still happens.

A misplaced, or ectopic, heartbeat is a common experience and is rarely due to any heart disease. Some people seem to have small areas in the heart that are more excitable than they should be, and respond to the normal electric control of the heart (and yes, your own body does generate a good deal of electricity) by causing an extra beat. The most common reasons for triggering off the excitable zones are over-use of stimulants such as caffeine or nicotine, lack of sleep and anxiety. So, if you tend to smoke a lot, drink a lot of strong coffee and get agitated and overtired, you will be likely to notice these extra beats. But as you have been told there is no disease of your heart, ignore them.

What causes palpitations? I keep getting them and my doctor takes no notice.

Experiencing palpitations is something which worries most patients dreadfully, and most doctors not at all. It is felt as a period of rapid, thumping heart-beats which can indeed be alarming. But there is rarely, if ever, any cause for the alarm. The phenomenon is similar to ectopic beat – an overstimulated person becomes aware of the beating of his heart (most of the time we ignore it) and becomes anxious about it, which increases the rate of beating and makes the palpitations seem worse. By all means check with a doctor the first time it happens to you, but if he reassures you that your heart is sound, believe him.

My son who is very athletic has a normal pulse rate of 40 beats a minute but mine is 80 beats. We've both been told we're normal. How can this be so?

The clue is your son's athleticism. A fit person, who spends a lot of time exercising his muscles, exercises his heart as well, gradually demanding more and more effort from it. As his leg and chest and other muscles get thicker and stronger, so does his heart muscle. This means that when he is at rest the heart can pump the blood just as far and just as efficiently with half the power that a less athletic person's heart must use. Then, when the athletic person wants to increase his muscle work, his heart can speed up, and double its output without difficulty, and so enable the leg and chest and other muscles to work twice as efficiently. So you are both healthy, but your son is much more fit.

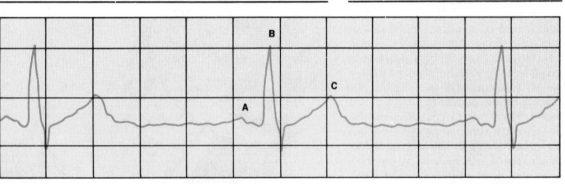

The heartbeat
This ECG is a record of electrical pulses in the heart. Wave **A** causes the atria to squeeze blood into the ventricles (*see* **1** *Below*). The 'spike', **B**, makes the ventricles contract (**2, 3**). Wave **C** marks the recovery before the next beat

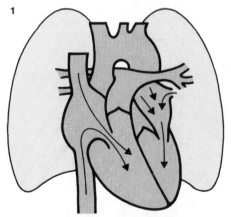

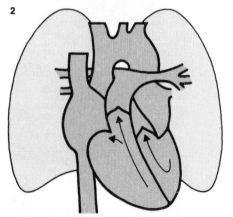

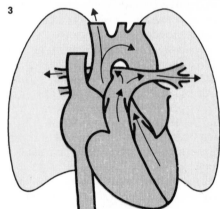

The right atrium, or upper chamber, fills with oxygen-starved blood from the upper and lower venae cavae, while the left atrium fills with oxygen-rich blood from the lungs through the pulmonary veins. Then the atria push the blood into the ventricles

The ventricles are filled and stretched by the blood pumped into them. Then their muscular walls begin to contract. The blood is prevented from returning to the atria, as the valves leading from them are pushed shut by the rising pressure

Finally the blood is forced through valves leading from the heart. The oxygen-starved blood from the right ventricle passes through the pulmonary artery to the lungs, while the oxygen-rich blood from the left ventricle travels via the aorta to the tissues

Heart and circulation

How does being overweight lead to heart disease?

There are several ways. Firstly, when you make extra fat and it is laid down in different parts of the body it may also be laid down in your heart. Having a lot of useless fat wrapped around the heart muscle makes it less efficient, and less able to move freely as it works.

Secondly, people who are fat may develop fatty plaques in the walls of their blood vessels, silting them up. This means that the arteries that supply the heart muscle (the heart, too, needs a blood supply for its own use, as well as having all the body's blood passing through it) are narrowed. Less blood reaches the heart muscle and it is deprived of essential fuel, especially oxygen. Not all fat people have fatty plaques in their arteries, and sometimes thin people have them, but there seems to be a greater likelihood of it happening to the obese.

Thirdly, the heart is put under extra strain when it has to provide the extra energy needed to push the blood around the heavy body and to carry it about. This is more likely to be a problem in people who have recently put on a lot of weight. Someone who has weighed 200 pounds all his adult life puts less of a strain on his heart than someone who has always weighed around 160 pounds and who goes up to 180 in a few weeks or months. The long-term fat person's heart will be in training, to an extent, rather like the athletic person's heart. But the recently fat man is definitely at a disadvantage.

Fourthly, fat people tend to be less active than thin ones. They use their muscles less than they should, so their hearts lack the training which the more active person's heart gets. Then, when the person needs to use a lot of energy in a hurry – running for a bus or train, for example – the heart just cannot cope.

From all points of view, losing weight is one of the kindest things you can do for your heart.

Structure of a blood vessel
The large arteries and veins consist of several layers, which have their own blood supply, just like other tissues. The muscular layers can expand or contract in order to regulate the blood flow

Why does smoking cause heart disease?

Nicotine, the drug that is in tobacco and for which people smoke because it stimulates them, is a vasoconstrictor, that is, it causes the smooth muscle walls of blood vessels to contract. This has the effect of narrowing the central channel and so reducing the amount of blood that can get through to the heart.

If the blood vessels are healthy this is not too much of a problem. However, if they are at all silted up, as they might be if there are fatty plaques sticking on the walls, or if they lack elasticity due to hardening of the arteries, this narrowing effect of nicotine can cause a total blocking of the throughway.

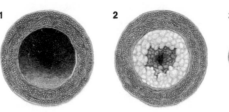
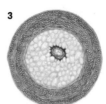

How arteries harden
An originally healthy artery (**1**) becomes coated with plaque (**2**), narrowing until it is easily blocked by a blood clot (**3**)

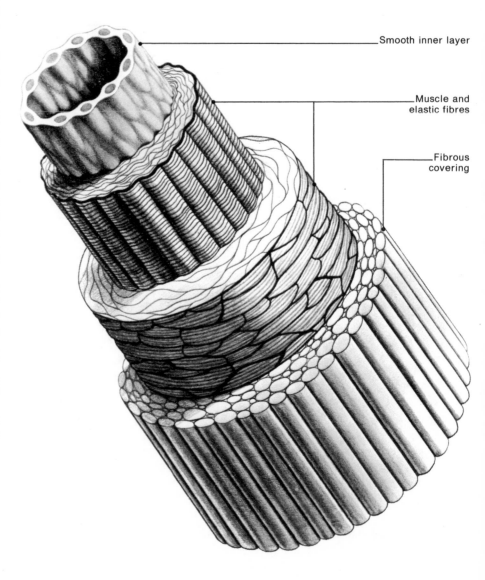

Smooth inner layer

Muscle and elastic fibres

Fibrous covering

What causes hardening of the arteries?

This term is usually applied to a condition which is actually made up of two components. First there is the creation of those plaques of fatty material which are laid down on artery walls. This is called atheroma. Then there is a thickening and hardening of the fibres in the walls of the arteries. This is called atherosclerosis.

The causes of atheroma/atherosclerosis are still being investigated. There is one school of thought that blames modern Western diet, with its high quantities of animal proteins, fats and refined sugars. It says that the high protein and fat content increase the quantity of fat in the blood, from which the wall plaques are made, and that refined sugar seems to encourage this tendency. It recommends a diet low in animal fats, high in vegetable fats (they are called poly-unsaturated fats because of their chemical structure), low in refined sugar and high in fibre (the largely indigestible part of grain and vegetable foods). The fibre is thought to scour excess fats from the gut, thus preventing them from reaching the bloodstream.

However, there are some doctors who dismiss this theory and say that diet control only matters in overweight people, who need to lose their excess fat.

Virtually all doctors agree that obesity is a common cause of atheroma/atherosclerosis. They are also virtually unanimous about the effect of nicotine.

It is also agreed that age has an effect; as we grow older all of us, thin or fat, smokers or not, develop less elastic arteries just as we develop less elastic muscles and tendons.

Probably the condition is due to many different causes. Almost certainly there is a genetic component – we inherit from our forebears a tendency to the condition and obesity, smoking habits and age all probably contribute to this.

I've heard that drinking water has an effect on hardening of the arteries. Is this true?

It has long been noted that there are marked regional differences in the incidence of heart attack and atheroma/atherosclerosis. Studies showed that one of the factors involved in the difference was the hardness or softness of the water. Areas where the water supply is hard – that is, it contains extra calcium among other things – showed a lower incidence of the diseases. In areas where the water is soft, the rate was higher.

The reasons are not fully understood. It could be that the extra calcium exerts a protective effect. It could be that soft water carries more soluble metals, such as lead, cadmium and mercury. Until we know for certain, it might be worth acting on the statistical evidence and seeking out hard water for drinking and cooking.

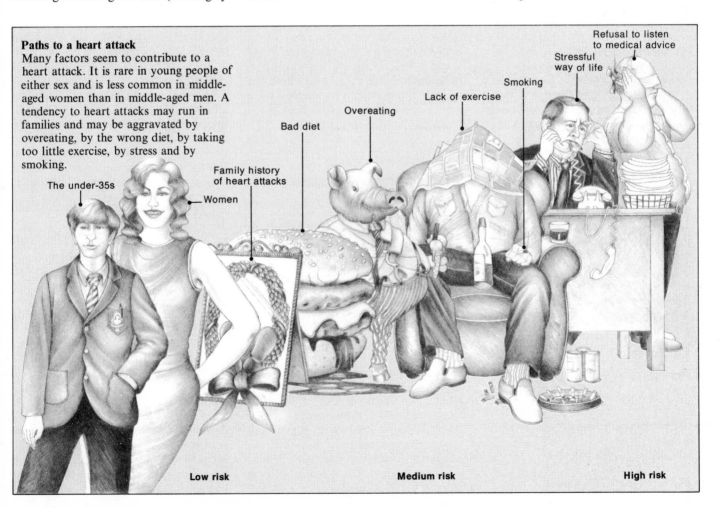

Paths to a heart attack
Many factors seem to contribute to a heart attack. It is rare in young people of either sex and is less common in middle-aged women than in middle-aged men. A tendency to heart attacks may run in families and may be aggravated by overeating, by the wrong diet, by taking too little exercise, by stress and by smoking.

The under-35s

Women

Family history of heart attacks

Bad diet

Overeating

Lack of exercise

Smoking

Stressful way of life

Refusal to listen to medical advice

Low risk

Medium risk

High risk

Heart and circulation

What has blood pressure to do with heart attacks? What is a normal pressure? And what happens if the pressure is low?

When blood is pumped out of the heart into the arteries, it presses on the walls, which, because they are elastic, resist the pressure. This resistance can be measured by seeing how high a column of mercury the blood vessel walls can support. The resistance is measured in two sections; first, the pressure on the vessel walls when the blood is pushed into them from the heart, and this is called the systolic pressure; and second, the pressure when the heart is refilling, and this is called the diastolic pressure.

The more important pressure is the diastolic. The systolic can be quite high during exercise – the heart sends blood spurting out hard and fast and this shows in the pressure on the walls – but that does not mean there is anything wrong. If, however, the pressure is high during the resting component of the beat, then that may mean that the arteries are hard and that the heart and kidneys can be under threat because of the high pressure (the kidneys filter poisons from the blood; if the pressure is consistently high, they cannot do their job properly, and are damaged).

The risk to the heart is failure of one of the arteries supplying the heart muscle. If they cannot expand enough to allow sufficient blood through, then the heart can be starved.

The range of normal pressure is considerable, but a healthy young adult will usually give a reading of 120 systolic, 80 diastolic. This is written as $\frac{120}{80}$. This reading is likely to increase with age, though not always. People with perfectly healthy arteries may maintain the same level all their lives.

A fall in blood pressure can be more damaging than a rise because then the brain is deprived of essential blood supply for a while. The brain needs to receive 750 cubic centimetres of fresh blood every minute of every day, all through a lifetime. A fall in blood pressure can diminish this quantity and the result is a faint.

Blood pressure is measured with a device consisting of an inflatable cuff which goes round one arm. It is then tightened until the artery underneath it is just obliterated, and the amount of pressure needed to do this is read from the attached scale. The pressure is then released, and the lower pressure reading is taken when the artery can just be heard again. The device used is called a sphygmomanometer, and was invented by an Italian named Riva Rocci. This is why in some European countries blood pressure is written not as BP but as RR.

What is the best way to treat high blood pressure?

Avoiding the precipitating causes comes first. So, lose weight, give up smoking and take regular exercise to protect your arteries as well as your heart.

People who already have a high blood pressure problem can nowadays be treated by medicines. There are several different ones which act by preventing 'constrict' messages from reaching the muscle walls of the blood vessels. These medicines can have unpleasant side effects, so they are best used sparingly, often in conjunction with other medicines which reduce the amount of fluid in the bloodstream, and so reduce the work load. Many doctors believe that the control of blood pressure with modern medicines is one of the greatest medical advances of this century.

When I told my doctor that I get pains in my chest he said that I had angina. I have to suck a tablet when it happens. He says I'm doing well, but I keep thinking I'm going to have a heart attack. Am I?

Angina means literally 'pain' (it comes from the same Latin word root which gives us words like anguish and anxiety). *Angina pectoris* means 'pain in the chest'. Another kind of angina is Vincent's angina – a painful inflammation of the mouth.

What happens in your case is that one of the arteries supplying your heart muscle is less efficient than it should be. Maybe it is narrow or partially silted up. If you make extra effort, and your heart works harder as a result, then it may not get enough blood from that artery, and the result is pain. In some cases it is little more than a dull aching tightness, in others it is a really nasty gripping sensation which goes from beneath the breastbone, across the chest and up into the neck and jaw and down the left arm. It depends on the degree of artery constriction and the amount of effort put out.

In a way, having angina is like having a monitor in your chest. If you overdo things and put your heart under strain, the pain comes on and warns you to slow down. Usually you will find that resting will stop the pain quickly – most attacks are over in under two minutes, and few last longer than 10 minutes.

The tablets your doctor gave you are useful both for taking before you intend to make an extra effort, for example climbing a flight of stairs, or when you have a pain. They dissolve under the tongue and their active ingredient then reaches the heart via the blood and causes the blood vessels to relax and allow more blood through, thus reducing the pain. When the pain comes, therefore, it actually prevents you from having a heart attack.

There is no reason why people with angina shouldn't live to a good old age, when once they learn to accept their disability and live within it. A life of controlled effort, free of excess stress – because anger and undue excitement bring on an attack – may not be dramatic but it is a happy and comfortable one.

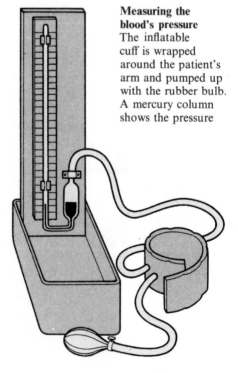

Measuring the blood's pressure
The inflatable cuff is wrapped around the patient's arm and pumped up with the rubber bulb. A mercury column shows the pressure

How can emotional shock and worry cause heart attacks?

When a person gets tense and worried or frightened the result is an outpouring of adrenalin from the adrenal glands. Adrenalin has the effect of speeding up heart action, and narrowing blood vessels. So, it can put an extra strain on a heart at risk.

One unfortunate effect of the realization that emotional triggers can lead to heart attack in vulnerable people is the way in which some heart patients' families get so frightened of upsetting the sufferer that he turns into a domestic tyrant. But it doesn't really help a person who has had a heart attack to have his every whim observed. It may make him fear that he is even more at risk than he is, and frighten him more. Good care for a person after a heart attack has been treated, and he has returned to ordinary living, involves everyone in the family behaving as normally as possible, even if that means occasional arguments and emotional scenes.

What actually happens in a heart attack?

Remember that the blood vessels supplying the heart muscle may get silted up and reduce the blood supply. If the supply is blocked altogether, for example by a clot of blood sticking to one of the fatty wall plaques, or by constriction of an already narrowed artery, the area of muscle supplied by the vessels is starved and may actually die. The heart then has trouble co-ordinating its pulses since all the muscle fibres are involved. The condition is called a myocardial infarct, or coronary thrombosis.

If the damaged area is small the patient survives if the normal beating of the heart can be restored quickly. If the damaged area is massive and the steady beat cannot be restored, then the result is death.

Prompt recognition of a heart attack and swift medical care are key factors in survival. That is why many countries have special Heart Flying Squads which are available to go to emergency calls.

I get a lot of heartburn. Does that mean I'll have a heart attack one day?

No. Heartburn is a popular name for the burning pain that comes when you have eaten too much or eaten foods that you know disagree with you. Some of the stomach contents rise into the gullet, and the acid juices from the stomach irritate its lining. This is felt behind the breastbone roughly in the same region as some heart pain, but has nothing to do with the heart.

But if you get heartburn because you overeat all the time, then you will get overweight and that certainly contributes to heart disease.

Three members of my family have had heart attacks. Does this make me a likely victim?

There does seem to be a family link – some people inherit a tendency to artery or heart disease. But this tendency is only one of many factors and it need not be more important than the others. Since you know your family history, you would be wise to control your weight, give up smoking, and follow a regular exercise pattern. Then you will be at no greater risk than most other people.

Incidentally, women appear to be less vulnerable to heart attack until they reach the menopause. Their hormone status appears to confer some protection. Once the menopause is complete, however, they seem to catch up with men as far as the risk is concerned. So women who have a family history of heart attack have more time in which to establish good habits.

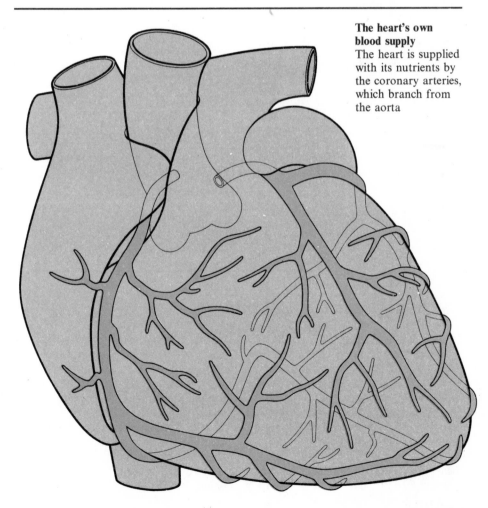

The heart's own blood supply
The heart is supplied with its nutrients by the coronary arteries, which branch from the aorta

Heart and circulation

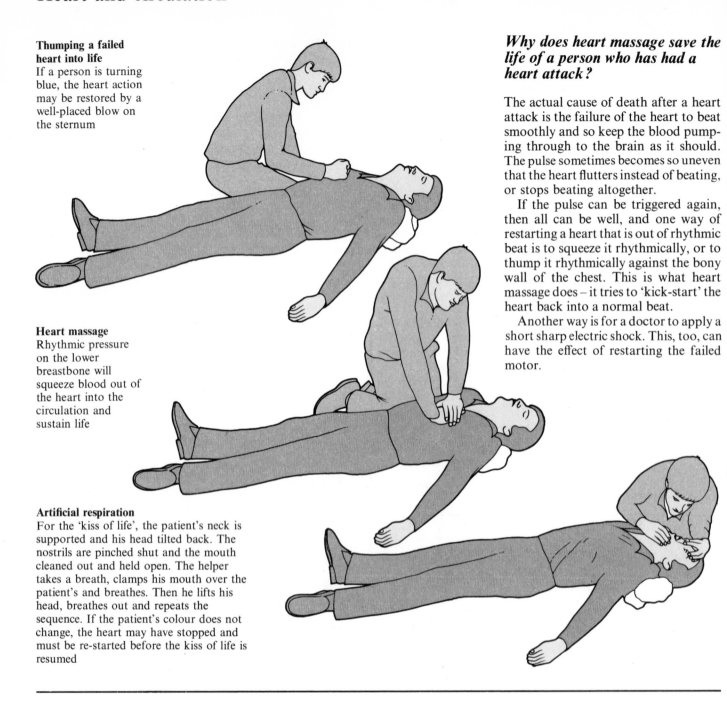

Thumping a failed heart into life
If a person is turning blue, the heart action may be restored by a well-placed blow on the sternum

Heart massage
Rhythmic pressure on the lower breastbone will squeeze blood out of the heart into the circulation and sustain life

Artificial respiration
For the 'kiss of life', the patient's neck is supported and his head tilted back. The nostrils are pinched shut and the mouth cleaned out and held open. The helper takes a breath, clamps his mouth over the patient's and breathes. Then he lifts his head, breathes out and repeats the sequence. If the patient's colour does not change, the heart may have stopped and must be re-started before the kiss of life is resumed

Why does heart massage save the life of a person who has had a heart attack?

The actual cause of death after a heart attack is the failure of the heart to beat smoothly and so keep the blood pumping through to the brain as it should. The pulse sometimes becomes so uneven that the heart flutters instead of beating, or stops beating altogether.

If the pulse can be triggered again, then all can be well, and one way of restarting a heart that is out of rhythmic beat is to squeeze it rhythmically, or to thump it rhythmically against the bony wall of the chest. This is what heart massage does – it tries to 'kick-start' the heart back into a normal beat.

Another way is for a doctor to apply a short sharp electric shock. This, too, can have the effect of restarting the failed motor.

Can people die of a broken heart?

If by broken heart you mean 'severe distress', then the answer has to be 'yes'. But not because the heart actually 'breaks' in any way, although people with damaged heart arteries may be in greater risk of a heart attack; and if that happens the heart could be said, in a sense, to be broken.

But unhappy people with healthy hearts have been shown to have a greater rate of early death than happy people. A study of some widowers a few years ago showed that they died prematurely from a range of causes, while other men of their age and about their health level, who had not been bereaved, survived. This is because of the way the body and mind work so closely together. Acute emotional distress can lead to a running down of the physical processes, even to the point of severe illness and death.

This is why it is so important that bereaved people should be given support and care for some time after their loss. Nowadays, most of us are so embarrassed by, and frightened of, death that we keep away from mourners, which adds dreadfully to their burdens. If we could be like the Victorians and treat death for what it is – a part of life – the bereaved would suffer much less.

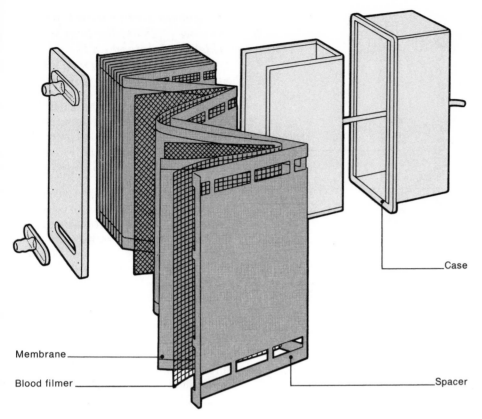

Membrane

Blood filmer

Case

Spacer

If your heart stops beating you die, so how can surgeons do heart operations?

It is not the passage of blood through the heart that is critical – it is the supply of blood to the brain. As long as this vital organ receives its regular 750 cubic centimetres every minute the heart can be as idle as a lizard on a hot stone.

So, to enable surgeons to operate on the heart, machinery to bypass it has been devised. Blood passes from the patient through a heart-lung machine, collecting vital oxygen and dumping carbon dioxide and going on its way to the brain, while the heart is stilled and repaired. With the aid of this machinery new valves, new arteries, even whole new hearts can be grafted into a human body. The operations have a variable degree of long-term success but usually the actual technique causes little risk.

An artificial lung
The blood is spread out, forming a thin film over the membrane, and oxygen passes into it as carbon dioxide passes out

Why do my finger tips go white in cold weather? Does it mean I have a bad circulation?

This is a common reaction in women – men are more likely to find their toes go cold and white in poor weather (no one knows why there should be this sex difference). It is not a sign of 'poor' circulation. It merely means that the smallest blood vessels at the extremities of the body are extra-sensitive and respond to cold by tightening up, sending the blood to the deeper tissues to keep warm.

The answer is to ensure that the fingers are covered with a light layer of fabric such as wool, which traps air (air is the best insulator there is) to prevent loss of warmth. Also, avoid smoking, which increases the likelihood of constriction of the blood vessels.

In some cases the constriction is severe enough to need medical treatment. A vasodilating medicine can then be used to relax the vessel walls. Incidentally, a chronic problem of this sort involving the finger tips is called Raynaud's disease and that involving the toes is known as Buerger's disease.

The blood network
The arterioles and venules can change size with changes in temperature. The capillaries have thin walls through which nutrients pass

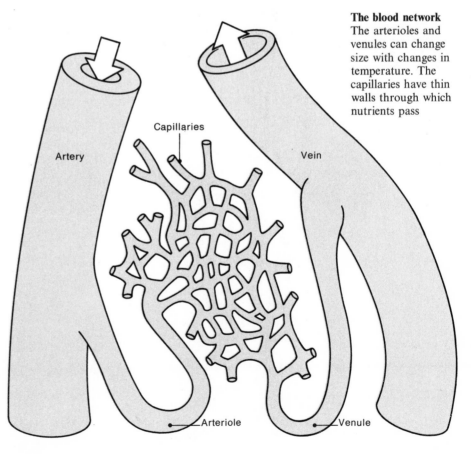

Artery

Capillaries

Vein

Arteriole

Venule

Heart and circulation

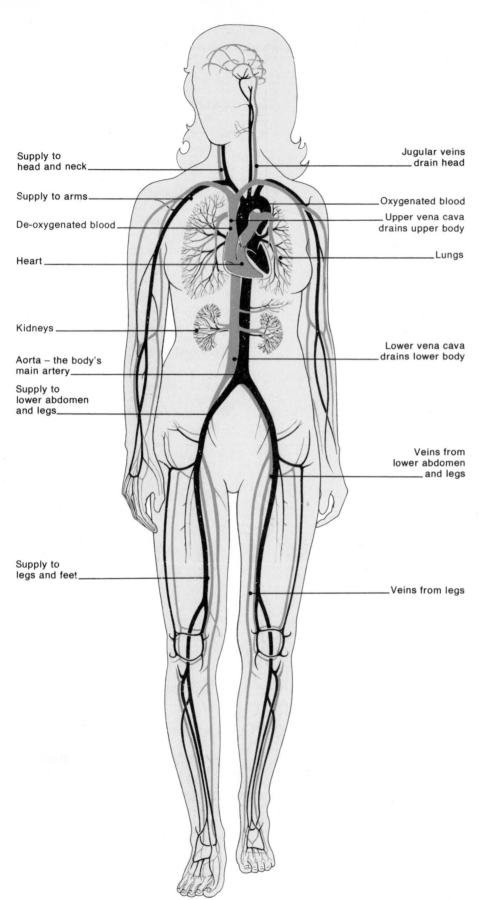

Supply to head and neck

Supply to arms

De-oxygenated blood

Heart

Kidneys

Aorta – the body's main artery

Supply to lower abdomen and legs

Supply to legs and feet

Jugular veins drain head

Oxygenated blood

Upper vena cava drains upper body

Lungs

Lower vena cava drains lower body

Veins from lower abdomen and legs

Veins from legs

Does blood always travel in the same way? What happens to athletes who stand on their heads, for example? Does gravity make the blood change direction?

Blood always travels the same way, through the right side of the heart into the lungs, back into the left side of the heart, down into the body through the central main artery (the aorta), on through all the arteries to every cell there is and back to the right side of the heart again via the network of veins. It is kept moving in this direction all through life by the powerful pumping action of the heart, and by valves at strategic points in the heart itself and in the veins, which prevent backflow whatever the body is doing and whatever its posture.

When there is backflow in the heart, which can happen when its valves are incompetent, the person can be quite ill and unable to live a normal life. Modern surgical techniques are now available to repair such valve failures.

Why does the blood you can see showing through your skin at your wrists look blue? Is it true that some people have bluer blood than others?

Blood is never blue. It is blood vessel walls that affect the colour that can be seen through the skin, not their contents.

The reason aristocrats were called 'blue bloods' was that they did not work in the fields as the peasants did, so they did not become tanned. Their skins remained white and translucent and allowed the blood vessels to show through more easily. Even the most tanned of people will have some white skin somewhere where the blood vessels show clearly. On women, for example, the veins on the breasts often create a blue tracery, and make them look very aristocratic indeed.

The body's supply lines
Thousands of miles of blood vessels supply the body. Only a very few of the main ones are shown here. The arteries carry oxygen and nutrients to the tissues, and the veins carry back carbon dioxide and other waste products

*My son had a heart murmur when he was born and it caused us much worry. He is now grown
up and quite healthy, but his daughter has a murmur. She is three weeks old.
Will she do as well as her father did? Her tests so far seem all right.*

Probably. About half of all new babies have a heart murmur, which is a sort of extra sound which can be heard through a stethoscope, and which sometimes sounds quite musical. Most of these murmurs disappear as the child grows, although sometimes they are heard for the first time in older children during routine school medical examinations. But these murmurs, too, are rarely a cause for worry, because any significant heart disorder would have shown itself long before school days.

If your grand-daughter has had some electrocardiograms done, which seems likely, and/or X-rays and you have been told that she is well then believe it because she is.

The height of these zig-zags represents the loudness of heart sounds. In this case the heartbeat shows a 'diamond' murmur. It increases in loudness and then diminishes between the two sounds of the normal heartbeat, shown by the 'spikes' **A** and **B**

The heart murmur shown below begins at the end of the normal heartbeat, **B**, and diminishes in loudness. Murmurs can be due to valves that are leaky, leading to backflow of the blood, or too narrow, leading to turbulence in the flow

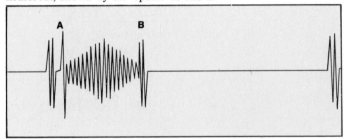

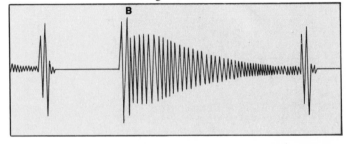

Why do some people get varicose veins? Are they at all dangerous?

Varicose veins are incompetent veins – they allow the blood that is pushed along them to surge backwards between pulse beats, because the valves which should prevent that happening have sagged out of shape. The causes are partly genetic – a tendency to varicosity runs in families – and partly acquired. Overweight people who stand a lot tend to get them as they put excess strain on the veins trying to return blood to the heart against the pull of gravity. They are common in pregnancy, partly because of the extra weight and partly because of action of the hormone progesterone which relaxes blood vessel walls. Tight garters which hold the blood back in the legs, and tight girdles, which hold it back in the trunk, may also contribute.

Varicose veins are not in themselves dangerous, though they are unsightly and uncomfortable. However, one of them may be damaged and start to bleed, and it can be difficult to stop the bleeding. This can lead to quite a severe haemorrhage and the vein may need tying up to stop the loss of blood continuing.

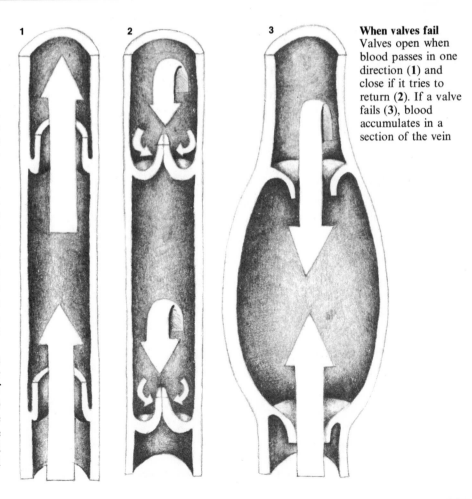

When valves fail
Valves open when blood passes in one direction (**1**) and close if it tries to return (**2**). If a valve fails (**3**), blood accumulates in a section of the vein

Nutrition

'It's a very strange thing, as strange as can be – whatever Miss T eats turns into Miss T' is an old rhyme which amuses children, but which is a clear statement of fact. People are indeed made of food. We are what we eat – and sadly many of us eat very foolishly indeed. For a large portion of humanity the problem is lack of adequate food. For far too many more, the problem is overeating, which can be as damaging a form of malnutrition as actual starvation. The current epidemic of coronary heart disease is believed to owe quite a lot to bad feeding practices. So, nutritionists, experts in the effects of foods on the human organism, are becoming more and more important in modern medical practice. Also, they have a vital role to play in encouraging good eating habits.

Principle nutrients and their functions

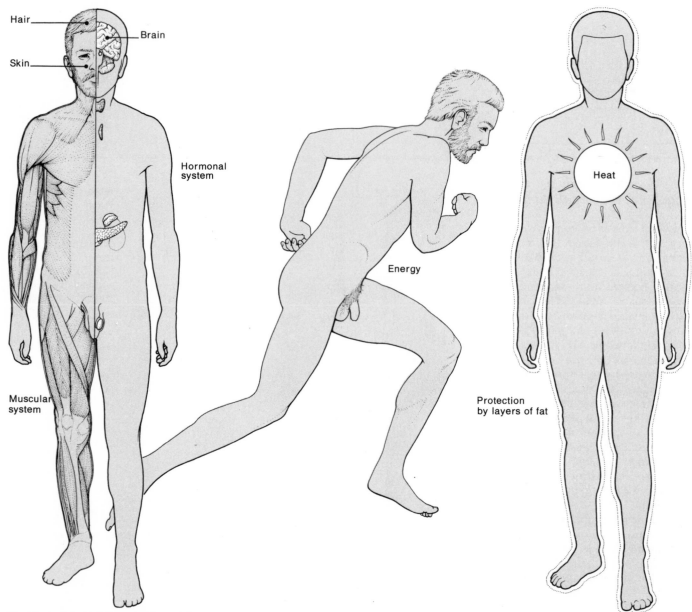

Hair
Brain
Skin
Hormonal system
Muscular system
Energy
Heat
Protection by layers of fat

Protein is essential for growth and tissue repair; any surplus is burned for energy

Carbohydrates are burned as fuel to give energy; any surplus is stored as fat

Fats are the greatest energy source; surplus fat is stored under the skin as insulation

Why do we have to eat so many different kinds of food when lots of animals are fine and healthy eating just one kind – grass?

Life is nothing if it is not adaptable, and over the millennia of evolution all the various life-forms have learned to survive on what is available. The grasses are the most widespread form of plant life, and large numbers of grazing species have developed digestive organs which enable them to extract from the grasses the protein, carbohydrates and fats that they need, and convert them into body muscle, fat and energy.

Humans, together with the other carnivorous and omnivorous species, learned to eat the grass-converting animals as a source of the foodstuffs they need, but when animal food is unavailable they can cope reasonably well on plant life. We do not in fact need to eat such a wide variety of foods; we just want to, which is a very different thing.

What we need is a regular daily intake of carbohydrate foods – the sugars and starches – to provide fast sugar in the blood as an energy source; protein, to provide the elements for building and repairing muscles and other tissues; fats, to provide energy (they are the richest calorie source) and as a food store against hard times; and a range of elements and vitamins to control various body processes. Most of these could be obtained from a simple diet, beans and rice, for example, and that is precisely what a large number of humans in the world today subsist on.

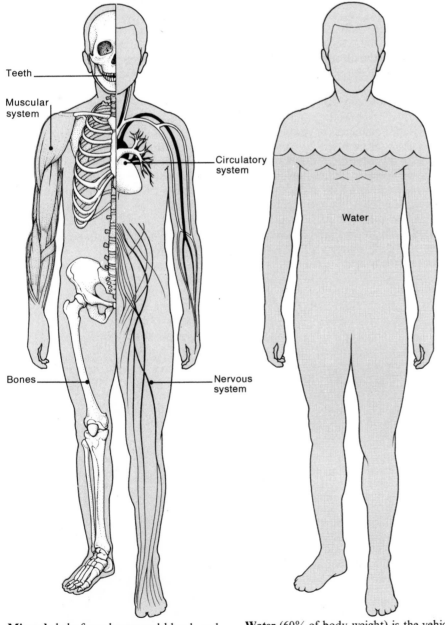

Teeth

Muscular system

Circulatory system

Bones

Nervous system

Water

Minerals help form bones and blood, and aid cellular energy transfer and enzymes

Water (60% of body weight) is the vehicle for chemical reactions and waste removal

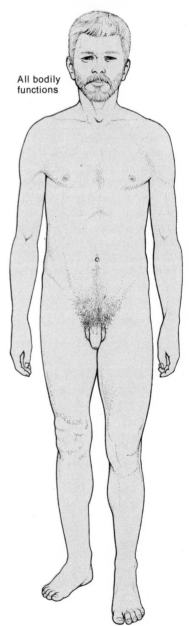

All bodily functions

Vitamins each have specific functions in regulating growth and all bodily processes

Nutrition

My doctor says I need a good, well-balanced diet, but how can I know what that is, when there are so many different kinds of food?

There is a theory which says that when people are presented with a wide range of foods they will instinctively choose those which they need. An experiment carried out with young children in Oslo seemed to confirm the theory. They chose the ideal breakfast, in nutritional terms, from lots of offerings including candy.

However, this does not seem to happen generally. Obesity is one of the major nutritional disorders of the Western world and this is because people do not choose the right foods or the right quantities from what they are offered. We have a tendency, in rich societies, to eat a great deal of sweet foods and a great deal of animal fats and proteins. We do not eat enough raw fruits and vegetables or 'rough' food, and consistently prefer the soft, the smooth and the bland.

This means that we not only put on debilitating ugly fat; we also lack certain vital substances. Fibre is the obvious one and we may also be short of certain vitamins and minerals, because their richest sources are raw fruit and vegetables.

To make an ideal diet, you need the minimum of sugars and refined starches, so take your carbohydrate food from whole cereals and vegetables. You need a daily amount of protein. The quantity should be in ratio to your other foods – protein should be about a quarter of the total volume and you are better off if you eat less rather than more protein and also if you select some vegetable protein. Beans, peas and lentils provide this, as do whole grain cereals. Fats, too, should be limited, and there is a school of thought that advises vegetable fats rather than animal-derived ones. At the present time, vegetable fats are said to be healthier although later research may dispute this. Meanwhile, an attempt to keep the fat intake fairly low – less than a tenth of the total day's diet – would be wise.

If the specimen day's diet shown in the next column is followed, there is no need to worry about minerals or vitamins; you will get them anyway.

This sounds Spartan and undeniably dull to a Western palate seduced by hamburgers, french fries and ice cream. But it is a healthy diet and if followed, as a general rule, the occasional indulgence in junk food will not matter. It is a diet made up entirely of junk food which is unhealthy.

Specimen day's diet

Breakfast
Orange/apple/grapefruit juice. Whole grain cereal. Fruit (apple, raisins). Nuts (hazel, almonds). Milk. Mild stimulant (coffee, tea). Slice wholemeal toast, butter/margarine and marmalade.

Mid-morning
Mild stimulant (coffee, tea).

Lunch
Portion cheese, *or* an egg *or* peas/beans. Mixed salad including lettuce, tomatoes, onions, celery, and dressed with vegetable oil, iodized salt, lemon juice. Slice wholemeal bread with butter/margarine. Fresh fruit. Wine, if liked.

Mid-afternoon
Mild stimulant (tea, coffee).

Dinner
Grapefruit or clear vegetable broth. Small portion meat *or* fish *or* poultry (season with curry powder occasionally – a rich source of dietary iron). Raw or cooked root vegetables – potatoes, parsnips, carrots, turnips, onions, *plus* leaf vegetables – cabbage, spinach, cauliflower. Dessert made with unrefined cereal, sugar, chocolate (also a rich source of dietary iron). A little wine.

What the different vitamins do

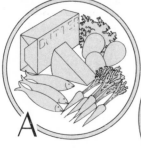

A — Essential to childhood growth, correctly functioning adult vision and the protection of skin and mucous membranes. A deficiency slows growth, leads to skin disorders and low resistance to infection; with a severe shortage (rare in developed countries) cells can dry and harden, harming the cornea and causing blindness

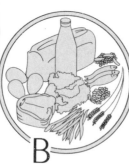

B — The B vitamins are involved in releasing energy from food, forming red blood cells and maintaining skin and mucous membranes. A deficiency causes loss of appetite, and slows growth and development

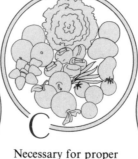

C — Necessary for proper formation of teeth, bones and blood vessels, and for healthy collagen (the protein linking the cells). A deficiency checks childhood growth, and severe shortage produces scurvy. Vitamin C is water soluble and not stored in the body, but half an orange a day is an adequate supply

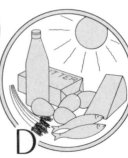

D — Regulates calcium and phosphorus in bone and tooth formation, so is important in childhood and pregnancy to ward off rickets and dental decay). Vitamin D is synthesized beneath the skin in sunlight

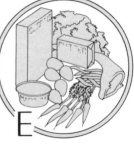

E — Important for normal reproduction in adults. It influences biochemical processes in the nuclei of growing cells, acting as an antioxidant and preserving other vitamins as well as preserving unsaturated fatty acids. It can also help skin wounds to heal

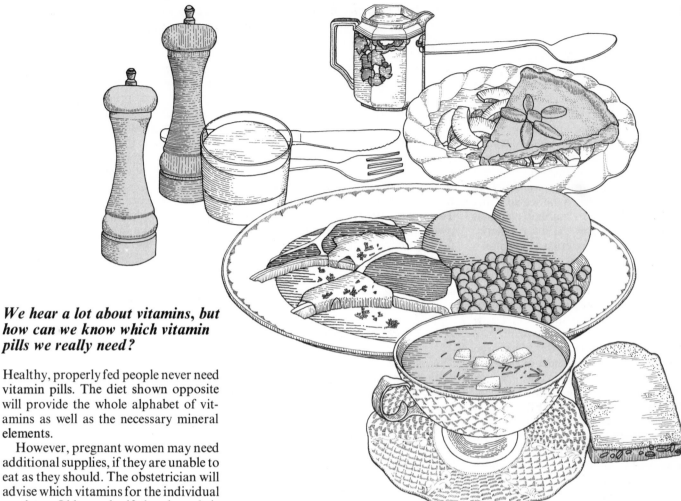

We hear a lot about vitamins, but how can we know which vitamin pills we really need?

Healthy, properly fed people never need vitamin pills. The diet shown opposite will provide the whole alphabet of vitamins as well as the necessary mineral elements.

However, pregnant women may need additional supplies, if they are unable to eat as they should. The obstetrician will advise which vitamins for the individual mothers. Old people, if they lose their interest in eating, may also need supplements. Ill people may need special supplements, too. Again, individual needs must be individually advised by doctors.

A typical main meal
This three-course meal contains nearly 1,500 calories – almost three-quarters of the 2,200 calories that the specimen diet (*opposite*) provides – the recommended daily intake for an average adult woman.

While such a meal might be suitable for the hearty appetite of a manual worker, for most people a smaller and more evenly distributed intake of food during the day would put less strain on the digestion

Do children need more vitamins than adults?

Body weight for body weight, children need more of all kinds of food than adults. They are growing at a great rate, and this demands lots of protein, and they are usually more active and this demands extra carbohydrate. If they eat enough of the right foods to satisfy these demands they will not need extra vitamin supplements.

The idea that all children needed extra vitamins arose with the spread of bottle-feeding for babies instead of breast-feeding. Breast milk is the comprehensive food for human infants and a well-fed mother provides her baby

with all he needs. A bottle-fed baby, however, may need extra vitamins if the milk he gets in his bottle lacks them – as it may.

In the UK, during World War II, a government policy of providing extra vitamins for all children was implemented to combat any deficiencies that food rationing might cause. In fact, it was found that the British public was never better fed, in purely nutritional terms, than during rationing. They complained that their diet was boring, of course, but it was undoubtedly adequate.

However, the use of vitamin supplements for babies and young children was maintained well into the 1960s when a less restricted diet was available, and then it was found that some children were getting too much, particularly of Vitamins A and D, which can be harmful if taken in excess. Vitamin C – the other widely used vitamin – appears to do no harm in excess of daily need; it is just excreted in urine.

Today, most doctors agree that the well-fed child – and that means taking the specimen diet shown opposite as a basis – needs no supplements.

Nutrition

Why do some diets make you lose weight faster than others?

If people are fat, they need to restructure their daily diet so that they take in less calories than they expend. This simple sum always equals weight loss.

However, this method tends to lose weight slowly, and many would-be slimmers get bored and discouraged. So they seek the faster systems often found in 'crank' diets. Eating nothing but oranges and peanuts for a week will take off weight, but it is a rather silly diet because as soon as normal eating is resumed, back goes the fat. Similarly, diets designed to restrict water intake may seem to lose weight at first, but as soon as normal drinking starts again, back goes the poundage.

So a good rèducing diet should be based on the specimen diet shown on the previous page. Just eat less of it than thinner people do. However, it has been found that a rearrangement of the diet's constituents may, in some people, increase the rate of weight loss. It seems that there are people who are less-efficient at converting fat and protein into energy. So, for them, a diet with little or no carbohydrate and made up entirely of protein fat and some unavoidable carbohydrate (that is, bran) will lead to a dramatic weight loss. However, to maintain that loss, they need always to severely control their intake of carbohydrate.

Why is it that my husband can eat twice as much as I do and not get fat, while I eat an ordinary diet and put on pound after pound? It seems so unfair.

Nature has never promised to be fair. It is an impossible concept in biological terms; what matters to Nature is survival of the fittest.

But even if you know that fact, it still rankles to contemplate people who have the sort of metabolism that permits them to take in a lot of food and not show the effect as obesity. However, there is nothing to be done about it. These lucky people are born with their own sort of internal economy, just as they are born with their particular eye colour and nose shape.

Some women have an added burden – their hormone balance seems to bend them towards a tendency to obesity. Estrogen and progesterone are very closely linked to fat deposits in the body (it is the way fat is laid down in women that gives them their classic curvy shape) so changes in their hormones may lead to changes in their fat stores, and of course vice versa.

It may also be that your husband eats less sweet foods than you do. Women seem to retain a taste for sweetness into adult life, while many men lose theirs. This, too, is thought to be linked to hormone balance.

Why do children have such a craving for sweet foods?

This is partly because they are using extra energy and need a fast replenishment; it is partly because they have a lower taste threshold for sweet things than adults and also – and probably most important – because adults expect children to crave for sweet things and so provide them. There is a whole mythology about the vital importance of giving candy to babies.

The hard fact is that children would do perfectly well if they never ate a piece of candy in all their lives. The need for fast energy can be obtained from sweet fresh fruits – they are high in fructose – or dried fruits such as raisins or sweet raw vegetables such as carrots.

Refined sugar in the form of candy is not only unnecessary, it is a health hazard, since it directly contributes to dental damage.

The cards (below) show the energy the average adult expends in different activities measured in kilocalories per minute

Calorie activity cards

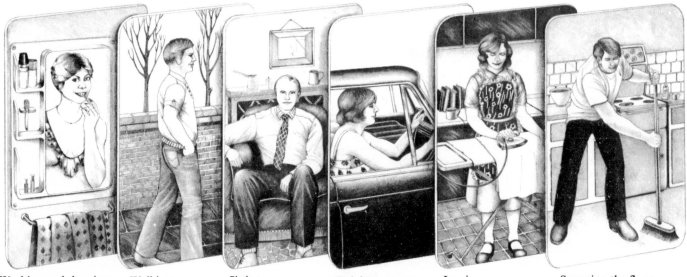

| Washing and dressing | Walking | Sitting | Driving a car | Ironing | Sweeping the floor |
| 2.9 | 4.0 | 1.7 | 2.8 | 4.2 | 1.7 |

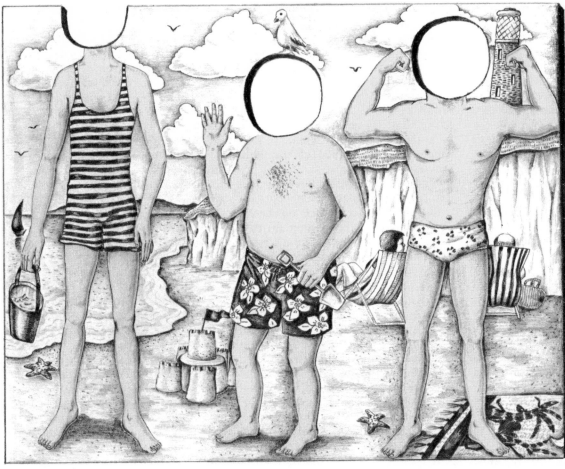

Somatotypes
These are extreme examples of each of the three different types of human physique – ectomorphs, endomorphs and mesomorphs. Somatotyping is a way of describing a body in terms of its tendency towards these three extreme types. A body is unlikely to tend *strongly* to more than one of them: an ectomorph, for instance, may have mesomorphic tendencies – be basically tall and thin, but have well-developed chest and shoulder muscles. Adults cannot actually *change* their somatotype with age, diet or exercise; although the body's shape can be modified or controlled, some people always have to cope with, say, an endomorphic tendency to store excess fat – while others burn it up easily

Ectomorphs are tall and thin, with narrow bodies and thin limbs. They do not tend to accumulate body fat or to have naturally well-developed muscles

Endomorphs have stocky, rounded frames with short necks and limbs. They tend to accumulate fat, particularly on the thighs and upper arms

Mesomorphs are strongly built and muscular, with little body fat. Ectomorphs and endomorphs do not become mesomorphs merely by developing their muscles

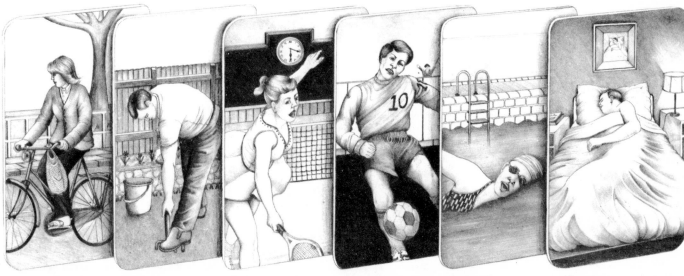

Riding a bicycle
7.8

Digging
8.6

Playing tennis
7.1

Playing football
8.9

Swimming
14.0

Sleeping
1.1

Nutrition

Why do food manufacturers put additives in food when everyone knows they are bad for you?

What 'everybody knows' is not necessarily true. The hard facts are very different. They need to be spelled out in order to counteract the hysteria which has been whipped up in recent years by some people who are less well-informed than they might be.

For centuries mankind has had to face the problem of ensuring a constant food supply from a fluctuating source. If the head of the family killed an animal one day, he needed to preserve its meat to eat on another day; he could not hope to kill every afternoon. The grains and vegetables he harvested in the autumn had to be preserved to see him through a hard winter.

Preservation is the key because food starts to change and rot very rapidly. Fats go rancid, and rancid food not only tastes foul (that's why we learned to use spices and fragrant herbs, by the way; to disguise the rotten taste of what we had to eat) it is also dangerous to health because it destroys essential Vitamin A. Proteins break down under the attentions of bacteria and become not only unpalatable but possibly dangerous to human health (toxic substances are made from the rotting protein; those spices only helped to cover the taste – they did not prevent some people from dying of food poisoning). Moulds grow on rotting foods and can produce toxins which are extremely unhealthy, since they can cause cancer (an epidemic of liver cancer in Africa a while ago was traced to peanuts on which a mould had grown but which were eaten, just the same, by turkeys which were then eaten by people).

So, humans invented methods of preservation. Salt and smoke were found to prevent food rotting. (But salt can be unhealthy. Heart, kidneys and blood pressure are all affected by it. And smoke can be carcinogenic – cancer causing). Drying and freezing helped, too, although sometimes the foods developed moulds or were grossly infected, which made people ill when they ate them. But, for a long time, mankind went on eating rotten, poorly preserved food and went without sufficient food during hard winters.

The development of methods of synthesizing anti-oxidants (to prevent rancidity), mould inhibitors and other preserving agents led to a greatly improved diet and reduced the incidence of food poisoning. However, as time went on, the food dealers became more ambitious and tried to swell their profits by adding all sorts of materials to food. Putting sand in sugar, water in milk, alum in flour for example, all these were the stock-in-trade of the 19th-century grocer.

Modern laws have put an end to all that. We have a system of control over food additives that protects our health far better than it could ever do in a 'natural' environment by eating 'natural' foods. It also keeps a close eye on greedy entrepreneurs trying to make money out of selling bad food.

But still, we do have one problem. Because food chemists do not rest on their laurels, but go on researching, from time to time they find that a food additive, be it flavour (and we demand lots of flavours in our food) colour (and virtually every eater is beguiled by food which is tinted prettily) or preservative, is not as safe as it was once thought. Then that substance is withdrawn, very properly, from use.

What happens after that is that an untrained outsider (untrained in chemistry, that is) hears that the substance has been withdrawn and makes an unjustifiable assumption – 'this food additive, once thought healthy, is now said to be unhealthy. That means that all food additives once thought to be healthy must be unhealthy. We must ban them all.'

This really is absurd, yet it is the thinking that prompted this question. All food additives are not bad; many of them are 'natural' in that they derive from plants or animals, and many are foods in their own right. Monosodium glutamate is a case in point. It is the sodium salt of one of the commonest proteins found in vegetables, it enhances the flavour of foods, and when swallowed is digested by the body as food. Some people have shown that they are highly sensitive to it, if they take it in large quantities, but that does not mean that it need be banned for all of us. That would be like banning all strawberries because some people are allergic to them.

Looking at the matter calmly, rather than emotionally, most sensible people now agree that the systems of control over food used by all advanced countries are protective. But it is difficult to be unemotional about food. It arouses passions and associations as imperative as the sexual drive. This is not surprising of course. Sex may be essential to survival of the species, but food is essential to personal survival.

Recommended maximum storage times in freezers			
Meat	Months	**Prepared dishes**	Months
Beef joints	8	Bread	1
Lamb, pork and veal joints	6	Meat dishes	2
Cutlets, steaks, minced or cubed meat and sausages	3	Mousses, soufflés	2
		Pastry, uncooked	3
Poultry		Pie cases and fruit pies, cooked	6
Chicken	12	Meat pies, cooked	3
Duck, goose and turkey	6	Pizzas, uncooked	3
Giblets and livers	3	Pizzas, cooked	2
		Sauces	3
Game		Soups	3
Gamebirds	8	Stocks	3
Hare and rabbit	6		
		Vegetables	
Fish		Most vegetables require to be blanched in boiling water and can then be frozen for up to 12 months. Courgettes may be blanched or sautéed before freezing. Mushrooms need to be sautéed and can then be frozen for up to 3 months.	
Whole or filleted	6		
Fruit			
Fresh	12		
Juices	6		
Purées	8		

There are always new theories coming up about what to eat, and how you should have naturally, organically grown food instead of synthetics and so on. How can I tell which are right and wrong?

Because eating is such an emotional business, there will always be food cranks and cults. Most religions include food cults as part of their structure after all, from the Christian Mass to the Judaic laws of Kashrus and Islamic fasting. This is unlikely to change.

All that any of us can do is to use our common sense when evaluating the latest craze. For example, take the 'organically grown foods' craze, which says that all synthetic chemicals are lethal. An element in fertilizer which matters a great deal is nitrogen and this occurs not only as a by-product of soil and animal metabolism but also can be made in a factory. Nitrogen is nitrogen, whether it is made in a factory retort, or comes from a cow's anus after she has digested grass. So claims that one kind of nitrogen is better than the other seem hard to validate. Being critical of all crazes and scares will help you steer a sensible middle course.

Is it true that some people can get unpleasant symptoms such as rapid heartbeat indigestion, sickness and diarrhoea and depression from being allergic to some foods? I had heard this, but my doctor said it was all rubbish.

There is a growing body of opinion among researchers that some people are indeed allergic to common foodstuffs and develop disagreeable symptoms as a result. Some allergies are well known, of course, for example those allergies to strawberries or shellfish which bring some people who eat them out in a rash. But it is in the region of less obvious food allergies that there has been recent controversy, with many doctors 'pooh-poohing' the whole concept.

The study of food allergies has suggested that there may be a link between allergy and addiction. A food which causes the body to react unfavourably also causes it to attempt to adapt to it. First, there is an alarm response in which heartbeat and breathing rates are speeded up and the person becomes tense, may sweat, turn pale, and certainly feels ill.

Second, there is a resistance stage in which the body overcomes the alarm and the person feels better as the symptoms subside.

Third, there follows an exhaustion stage – but there is a point as the body moves from resistance to exhaustion when taking the food again can actually make the person feel better.

This is just like 'the hair of the dog' treatment which some alcoholics try; as the effect of the alcohol they first took wears off and they begin to feel ill, a little more alcohol can restore them to the resistance stage in which they feel better.

This is why there is this extra-ordinary paradox of people having an addiction to a substance that actually makes them feel ill.

Why do some people show such a wide range of symptoms to common foods? According to some researchers there may be a genetic component. They say that an inability to tolerate a certain type of food – for example, an allergy to carbohydrate – can run in a family. The researchers have found that there are people who are addicted to bread, sugar, biscuits and so on, who continue eating them even though the result is obesity. In the past it has been said that when several members of one family are obese it is because they all have bad eating habits.

Yet that same family can include people who are able to eat as much carbohydrate as they like and not get obese. These people have a different genetic pattern inherited from different forebears. This suggests that obesity could in fact be due to a carbohydrate allergy, and that people who are addicted to such foods eat them because they are allergic to them.

If they can realize how much better they feel when they banish them from the diet and give them up altogether, they lose weight – but that is a side effect. It is more important for them to be rid of the depression, the abdominal pain, the attacks of rapid heartbeat. And that is why they abandon the foods that have caused the symptoms.

Clearly, whoever coined the term 'foodaholic' for the person who goes on carbohydrate-eating binges, was more accurate than he knew. People with this sort of addiction are in just the same situation as alcoholics. And, interestingly, many experts in the field of alcoholism are coming to the conclusion that people with this problem are actually allergic to the stuff. A similar reaction – allergy linked with addiction – can be shown to caffeine. There are many people 'hooked' on coffee, tea and cola drinks who show severe symptoms which are relieved when they stop taking the caffeine.

Why has the medical profession as a whole resisted the idea that food allergies can cause illness?

The trouble is that the symptoms are so diverse – there are so many different types – and the foods which cause the problems are so varied, it is very difficult to actually prove the links. Yet there are a number of food allergies that have been definitely proved.

There are people who always get attacks of migraine headaches if they eat cheese or chocolate. There are babies who are allergic to cow's milk and many people cannot tolerate the gluten in wheat. If the latter group of people take gluten in infancy, they suffer from coeliac disease in which there is dry hair, a swollen belly and matchstick limbs and severe digestive disorder. In older people, there can be diarrhoea, weight loss and mouth ulcers. Some people are even suggesting that there may be a link between the eating of gluten and symptoms of such diverse illnesses as multiple sclerosis and schizophrenia. None of this is proved so far. Until it is, many cautious practitioners will go on dismissing the allergy theory as nonsense. And they might be right, of course.

113

Food composition chart

Meat, Fish and Poultry	Protein	Fat	Carbohydrate	Vitamins	Minerals	Fibre
Pork	H	H	L	B	calcium	L
Bacon	H	H	L	B	calcium/iron	L
Beef	H	M	L	B	calcium/iron	L
Liver	H	M	L	A B C D	iron	L
Lamb	H	H	L	B	calcium/iron	L
Veal	H	L	L	B	calcium/iron	L
Tongue	H	H	L	B	calcium/iron	L
Sausages	M	H	M		calcium/iron	L
Chicken	H	M	L	B	calcium	L
White fish (e.g. plaice)	H	L	L	B	calcium	L
Dark fish (e.g. herring)	H	H	L	B D	calcium	L
Tinned fish (e.g. sardines)	H	H	L	A B D	calcium	L
Vegetables						
Cabbage	L		L	A C	calcium/iron	H
Cauliflower	L		L	C	calcium	H
Carrots	L		M	A C	calcium	H
Potatoes	L		M	C	calcium	H
Lettuce	L		L	A C	calcium	H
Onion	L		M	C	calcium	H
Mushrooms	L					H
Pulses (e.g. peas, lentils)	M	L	M	B C	iron	H
Canned sweetcorn	L		M			H
Green peppers	L		L	C	calcium/iron	H
Fruit						
Apples, pears	L	L	M	C		H
Oranges	L	L	M	C	calcium	H
Tomatoes, strawberries	L	L	M	A C	calcium	H
Blackcurrants	L	L	M	A C	calcium/iron	H
Dried fruit (e.g. sultanas)	L		M		iron	H
Nuts	H	H	M	B C	calcium/iron	H
Canned fruit	L	L	H	traces	traces	M
Bananas	L	L	M	C		H

Food composition chart
A well-balanced diet requires a wide variety of nutrients. Check the nutritional value of the things that you like to eat in this list to find out which foods do you the most good

Key
L – low   M – medium   H – high

Dairy	Protein	Fat	Carbohydrate	Vitamins	Minerals	Fibre
Cheddar cheese	H	H	L	A D	calcium	
Cream cheese	L	H	L	A B D	calcium	
Cottage cheese	H	L	L	B	calcium	
Butter	L	H		A D	calcium	
Margarine	L	H		A D		
Milk	M	M	M	A B C D	calcium	
Cream	L	H	L	A D	calcium	
Yoghurt	M	L	M	A (trace)	calcium	
Eggs	H	M	L	A B D	calcium/iron	
Cereals						
Bread (wholemeal)	M	L	H	B	iron	H
Bread (white)	M	L	H	B	calcium/iron	M
Breakfast cereals	L	L	H	B	calcium/iron	H
Sweet biscuits	L	H	H		calcium	
Rice (brown)	L	L	H	B	traces	H
Rice (white)	L	L	H			
Pasta	M	L	H	B	calcium	L
Flour (white)	M	L	H	B	calcium/iron	M
Rusks	M	M	H	B	calcium/iron	
Oatmeal	H	M	M	B	calcium/iron	M
Miscellaneous						
Popcorn	L	H	H	traces	traces	
Chocolates	M	H	H		calcium/iron	
Boiled sweets			H			
Ice cream	L	H	H			
Crisps	L	H	H	traces	traces	
Golden syrup			H			
Jam			H			
Cocoa	L	M	H	B	iron	
Orange squash			H			
Sugar (white)			H			
Canned tomato soup	L	L	M	A	calcium	

Stomach and gut

Of the two systems which give us the most pleasure in life (the other, of course, is the reproductive) the alimentary is the larger. It runs from the mouth to the anus, is around 25 feet long when unravelled and deals with some 40 tons of food during the average lifetime. Any diseases which attack it will obviously cause its owner considerable anxiety. The science of gastro-enterology deals with such diseases and the symptoms they cause. However, gastro-enterologists usually leave the last few inches of the alimentary canal to their colleagues, the specialists in rectal diseases.

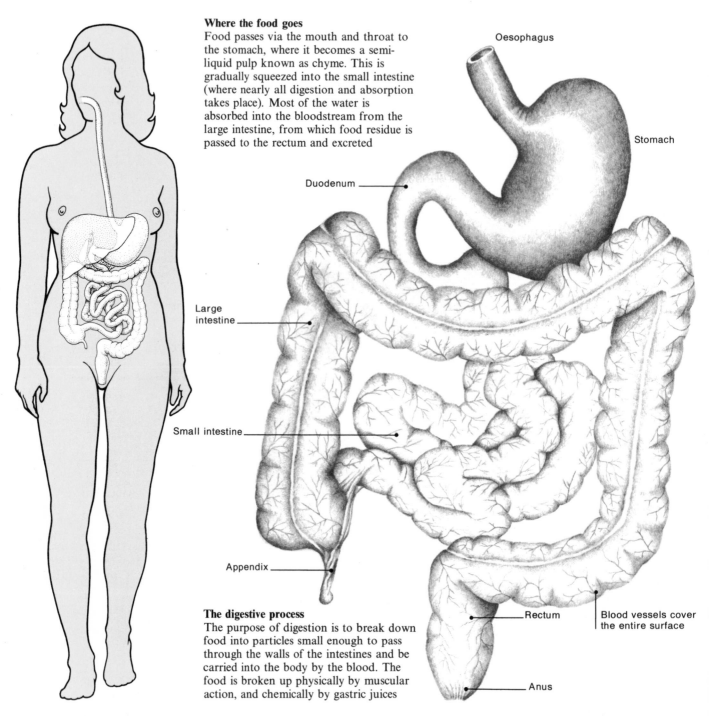

Where the food goes
Food passes via the mouth and throat to the stomach, where it becomes a semi-liquid pulp known as chyme. This is gradually squeezed into the small intestine (where nearly all digestion and absorption takes place). Most of the water is absorbed into the bloodstream from the large intestine, from which food residue is passed to the rectum and excreted

Oesophagus

Stomach

Duodenum

Large intestine

Small intestine

Appendix

Rectum

Blood vessels cover the entire surface

Anus

The digestive process
The purpose of digestion is to break down food into particles small enough to pass through the walls of the intestines and be carried into the body by the blood. The food is broken up physically by muscular action, and chemically by gastric juices

What causes indigestion?

Dyspepsia is one of the more common of the symptoms which people take to their doctors, yet often these worried people have perfectly healthy stomachs and guts.

Quite a lot of them are tense and anxious about their digestion. They seem always to be aware of what is going on inside them, especially after eating, and are rather given to belching and complaining of feelings of fullness. This sort of behaviour can run in families, and individual members will say with melancholy pride that they have inherited a weak digestion. But, in fact, this is rarely the case. It is simply that they have learned to be intense about the perfectly normal sensations they get

from their stomachs, and automatically misinterpret them as 'bad'. These same people are also likely to swallow a lot of air, and therefore to belch a lot. There are some families which do this all the time and, of course, some societies actually practise it. In parts of the Middle East enthusiastic belching is expected after a meal.

Indigestion which signals underlying disease is not so easy to identify. The range of pain complained of is wide, from gnawing sensations after eating or when the stomach is empty, to dull aching between the shoulder-blades at the back, via heartburn (the burning discomfort felt behind the breastbone) and nausea and bloating. Pain of any

kind in the epigastrium (the area just below the ribs, across the middle) may be due to a peptic ulcer, in which a section of the stomach or duodenum (upper gut) lining has been eroded, or gallstones or even an impending coronary thrombosis. People with the early symptoms of a threatened heart attack may complain of 'wind' pains because the sensations affect the same area.

People who regularly get pain in this area and who find themselves using a lot of proprietary antacid medicines should seek medical advice. Self-treatment for occasional dietary indiscretions is commonsense, but continued self-treatment, when you are not sure what it is that you are treating, is not.

The stomach digests all the food that is put in it, so why doesn't it digest itself?

The stomach does not actually digest all food. It is a staging post on the way to total digestion which starts in the mouth, where the teeth break food into pieces and some of the food constituents are taken apart by enzymes in the saliva, and it goes on for long hours in the gut, notably in the upper part of the small intestine. But of course the stomach is very important in digestion, and it does its two jobs very well. First, it churns the food up into a thick gruel-like mixture, using its powerful muscle walls to do so. Second, it mixes in powerful digestive juices, which it makes in its own lining, and which carry on the work, started by the enzymes in the saliva, of the splitting apart of the food into basic materials.

One of the digestive juices produced is hydrochloric acid, which is an extremely powerful acid – it can burn holes in planks of wood.

The reason it does not burn holes in the stomach itself is the stomach's special protective lining. It produces a thick mucus which coats the whole area and allows food to be attacked by hydrochloric acid, but keeps it away from the living stomach walls.

How the stomach works
After reducing food to a pulp, wavelike motions of the stomach pass it through to the small intestine for further digestion

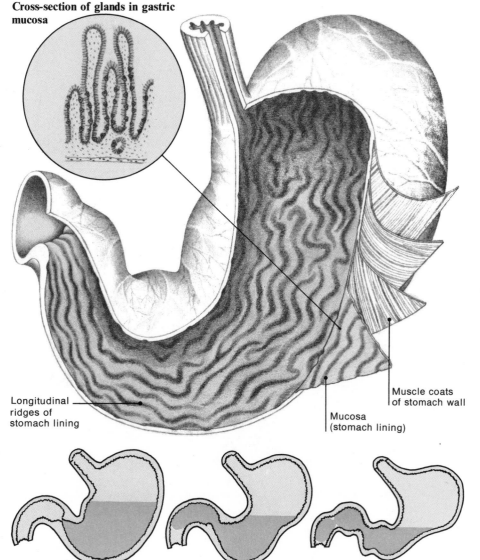

Cross-section of glands in gastric mucosa

Longitudinal ridges of stomach lining

Muscle coats of stomach wall

Mucosa (stomach lining)

Stomach and gut

Whenever I get sick, my mother says it's a liver attack. Just what is a liver attack?

The liver is the biggest and one of the most vital internal organs that we possess. It has a very large work load indeed, being intimately involved with the metabolism of all types of food; the storage of food, especially sugars, and fat and probably some proteins; the making of plasma (blood) proteins and blood-clotting substances; the making of bile – a vital digestive substance – from broken-down old red blood cells; the detoxification of poisons, and, in the unborn, the making of new red cells. This is a formidable list indeed.

With so many functions it would seem that the liver would be likely to be an organ which would go wrong, but in fact liver disorder is rather rare, although in some European countries there is a tendency to blame it for all sorts of symptoms (the French constantly complain of their livers). 'Liver attacks' are more likely to be due to mild gastro-intestinal upsets than to the liver.

Liver disorders, when they occur, do not always show themselves as periods of nausea and vomiting. A more significant symptom is jaundice – yellowing of the skin, and possibly the whites of the eyes. This happens when there is an excess of bilirubin in the blood plasma. Bilirubin is the colouring substance which is made by the liver when old red blood cells are destroyed, and it usually goes into the bile which is stored in the gall bladder, a little bag which lies just under the liver. If there is a breakdown in the liver's system for storing bile, for example a blockage in the ducts which allow the bile to get out of the gall bladder and into the gut where it is needed to digest fats, then the bilirubin can escape into the blood, and so discolour the skin and the eye whites.

Jaundice may be accompanied by dark urine, as the kidneys excrete some of the unwanted bilirubin, and very pale offensive stools, which are usually darkened and deodorized by the bile which is no longer reaching the gut. This happens in obstructive jaundice, when the liver is making its bile normally, but there is a blockage somewhere along the line liver – gall bladder – bile duct – gut.

Other forms of jaundice are due to liver infection (hepatitis), or cirrhosis (liver damage), which is often due to alcohol abuse. There is also a type of jaundice which occurs in new-born babies, but which is not at all significant or dangerous. It does not mean that the baby has a damaged liver or any blockage in its gall bladder ducts. It happens as a result of the breakdown of extra red blood cells the baby had in its prebirth life, but which it no longer requires. This sort of jaundice usually fades in a few days and need worry no mother.

People who have had attacks of hepatitis are not able to be blood donors, because the causative organisms can go on living in their blood for many years, and they may pass the disease on to a recipient. This is why doctors always check whether a blood donor has had jaundice before taking the person on the list. It is only the type of jaundice that is due to infection which excludes a potential blood donor.

Women who have had jaundice are also advised not to use the Pill because it, too, can affect the liver by causing obstruction in small branches of the bile-carrying tubes that come from the liver. Certain drugs can also have this effect. People who have jaundice are advised not to drink alcohol.

The digestive system has two complementary sets of organs. The oesophagus, stomach and intestines are directly involved in the passage of food, while the liver, pancreas, gall bladder and blood supply help to break down and absorb the food

The accessory digestive organs

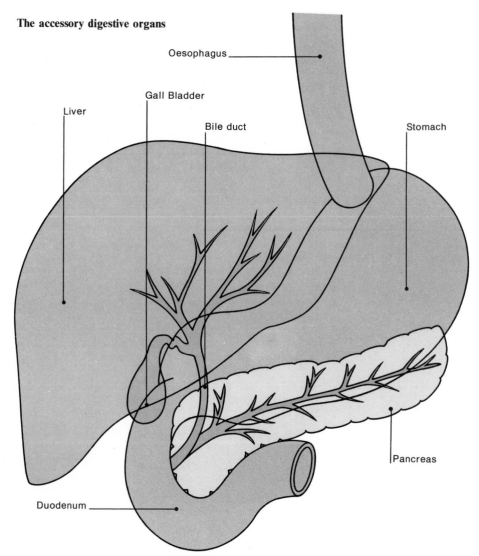

Oesophagus

Gall Bladder

Liver

Bile duct

Stomach

Pancreas

Duodenum

What are gall stones? Why do they happen?

They are not really stones as such but are hardened pebble-shaped collections of materials precipitated from the bile in the gall bladder. The commonest stones are made of cholesterol, a fatty material derived from food, notably saturated (animal) fats derived from meat, eggs and milk fats. Unsaturated fats derive from vegetables, for example, beans, corn and sunflowers.

Most gall stones are quite symptomless (one large post-mortem study showed that fully 55 per cent of women and 25 per cent of men had undetected gall stones) but sometimes they can cause pain, inflammation and jaundice as the stones block the outlet from the gall bladder. Symptoms may be obvious, such as the pain and jaundice, or less so, such as flatulence, vague nausea or some pain behind the breastbone. The trouble with these symptoms is that they can be caused by other things, such as a peptic ulcer, or 'nervous dyspepsia'. So, sometimes people are diagnosed as having gall stones when their stones are in fact silent and causing no symptoms, have an operation, and then go on having their symptoms afterwards. One study of patients who had had their gall bladders removed (cholecystectomy) showed that only half of them benefited. Today, attempts are made to use medicines which make the stones dissolve.

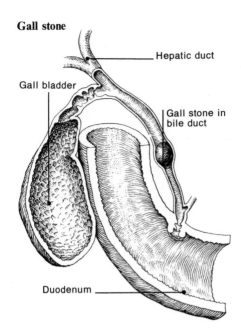

Gall stone

- Hepatic duct
- Gall bladder
- Gall stone in bile duct
- Duodenum

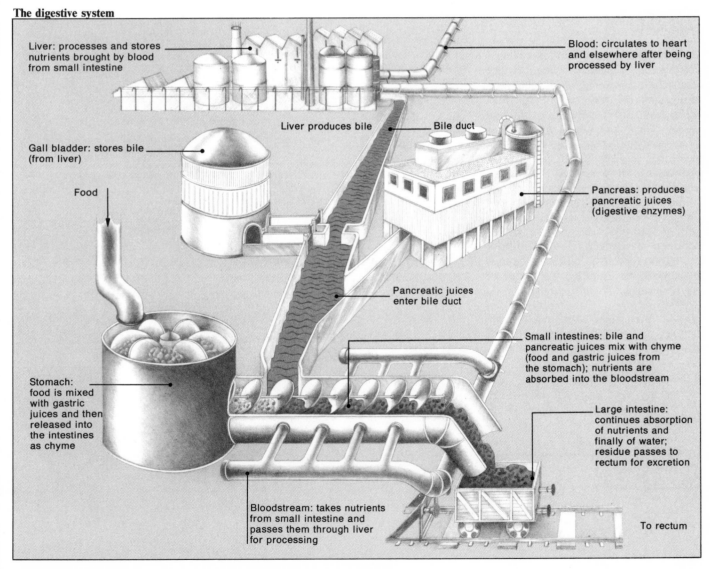

The digestive system

- Liver: processes and stores nutrients brought by blood from small intestine
- Blood: circulates to heart and elsewhere after being processed by liver
- Liver produces bile
- Bile duct
- Gall bladder: stores bile (from liver)
- Pancreas: produces pancreatic juices (digestive enzymes)
- Food
- Pancreatic juices enter bile duct
- Small intestines: bile and pancreatic juices mix with chyme (food and gastric juices from the stomach); nutrients are absorbed into the bloodstream
- Stomach: food is mixed with gastric juices and then released into the intestines as chyme
- Large intestine: continues absorption of nutrients and finally of water; residue passes to rectum for excretion
- Bloodstream: takes nutrients from small intestine and passes them through liver for processing
- To rectum

Stomach and gut

My doctor said I had a hiatus hernia. What is that?

The word hernia means simply displacement – the protrusion of a body part into an area it should not occupy. Thus, an inguinal hernia means that a loop of gut has pushed through a weak place in the muscles of the groin; an umbilical hernia means that a loop of gut has pushed through the weakened navel area; and a hiatus, or diaphragmatic, hernia means that the upper portion of the stomach has pushed through the hiatus (or gap) in the sheet of muscle which separates the chest cavity from the abdomen.

The condition is not usually permanent; that is, the herniated stomach moves up and down. When a person is upright and has not eaten, the stomach will probably lie below the diaphragm. When he has eaten and is lying down, it will slide up. The problem tends to be most common after middle age, in overweight people (the extra fat inside the abdomen exerts an upwards pressure on the stomach) and in women who have had several pregnancies.

The symptoms vary. In some people there are none at all. They only discover they have a hiatus hernia following an abdominal X-ray for other reasons. In others there is breathlessness, rapid heartbeat after eating, difficulty in swallowing and 'heartburn' – burning pain behind the breastbone. Some people have pain behind that radiates up into the jaw and left shoulder and arm, so mimicking the pain of heart disorder. There may be frequent regurgitation into the mouth of stomach contents. Some people have one or two of these symptoms, others have all of them.

Treatment is at first conservative – the patient is advised to lose weight if necessary, and to eat a little at a time. An overloaded stomach is more likely to herniate. Also, sleeping semi-upright helps to prevent breathlessness, pain and regurgitation. In a few cases if the symptoms persist despite medical treatment, surgery can prevent the stomach from migrating upwards.

Why does my belly rumble sometimes?

Stomach and gut are both exceedingly active pieces of digestive apparatus. The stomach churns food, the gut squeezes it along, and the result of all this busy activity is to produce slurping, rumbling noises. These happen all the time, as listening over the belly with a stethoscope will show you, but usually you cannot hear them without that sort of amplification. However, sometimes the sound is extra loud, for example when there is a great deal of air in the stomach, perhaps because of air swallowing (a common nervous habit) or because there is no food in it. Then the sound is clearly audible. A rather elegant name for the sound is borborygmus.

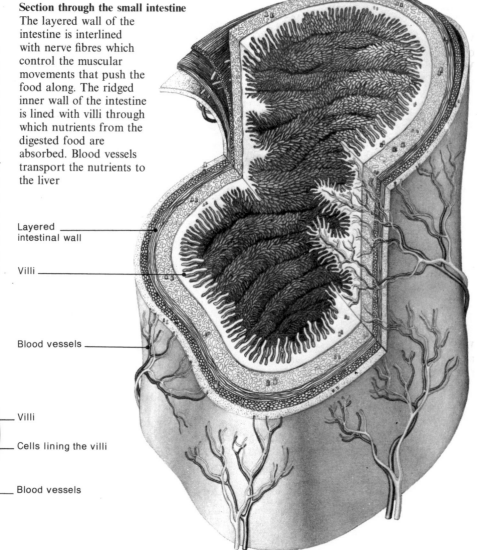

Section through the small intestine
The layered wall of the intestine is interlined with nerve fibres which control the muscular movements that push the food along. The ridged inner wall of the intestine is lined with villi through which nutrients from the digested food are absorbed. Blood vessels transport the nutrients to the liver

Layered intestinal wall

Villi

Blood vessels

Section through the villi

Villi

Cells lining the villi

Blood vessels

What actually happens when you vomit? And why do children do it much more than adults?

In very simple terms the stomach works backwards, pushing its contents up towards the gullet, instead of down towards the gut. But it is rather more complex than that.

There is a 'vomiting centre' in the brain that can be triggered to set off the complex muscular movements which are involved – the muscles of the belly wall, the diaphragm and the stomach itself interact to make it possible for the stomach contents to be forced upwards and outwards. The vomiting centre can be triggered by a number of things – the presence of dangerous poisons in the blood, irritants in the stomach itself, fever and general illness due to a number of different causes (as in sea-sickness), or even, it has been found, by a direct effort of will. Some children learn how to induce vomiting deliberately, and it is a most useful little trick if you don't want to attend a particular school lesson or follow a particular adult wish. Vomiting is the sort of spectacular symptom which everyone takes seriously.

It tends to be more significant in adults than in children who do seem to vomit more easily. Even a simple cold can be enough to make a baby vomit, and just a mild fever can make an older child throw up. Many children have travel-sickness, too, seeming to find their balance disturbed more easily than an adult's.

In the vast majority of cases children outgrow the vomiting tendency before they reach puberty, and thereafter show an adult pattern, in which the symptom should be taken seriously, unless there are obvious causes, like drinking or eating too much.

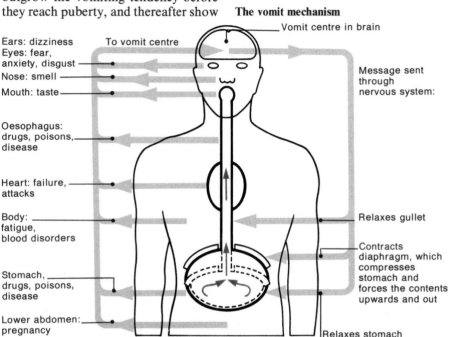

The vomit mechanism

Vomit centre in brain

Message sent through nervous system:

Ears: dizziness
Eyes: fear, anxiety, disgust
Nose: smell
Mouth: taste
To vomit centre

Oesophagus: drugs, poisons, disease

Heart: failure, attacks

Body: fatigue, blood disorders

Stomach, drugs, poisons, disease

Lower abdomen: pregnancy

Relaxes gullet

Contracts diaphragm, which compresses stomach and forces the contents upwards and out

Relaxes stomach

Why can some people eat with pleasure something that makes others really sick – like high game, or sheep's eyes?

Taste in food is infinitely variable, depending far less on the messages sent to the brain by the buds on the tongue and the smell receptors in the nose, than on training and experience.

These, of course, are governed by what happens in childhood. A baby can accept any food of any taste, and learn to like it. Even if he rejects a new flavour when it is first presented to him, if adults persist in giving it he will learn to like it. Also, he will pick up food flavours from his mother's milk, and food scents from his environment, and learn to associate those with the good feeling of being full after feeding, and so come to like them. Thus, an Indian child whose mother eats spicy curries will be 'primed' to enjoy curry in his turn, and the child of a garlic-eating family will take to garlic-laden food with glee, while children

reared on a bland, less aromatic diet will refuse such foods with sheer revulsion when they are offered. Such a child may do more than refuse – he may trigger his vomiting centre and retch and actually vomit when introduced to foods that are totally foreign to him.

Much of our attitude to what is wholesome and edible depends on colour and texture. Most people presented with meat that has been dyed bright blue would reject it as inedible, even if the dye used was totally harmless. Similarly, slippery food is likely to create revulsion in people unused to it, while crisp food seems to attract almost everyone.

The source of food matters a great deal, too, because we have vivid imaginations. If you tell a person that a piece of meat which he might have swallowed

happily if he were ignorant of its source is actually a sheep's eye or a bull's testicle, he is very likely to gag, no matter how foolish that would be. An eye is made of similar materials to a steak, and if you are willing to eat a hen's egg or drink a cow's milk, why be disturbed by bull's testicles? But that is the effect, unless hunger supervenes, and then we will eat anything. In Paris, during a siege, people ate rats and cats and were glad to get them, and after a plane crash in the Andes those who survived ate those who did not.

There are also, of course, religious rules about food which profoundly affect appetite. Devout Jews may be sickened at the thought of pig meat and practising Hindus are revolted by the idea of beef. Yet there is nothing inherently sickening in these foods.

Rectum and anus

The rectum is the last few inches of the alimentary system, and is really little more than a containing area for waste food and the other products of digestion. But we all tend to give the rectum a great deal of attention, worrying about its activities – or more especially any lack of activity – perhaps more than we need. Some rectal disorders which need surgery are dealt with by general surgeons, and are dealt with very well; but there are some surgeons who only look after diseases afflicting the rectum.

The rectum

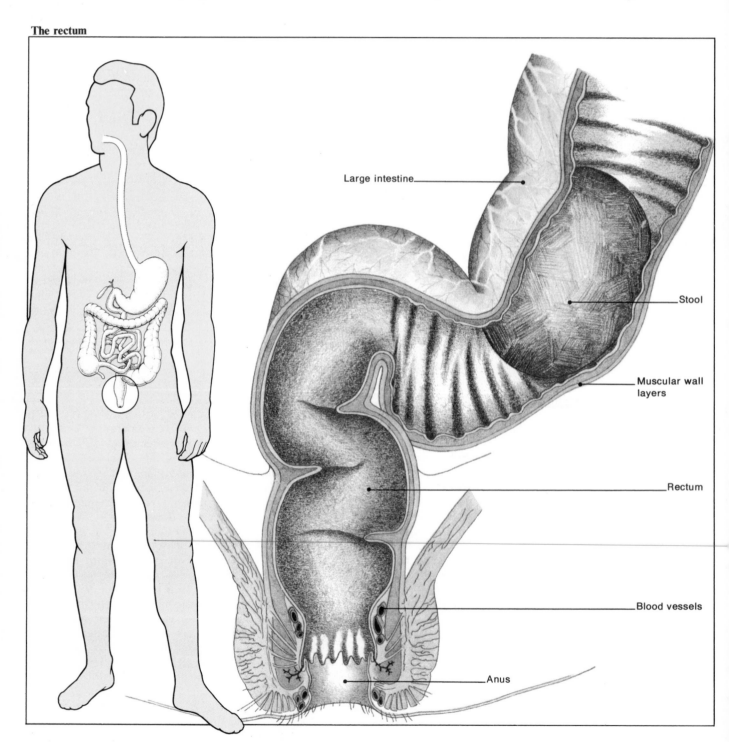

Large intestine

Stool

Muscular wall layers

Rectum

Blood vessels

Anus

What causes constipation? Why is it so bad for you?

The idea that constipation is a dread disease that leads to everything from pimples to imminent demise was invented by 19th-century purveyors of laxatives. In fact, it is not a disease at all, and rarely all that important. It does not cause bellyache, bad breath, furred tongue, headache, depression or spots. If you have these problems, they have other causes.

The word constipation means simply 'delay in the passage of a stool', but it tends to be interpreted in many different ways. There are some people who will say they are constipated if they do not have a bowel action every day at the same time; others who reckon they are constipated if they feel a bit off colour even if they are having their usual bowel actions; others who think they are constipated unless their stools pass without their making any expulsive effort.

None of these is accurate. True constipation can only be diagnosed in the context of what is normal for an individual. Surveys have shown that the range of normal is extremely wide, varying from two or three bowel actions a week, to three a day. As long as a person is healthy and functioning normally in every other way, then whatever is normal for him is normal.

Diet obviously plays a part. Stools are made up of undigested food waste (the so-called fibre derived from cell walls of plants and some protein foods – wheat leaves some indigestible fibre behind, though not as much as vegetables and other grains); dead bacteria, which account for a third to half of the total dry matter; secretions from the intestine and, of course, water.

The amount of stool produced depends largely on how much fibre is eaten. A rich vegetable diet is said to produce about 13 ounces a day and a starvation regime, during which stools still go on being produced, less than an ounce. Children tend to produce more than adults, weight for weight.

But it isn't only volume that matters; texture comes into it. This is governed by the water content. During digestion, water is constantly being extracted from the material inside the gut, and passed back into the body's general supply. It takes four to six hours for the food that enters your stomach to be pushed out into the small intestine, in a highly liquid state. It spends five hours in the small intestine, still very moist, and up to 24 hours in the large gut, where it becomes progressively drier. The longer it spends in the large gut, the more it is going to dry out, and hard dry feces can be painful to pass. People who have them tend to try to hold on to them longer, because it is so uncomfortable to pass them, and this makes them drier and harder than ever. These people can truly be said to be constipated. Their only symptom, however, is pain at passing stools.

In a few cases – few, that is, compared with the number of people who complain of the problem – constipation is an indication of significant disorder. There may be a blockage of the gut, due to a growth, either benign of malignant, or kinking of the tube (this may sometimes happen in small children under one year and is called intussusception) but both of these will be signalled by other symptoms, apart from constipation. There may be blood in the stools in the case of a growth (black and sticky stools if there is bleeding high in the gut, brighter red when it comes from lower down) and a baby with intussusception will be obviously ill and in pain as well as possibly having a distended belly.

In some general illnesses, such as disease affecting the central nervous system, or hypothyroidism (myxedema) true constipation may be one symptom among many. It may also be present in certain psychiatric illnesses; severely depressed people, for example, are often constipated. It seems that the entire body as well as the mind is 'flattened' and slow.

There is also a fairly rare disease, with which some babies are born, called Hirschsprung's disease (or megacolon) in which there is severe constipation. But it is rare and rapidly diagnosed in early infancy.

So, generally speaking, constipation is a symptom which does not deserve the years of attention it has had, nor the vast sums of money spent on dealing with it.

My elderly father who had diarrhoea was told by his doctor that the real problem was constipation! How could that be?

Sometimes a mass of feces can become impacted in the rectum, possibly because of a narrowing of the gut at that point, caused by a blockage of some sort, perhaps due to a tumour (which is not necessarily malignant). What then happens is that there is an 'overflow': feces continue to arrive in the gut, behind the impacted mass, as food is put into the stomach, but can get no further. Because it is still liquid the feces can to a certain extent seep past the blockage. So, some forms of diarrhoea can in fact be due to constipation.

Once your father's doctor has diagnosed the cause of his constipation and has dealt with that, the diarrhoea will cease, too.

Can constipation lead to general illness?

No. Anxiety about it can make some people feel ill. But otherwise the symptom itself can do no harm.

However, if it is due to an underlying illness, that is different. The illness can get worse, but that is not because of constipation: the constipation is because of the illness.

Rectum and anus

Why do doctors nowadays say that laxatives are bad for you, when at one time they used to recommend them frequently?

Doctors were once as affected by anxiety about constipation as less well-informed individuals. They, too, fostered the erroneous belief that stools inside the body were 'poisonous' and 'dirty' and must be expelled as fast as possible. It could be that they were as unaware as their patients of the underlying sexual significance of the anxiety about constipation, certainly before Freud and his followers arrived to explain our hidden drives to us. So doctors prescribed appalling concoctions of jalap (from which we get the slang term 'jollop' for any foul-tasting medicine), castor oil, Epsom salts and other disagreeable materials which caused painful and extremely enthusiastic purgation.

These were in time replaced by so-called 'gentle' aperients such as senna infusions, vegetable laxatives such as cascara, liquid paraffin and magnesium mixtures (like Epsom salts but less violent).

But these were in their effects no better than the old-fashioned blunderbuss methods. They all do the same thing; they force the gut to expel its contents by unnaturally hurrying the gut action. This means that the bowel is thrown out of its normal synchrony. The stool that was meant to be produced tomorrow, as a result of laxatives appears today; which means when tomorrow comes there is no stool, and the anxious 'I-must-go-every-day' type resorts to another dose, and prolongs the problem to the next day. And then the next day the same thing happens, and so it goes on until the bowel is stunned by the constant application of the medicines, and can't operate without them.

This is how otherwise healthy people get 'hooked' on aperients, and are convinced they have the disease of constipation.

Children above all should never be given these medicines: they will make them ill, in the long run. Nor should people with bellyaches ever be given aperients. Normal digestion is painless, and even a grossly distended rectum full of feces rarely causes pain. Giving a laxative may cause more illness than it relieves if, for example, the pain is due to an infection such as appendicitis. The laxative will make the gut more active, increase the pain and possibly cause the appendix to rupture and so cause peritonitis – a widespread infection of the abdomen which is a life-threatening condition.

Movement through the intestine

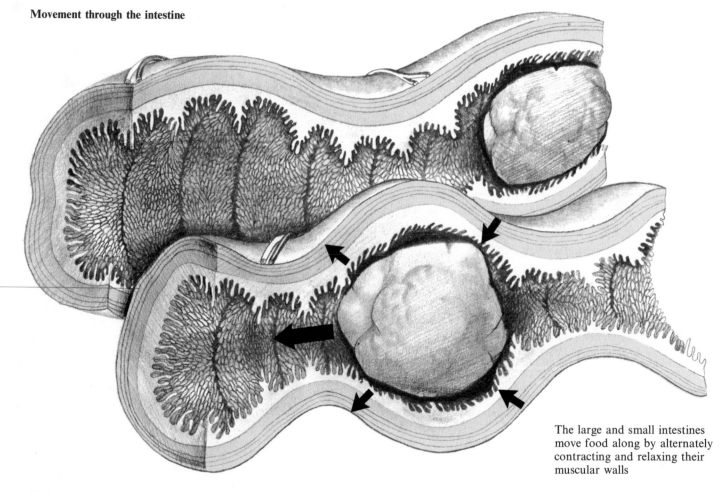

The large and small intestines move food along by alternately contracting and relaxing their muscular walls

Why is it said to be best to eat food with a lot of fibre in it?

Doctors now know that the only way to deal with the all-too-common self-induced (or doctor-induced) constipation resulting from laxatives is to withdraw all aperient medicines and start on a diet rich in fibre – raw fruits and vegetables, wholemeal bread, added bran if it is liked, and ample fluids.

This regime will, within three weeks (during which there may be some discomfort due to extra wind and slight distension, as the gut learns to regain its old self-control) lead to a comfortable regular stool and no need ever again for laxatives.

This is because fibre, being indigestible, passes through the digestive process and creates a bulky soft stool which holds water. It is easy to pass and being large, demands frequent bowel opening which gives considerable psychological comfort to those who, despite reassurance to the contrary, cannot lose the belief that a daily evacuation is vital to health and comfort.

That a high fibre diet ensures large, frequent, soft stools is beyond doubt. Less certain are some of the other claims made for a high fibre diet.

For example: one, that it reduces weight both by preventing a too-high calorie intake (you feel so full of fibre you can't overeat other foods) and by carrying more fats out of the body, before they can be absorbed into the tissues; two, that it reduces heart attack incidence because it carries out the fats that are said to contribute to heart attack; three, that it prevents malignant disease of the gut which some (and only some) theorists think may be linked with stasis of gut contents; four, that it limits the likelihood of appendicitis which is said to be due to back-pressure from a gut struggling to excrete small quantities of hard stool; five, that it prevents diverticulosis, a painful condition in which small 'pockets' form in the gut wall and become inflamed and cause pain and diarrhoea; six, that it reduces the risk of piles by ensuring that there is no undue pressure at the anus from hard stools; seven, that it prevents the formation of fissure-in-ano, again by creating stools that are easy to pass.

That is a considerable list, of which the last two claims seem to be indisputable, while the others (except perhaps for the weight-loss one which makes a lot of sense) remain in the realms of conjecture at present.

However, the evidence overall is that a fibre-rich diet can do no harm and may well do good, so it is worth following. It has the added virtue of being an ecologically sound regime. To rear enough animals to satisfy the typical Western appetite with its preponderance of animal protein and fat, much land and agricultural effort is needed. To raise vegetables and beans instead, is cheaper and simpler.

Is it true that swallowing cherry pits can cause appendicitis?

No. This idea arose because in the early days of this operation surgeons discovered little hard pits that looked like cherry pits inside the swollen appendices which they had removed. They jumped to the conclusion that that was precisely what the pits were. In fact, they were fecoliths – small, stone-hard bits of feces that had got trapped there because the appendix is a dead end. What usually happens when pits from fruit are swallowed is simple excretion at the anus.

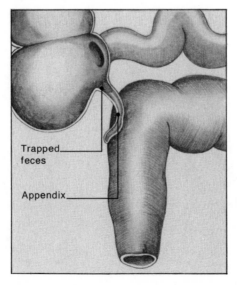

Trapped feces

Appendix

I pass a lot of wind and it's very embarrassing.
What can I do to prevent it?

The amount of gases entering or forming in the large bowel each day is between seven and 10 litres. Some of it comes from swallowed air; we all take in a great deal with our food, as well as swallowing a lot of air if we are tense or nervous. Much of this is disposed of by burping, but some is passed on from the stomach to the small intestine and so on to the large one.

Some of the gas comes from chemical changes as food is digested, and this has been analyzed and shown to consist of mostly nitrogen (59 per cent), some hydrogen (21 per cent) and the rest carbon dioxide, methane and oxygen with occasionally a little hydrogen sulphide.

Usually most of that seven to 10 litres of gas is re-absorbed into the body as the stools make their slow progress to the anus – the emptying point – so that only half a litre or so is actually expelled, and most of that at the same time as stools. But some people have active large intestines which hurry the gas along to the anus and they are the ones who suffer from a 'wind problem'.

Sometimes intestinal gas is due to anxiety. Fear tends always to cause speeding up of the gut and anxiety is low grade fear. Learning to relax and cope with life more calmly can cure the problem.

Sometimes the fault is dietary. A diet very rich in meat and fats is likely to produce extra intestinal gas and a change to less of such foods can reduce the volume. A high fibre diet, for the first few weeks after switching to it, can also cause extra gas; but most people find that this settles down as the gut becomes accustomed to its new food. However, some people always find that certain forms of vegetable protein, such as the infamous bean, create extra wind in them. It doesn't happen to everyone however; some people can eat masses of beans and suffer no problem.

If learning to relax and changing diet are no use, taking charcoal might help. Charcoal can absorb gases; it is available as biscuits.

Rectum and anus

I have been told by my doctor that I have piles. What exactly are they?

Blood should follow a one-way route, being pushed along the vein by each heart pulsation that reaches it through the blood vessel network, and prevented from being sucked back between pulses by valves. Usually the blood does this, but varicose veins may arise where there is just too much back pressure for the valves to cope with. They fail, the vein bulges outwards in lumps, and the blood flow is impeded.

This happens commonly in the legs, where the veins have to work extra hard to do their job against gravity (the blood has to be pushed a long way up to reach the heart from these lower ex-tremities) and at the opening of the anus. It can happen elsewhere in the body, though fairly rarely.

There are two kinds of haemorrhoid, which is their proper name. One arises in the part of the anal canal covered by skin; these are called external piles. Then there are those which occur in the part of the canal which is covered with mucous membrane, and these are called internal piles.

They tend to be fairly painless, though they may irritate when a hard stool is passed, and there may be some aching. Really sharp pain in the anus usually has other causes, including fissure.

However, piles are distressing because of the itching and also because they tend to break down and bleed from time to time. A good deal of blood can be lost over a long period from this source, and the result can be an anaemia that leaves a person tired, breathless, low in spirits and generally 'run down'.

So treatment should always be sought, not least because bleeding from the anus may be due not to piles but to a treatable cancer of the rectum. Too often people have gone on tolerating self diagnosed 'piles' long after they should, and a curable rectal cancer has been missed until it is too late.

My mother told me I'd get piles from sitting on hot radiators, or on cold concrete. Is this true?

The cause of piles is not fully understood, any more than the cause of varicose veins. There seems to be an inherited tendency to varicosity – if a parent had varicose veins and/or piles you are a likely candidate. Pregnancy definitely seems to contribute, possibly because of the rise in intra-abdominal pressure from the developing weighty uterus, and possibly because of hormone action on the muscular walls of the blood vessels. Also, it is thought that overweight people are more prone to the problem, because of increased pressure on the area.

The only proven cause of piles is the frequent passage of hard painful stools, which press on the area and distend the blood vessels. A high fibre diet is likely to prevent this.

There is no evidence that local heat or cold have any effect.

I have to go into hospital soon to have a fissure operation. What is a fissure and what is the operation?

In simple terms, a fissure is a crack which when it occurs in the anus, for reasons no one fully understands, will not heal. It sometimes causes appalling pain on bowel movements, sharp at the time the stool is passed, and heavy aching for long periods afterwards.

No one knows why they happen, though the most likely cause is the

Piles

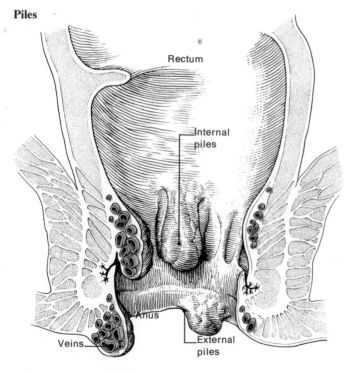

Rectum

Internal piles

Anus

Veins

External piles

Fissures

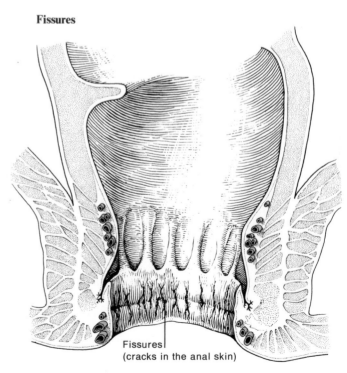

Fissures (cracks in the anal skin)

Are the different colours of stools significant?

Obviously what you eat will to an extent determine the colour of what you excrete. A diet rich in carrots can produce stools glowing like a sunset, and an excess of beets can have an almost alarming effect. Most people, however, will not be worried by such colours when they recall what they have eaten in the previous 24 hours.

More significant are marked changes from the norm unconnected with diet. A range of browns from pale to very dark is average, and depends on the bile content of the stool. Bile, which is made in the liver from breakdown products of red blood cells, both deodorizes and colours the stools. If there is a shortage of bile, due perhaps to obstruction of the bile duct, which carries bile from the storage sac (the gall bladder) or if there is disorder of the liver resulting in low bile production, the result is a pale, foul-smelling stool. If there is excess bile then the result is a very dark stool. So, changes like this, especially if associated with other symptoms such as a feeling of general ill health, nausea and vomiting and changes in skin colour, especially yellowing (jaundice), need medical attention.

A black tarry stool should also be treated as significant, unless you are taking an iron supplement by mouth. This medicine colours the stool jet black. Otherwise, the colour can be due to the presence of digested blood, and that means there is blood loss somewhere high in the digestive tract that deserves attention.

Babies' stools vary in colour and may alarm their mothers, but this variation is rarely important. But a greenish, frothy, offensive stool in a fretful baby could be due to gastro-enteritis and needs swift medical care, especially in a bottle-fed baby. Greenish stools in an otherwise well baby could be due to hunger; a little more milk could remedy this.

---

passage of small hard stools. The trouble is that this tends to be a self-perpetuating problem; because it hurts to pass the stool, the sufferer holds on, the stools get harder and drier and eventually when they are passed they make the fissure worse.

Most people see their doctors about their fissures complaining of 'a painful attack of piles' but, in fact, uncomplicated piles do not hurt (they just itch and occasionally ache mildly) so this complaint should alert any doctor to the possibility of a fissure.

In a fairly new case of fissuring – and some people go on for years with one, failing to see their doctors about it when it first starts – it may be possible to manage a cure with the use of a high fibre diet to soften the stool and a local anaesthetic cream to relieve the discomfort while healing takes place. More usually, however, surgery is needed to open out the afflicted area and give it a chance to heal properly.

If there are haemorrhoids present, the surgeon will usually deal with them at the same time.

Many people think that such an operation is very painful to recover from, but, in fact, the fissure is much more painful, and most people who have surgery for it report blissful comfort afterwards.

Why do the smells of wind – and stools, of course – vary so much?

Diet is all important. Stools and gases smell most pungent with a high meat and fat diet, because excess hydrogen sulphide seems to be made (this is the classic 'rotten eggs' smell). A vegetable diet is less odorous, unless it contains a great deal of vegetable protein, and a milk diet, despite its comparatively high fat content, smells least of all.

Babies' stools also vary in odour depending on their diet. A breast-fed baby produces small stools and they smell quite pleasant. Once babies are put on solid foods their stools smell more.

Why do doctors use such a disagreeable treatment as an enema? Is it really necessary these days?

In the bad old days when doctors and patients shared the same delusions about the importance of constipation, *enemata* were a common feature of a doctor's treatment. They were used to empty a reluctant bowel, by pouring in irritant material from outside. Soap and water was a popular choice.

Now, if it is felt necessary to empty a bowel in this mechanical way, it is simpler to use a much less uncomfortable procedure, a suppository. This is a small pledget of material which can be eased into the rectum through the anus by the patient. The best kind to ensure a bowel action is glycerine which softens the stool, and also attracts water from nearby tissues, so bulking up the stool, and making it easier to pass.

The reasons for giving enemas or suppositories to empty the bowels these days are few. They may be used for very old people who have developed impacted feces because their guts are just not working as they should; they may be used for a baby who needs similar help; they are used before abdominal surgery, to ensure as comfortable an operating area as possible (a full rectum occupies a lot of abdominal space and is awkward for a surgeon to manipulate), and before childbirth, because the expulsive efforts the mother makes to push out her baby will also push out the contents of her rectum. That not only gets in the way; it is dispiriting for the mother who would rather maintain as much dignity as she can.

Genitals, kidneys and bladder

Because the reproductive system and the urinary system – kidneys, bladder and associated tubes – are so intimately involved with each other, even though they have two quite separate functions, it is inevitable that doctors who specialize in the care of one of them tend to specialize in the care of the other. This is particularly the case for men; a woman's reproductive system is so complex that there is a special group of doctors who look after it. So a man who is having problems with passing water or with his sexual organs will be sent to see a genito-urinary specialist. A woman who is having bladder problems may be sent to him, too, or possibly to a gynaecologist. These specialities, like so many others in the field of medicine, overlap a good deal.

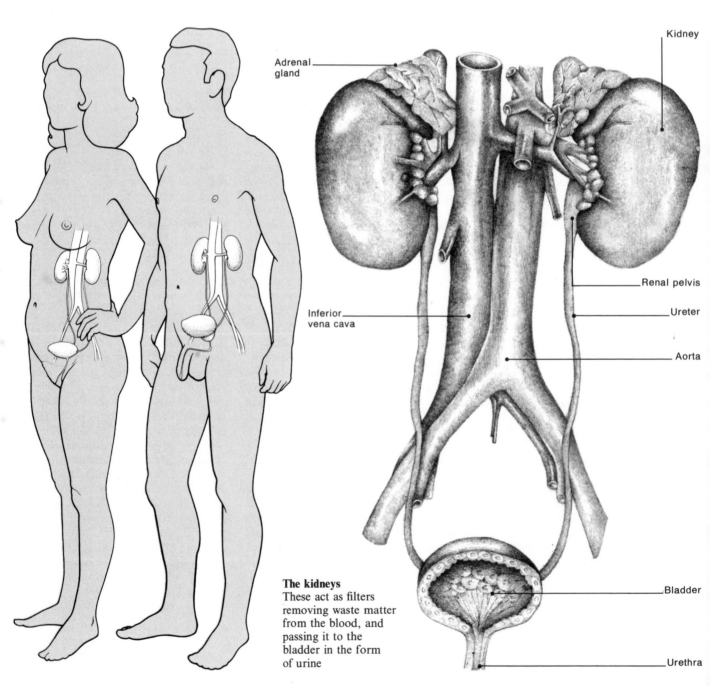

Adrenal gland

Kidney

Renal pelvis

Inferior vena cava

Ureter

Aorta

Bladder

Urethra

The kidneys
These act as filters removing waste matter from the blood, and passing it to the bladder in the form of urine

Why is my urine so different in colour sometimes? In the morning it's very dark, but during the day it is quite pale.

Urine is not a constant substance; its contents vary considerably from time to time. It depends on what you have been eating, on what you have been drinking and how your body has been functioning. There will be times when you use up more water than usual (for example, if you have a fever and have been sweating heavily) and then there is less water to dispose of. So, your urine will be dark because it is concentrated. It is often dark and concentrated in the morning because the kidneys produce less urine at night. If you have been drinking a great deal more fluid than usual, then your urine will be more pale because it is more dilute.

I've always understood that all the body's vital functions went on all the time, waking or sleeping. Yet at night I can go 12 hours without emptying my bladder, but during the day I have to several times.

It is true that organs such as the brain, kidneys and heart function continuously, but they do so at different rates of output. A sleeping heartbeat, for example, is much slower and less forceful than the beat in an awake and active person. Similarly, the kidneys respond to the overall level of body activity. When the heart is beating harder and faster because of busy muscle activity, then the blood moves more rapidly through the kidneys, and they work more busily, too, and produce more urine.

There is also the effect of digestion. Taking in food and drink triggers the body to more rapid metabolism so this also affects daytime kidney activity.

The bladder is involved as well. The bladder is a very distensible organ and can hold much more urine than we usually require it to do, during the day. As we move busily about we are more likely to trigger the bladder-emptying reflex (this is why it is uncomfortable to travel on a bumpy bus with a half full bladder – you keep wanting to empty it, even though you could hold on much longer if you were in a more serene situation). At night the bladder is left in peace to hold more.

And, of course, training comes into it. We train ourselves from an early age not to empty the bladder during sleep, although we do so in infancy with happy abandon.

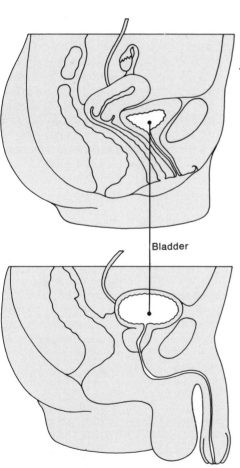

There is little difference in capacity between the male and female bladders. Both are muscular containers which can stretch to accommodate urine

Why is it harder for men to control their bladders than women? It obviously is, because there are so many more public lavatories for men, and anyway, everyone knows women can hold on longer.

What everyone knows is what everyone expects, rather than what is actual fact. There is no difference between male and female bladder capacity. Both are capable of holding roughly the same amount of urine for roughly the same amount of time. However, there are two reasons why women are thought to be more continent.

One is the fact that traditionally men have drunk much more alcohol than women. This is becoming less and less true in Western societies, but there are still areas of the world where men take alcohol and women never or rarely do. So, men needed to urinate more often than women because of the effect of the alcohol they had imbibed *(see the next question)*.

A second point is that the connection between the sex organs and the excretory organs has always meant more to women than to men. For a modest woman with any pretensions to respectability to admit that she had any sex organs at all was unthinkable in the polite society of a century or so ago; so she also could not admit that she had any lavatory needs. She taught herself to control her bladder for as long as she could in public places, because of the 'shame' of admitting that she actually possessed such an organ. Hence, no public lavatories for women.

Also, it was much easier to provide lavatory accommodation for men – they need little more than somewhere to stand and aim. Women, with their different arrangements, need room to squat which, in times when women wore large flowing skirts, demanded a great deal of expensive space. Hence, again, the lack of public lavatories for women, and the female need to learn control.

Interestingly enough, women did find an answer to their needs in Victorian and Edwardian times. It was considered vulgar then to wear drawers – polite women wore chemises and petticoats under their spreading skirts but the genital area was unencumbered. So, when women went strolling in parks and gardens, all they had to do when their bladders insisted on attention was to stand somewhere soft – on grass or earth – straddle their legs and quietly go ahead. Then, in due course, they strolled away, leaving little evidence behind them. (Havelock Ellis, the writer on sexual matters, in one of his books described such an episode with his mother.)

Genitals, kidneys and bladder

*If I take an alcoholic drink I need to pass urine much more often than usual,
but I produce much more than can be accounted for by the amount
I have drunk. If I drank pints and pints I'd understand it,
but why does this happen after just a few ounces of whisky?*

Alcohol is a poison. The body doesn't really like it, and that is why we get the responses that we do – the giddiness, the loss of balance, the loss of control of certain intellectual functions. We like some of these effects – that's why we drink alcohol. But there are other effects we usually do not like quite so much. Alcohol stimulates the heart to beat faster, dilates blood vessels – hence the reddening of the face that some drinkers get – and stimulates the kidneys. It acts as a diuretic – it makes the kidneys make more urine to the extent of removing from the body water that it actually needs. That is why we get hangovers – we become dehydrated – and the result is dryness of the mouth and headache as the water-depleted brain cells complain. (This dehydration is made worse if the amount of alcohol was enough to make the stomach protest and cause vomiting.)

So, the reason for the large quantities of pale dilute urine you produce when you drink alcohol should be obvious – as should be the way to prevent the more unpleasant effects of a hangover. Drink a great deal of extra water after or during drinking alcohol.

Why do some children learn bladder control so much faster than others?

Some of the differences are constitutional, some are due to learned behaviour.

The constitutional differences are inborn – children inherit a nerve-control pattern from their parents. It is known that children with parents who themselves had a bedwetting problem are much more likely to experience the same problem.

Also there are some rare conditions in which conscious control of the bladder is faulty, some of them congenital (present at birth), others developing later because of disease. For example, people with damage to the spine may have no bladder control at all.

More common is the problem of the child who is mismanaged. A baby is incapable of exercising conscious control over his bladder much before the age of 15 to 18 months. He becomes aware of an ability to control his bowels a little earlier.

Before this age, he has a simple reflex – his bladder is full and he empties it. However, he can be triggered by other stimuli. For example, the pressure of a cold object against the skin of his buttocks may make him pass urine.

This effect has been used by a great many mothers who want to 'train' their babies to urinate into a pot from an early age. In fact they are not 'training' the child at all. They are merely training themselves to make use of a normal reflex. They may use other reflexes, too, and learn to recognize signs that a baby is about to pass urine (or a stool) perhaps from his wriggling or the change of the colour in his face. Then they run for the pot, and fondly imagine they have a 'clean' baby.

But, once the child begins to identify the sensations he receives from his bladder and realizes that he can control them at his own will, he may well rebel against his mother's control. It is more agreeable for him to use his own control. Then the mother complains bitterly that her 'clean' child is now a 'naughty' one who refuses to do what he should, and she displays anger and administers punishment.

This confuses the child, makes him begin to feel that these pleasant body sensations he has been getting are somehow wicked, and he tries in his own way to deal with the confusion. The result can be failure to develop socially acceptable lavatory habits and can create a problem which lasts well into the fourth or even fifth year, long after the child whose mother had cheerfully left it to him to choose for himself when he would exercise control has forgotten all about nappies.

Sensible non-fussing mothers, who allow their children time to develop at their own rate, may still have children who go on bedwetting at night for some time. It used to be thought that children who bedwetted always had a deep psychological problem, and much effort would be put into analyzing what had frightened them and caused the problem. However, it is now accepted that about 10 per cent of all children will be late in gaining control, however perfect their psychological care, and that boys suffer from the problem more commonly than girls. Oddly enough, statistics vary around the world; Australian and American schoolchildren are 10 times more likely to have a bedwetting problem than Swedish or British children.

Bedwetting is best treated by simple training methods aimed at giving the child a conditioned reflex. A simple device has been developed, consisting of two metal mesh pads which are placed in the bed, between the sheets. The pads are wired to a battery-operated box equipped with a light and a buzzer. If the sleeping child wets, the wire meshes make a connection, which activates the light and the buzzer and wakes the child. It has been found that this device can, in a child who wants it to work, create a conditioned reflex within a matter of a few days. The first time the child passes a plate-sized wet patch, the second a hamburger-sized one, than a penny-sized one, and finally he wakes before the buzzer and light are activated.

Prevention of bedwetting
A simple but effective kit can be used to train a child to wake when he feels the need to urinate. A pad, which is placed between the sheets, is connected to an alarm beside the bed. If the child wets the pad the moisture completes an electric circuit between the top and bottom halves of the pad, which activates the alarm. By waking the child as he begins to wet the bed, a conditioned reflex is formed, so that after a few nights he will wake when he feels the urge to urinate

Why do some people always suffer from bedwetting?

People who have never had adequate help in childhood to cope with the problem may become inaccessible to retraining in later life – these are the ones who do have an emotional problem underlying their difficulty. Tragically, these individuals may become so ashamed of their situation that they fail to seek help, deny themselves all sorts of normal activities, such as going on holiday, visiting other people's houses and so on, and become social recluses. Others seem to slip farther and farther and drop out of normal life altogether. It is known that many of the hoboes who are to be found in affluent Western societies have this problem. Yet often it is quite unnecessary for it to have become such a handicap; a great deal can be done to help this sort of in-continent person, if only to equip him with easy-care disposable bedding.

I can sleep through a thunderstorm, but the need to pass urine always wakes me. Why is it so much stronger than the effect of outside noise?

You have a deep-seated training which ensures that you wake when your bladder is full, and this is so powerful that you have no control over it. You have, however, control over other experiences; your brain can choose to ignore sounds coming in during sleep, though you do in fact hear them, and so allow you to sleep on. But the desire to empty your bladder by-passes your conscious mind, and so you wake to empty it.

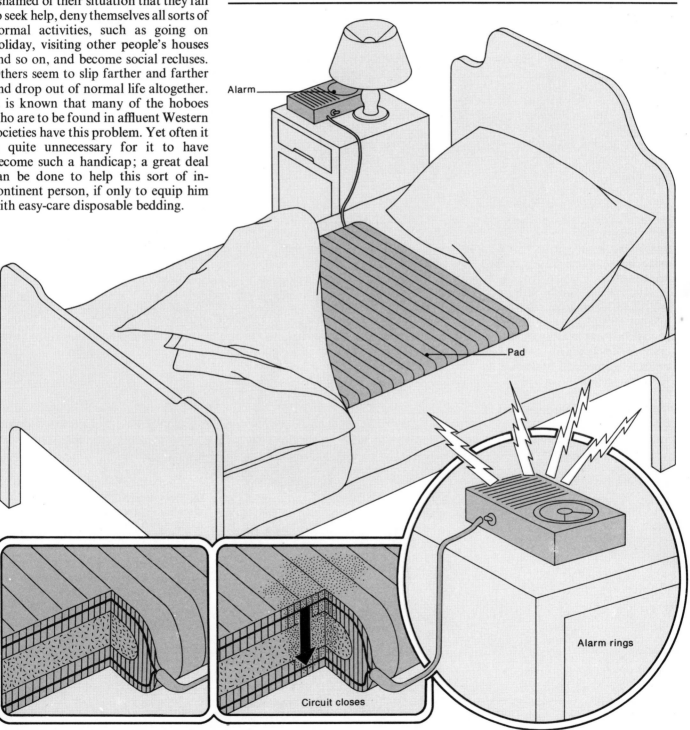

Alarm

Pad

Circuit closes

Alarm rings

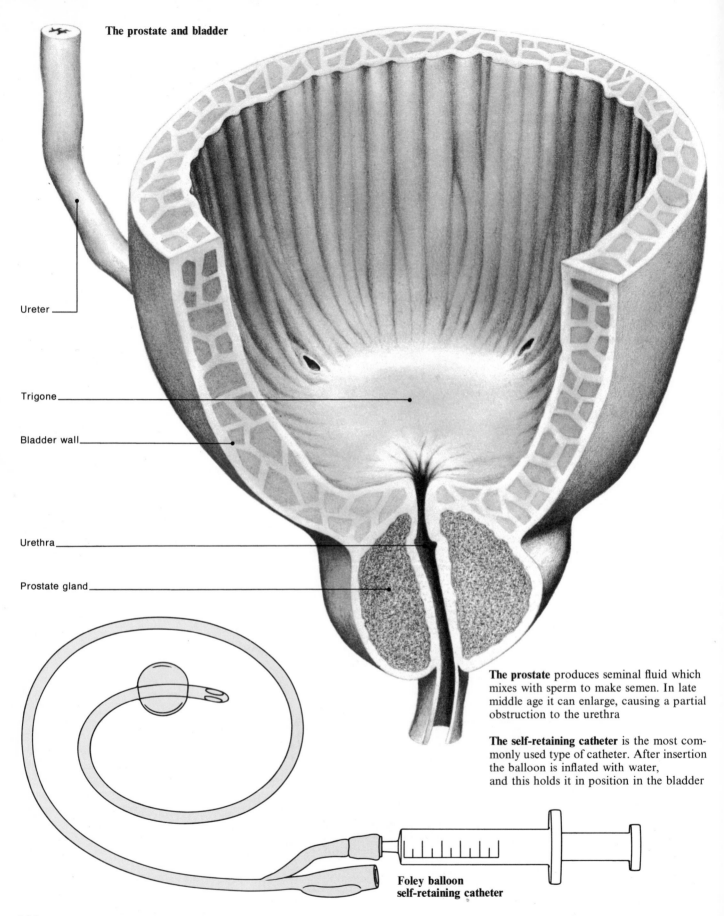

The prostate and bladder

Ureter

Trigone

Bladder wall

Urethra

Prostate gland

The prostate produces seminal fluid which mixes with sperm to make semen. In late middle age it can enlarge, causing a partial obstruction to the urethra

The self-retaining catheter is the most commonly used type of catheter. After insertion the balloon is inflated with water, and this holds it in position in the bladder

**Foley balloon
self-retaining catheter**

Why do so many men have prostate problems?

The prostate gland is one of the male sex organs. It is a little mass of gland tissue and muscular fibres surrounding the opening from the bladder. It has the job of making some of the liquid (semen) in which sperm are transported. After the age of 50 or so there is a tendency for the gland to enlarge; this physical change is the nearest a man gets to experiencing a form of mid-life climacteric – it is called the menopause in women – and is probably due to a change in his hormone balance.

Whatever the cause, it is the effect that matters. In some men, this enlargement may cause a partial obstruction in the bladder outlet, causing difficulty in passing urine. There may be delay in starting and some difficulty in emptying the bladder completely, which means that urine is left behind to stagnate and become infected. There may also be frequency problems – the man feels almost all the time that he needs to pass water because of the pressure of the gland on the bladder outlet.

If the obstruction is complete, then he can pass no urine, the bladder fills to the point of causing severe pain, and there is potentially damaging back-pressure on the kidneys. This constitutes an acute emergency, and the sufferer needs to have a catheter passed to empty his bladder at once.

The treatment is to reduce the enlarged prostate gland, and this can be done by surgery. The results of modern prostate operations are excellent and need have no effect on a man's sex life.

Does circumcision make a man more sexy?

No. It does not, as is widely believed – unless the man is determined to believe it. The power of the mind over the penis is such that deeply held beliefs act very strongly upon its reactions. But in purely physical terms, circumcision does not confer a greater sex drive. Indeed, it may have the reverse effect. If the glans is always exposed, and not only when it is erect, it may lose some of its sensitivity because it is always being stimulated by friction from clothes.

Why do some religious groups insist on circumcision?

The whole question of circumcision is bedevilled by myth. It has long been the practice among some groups to circumcise their baby boys, using an exceedingly ancient ritual. Modern adherents of the practice tend to regard it as healthy and give this as a reason for continuing it, but there seems to be little doubt that it is rooted in ancient fertility rites rather than in hygienic ones. The circumcised penis, with the glans exposed, looks like an erect and therefore potent one; probably most circumcising societies began to perform the operation on the pubescent boy in order to prove he had moved from dependent infancy to virile manhood. The shifting of the ritual to infancy in ancient Judaism may have been partly for humanitarian reasons (it hurts 13-year-olds more than it seems to hurt infants) and also to make clear that the Jews were different.

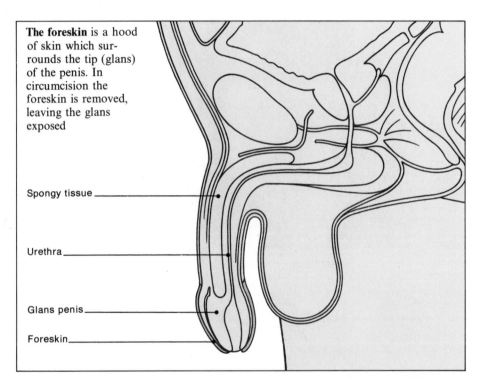

The foreskin is a hood of skin which surrounds the tip (glans) of the penis. In circumcision the foreskin is removed, leaving the glans exposed

Spongy tissue

Urethra

Glans penis

Foreskin

Why is circumcision healthier for men?

There is no hard evidence that it is. The penis is born equipped with a hood of loose skin, the prepuce, or foreskin, which has the function of protecting the sensitive *glans penis*, the acorn-shaped cap at the tip of the organ. In the infant, it is fairly closely fixed and cannot easily be slipped back. But as the child grows so does the foreskin and in time this can easily be moved back along the shaft of the penis. Then it is possible to wash away the thick whitish material, called smegma, that is secreted under it.

Smegma, if it is allowed to collect, may in some people become carcino-genic, that is, carry the risk of causing cancer. Cancer of the cervix is rare in sexually inexperienced women, such as nuns, and in Jewish women whose husbands are circumcised and it is thought that this is because neither group is exposed to smegma.

However, it seems a little extreme to deal with smegma by surgery when simple washing would be enough.

So there is no health reason for circumcision today unless there is real tightness of the foreskin which obstructs the passage of urine, and this is comparatively rare.

Genitals, kidneys and bladder

Why do some people, especially babies and children, have urine that smells of ammonia?

Freshly passed urine never smells of ammonia. However, shortly after it is passed it is attacked by organisms which are everywhere in our environment. They break down the urea – one of the main waste products in urine – into its basic chemical parts, one of which is ammonia.

The smell of ammonia that comes from a baby may be due to the use of inadequately sterilized fabric diapers, or to leaving the child too long unchanged. This not only smells unpleasant – it can irritate the skin badly and cause an ammonia rash.

In older people the cause is usually a loss of control, leading to urine dribbling into the clothing. This can happen to men with prostate problems, or to women with stress incontinence – weakness of the bladder walls which results from their excess stretching during childbirth.

If freshly passed urine has a strong, offensive, fishy odour this may indicate the presence of infection which will require treatment.

Urine is formed within the kidneys by filtering off the organic wastes and excess salts and water carried in the blood. There are over 1,000,000 filtration points in a kidney and about 2,500 pints of blood are filtered each day

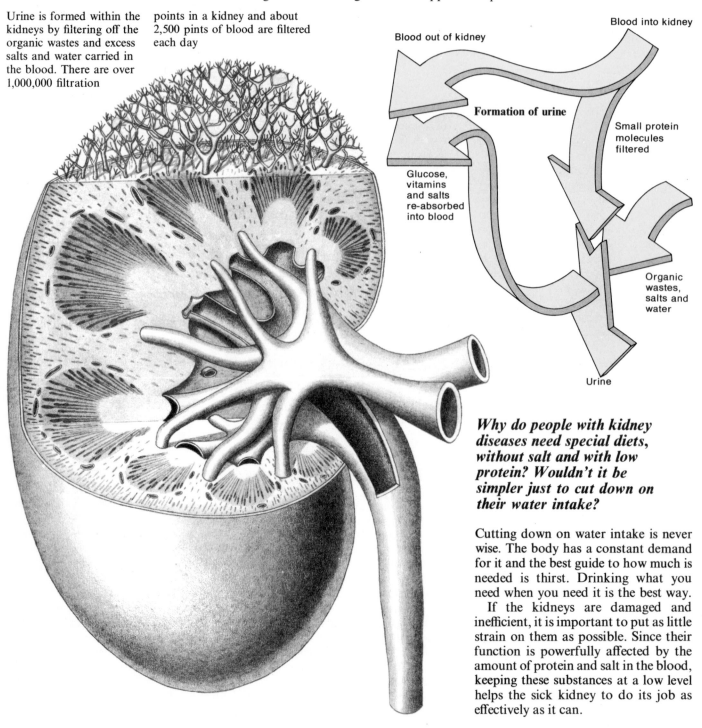

Blood out of kidney

Blood into kidney

Formation of urine

Small protein molecules filtered

Glucose, vitamins and salts re-absorbed into blood

Organic wastes, salts and water

Urine

Why do people with kidney diseases need special diets, without salt and with low protein? Wouldn't it be simpler just to cut down on their water intake?

Cutting down on water intake is never wise. The body has a constant demand for it and the best guide to how much is needed is thirst. Drinking what you need when you need it is the best way.

If the kidneys are damaged and inefficient, it is important to put as little strain on them as possible. Since their function is powerfully affected by the amount of protein and salt in the blood, keeping these substances at a low level helps the sick kidney to do its job as effectively as it can.

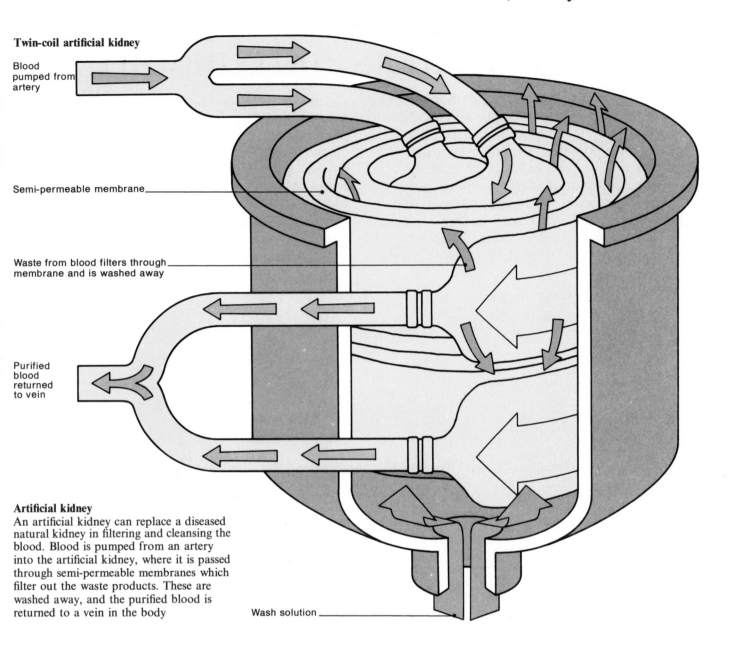

Twin-coil artificial kidney

Blood pumped from artery

Semi-permeable membrane

Waste from blood filters through membrane and is washed away

Purified blood returned to vein

Wash solution

Artificial kidney
An artificial kidney can replace a diseased natural kidney in filtering and cleansing the blood. Blood is pumped from an artery into the artificial kidney, where it is passed through semi-permeable membranes which filter out the waste products. These are washed away, and the purified blood is returned to a vein in the body

Why do some people have to have kidney machines, and others transplants?

If the kidneys are damaged enough to stop working altogether, then the patient slowly succumbs to poisoning as breakdown substances from metabolism build up in the blood. In the past, kidney failure inevitably led to death. Today, however, we have technology that enables a person with dead kidneys to go on coping reasonably well, as long as he is attached from time to time to a machine through which his blood can pass and be filtered of waste products, in the same way as the kidney filters. The machines have saved many lives and no doubt will continue to do so.

But obviously it is inconvenient to have to live always close to a large machine. Replacement of a dead kidney by one from a living donor offers a much more normal life to patients in whom the technique is successful. However, not all patients with kidney failure can benefit from transplant. It depends on the cause of the kidney failure, as well as the individual patient's basic constitution. And there are many problems still to be solved, not the least being the available supply of donors. Each human body has its own immune system; it rejects foreign invaders such as bacteria

and viruses, and also foreign tissue such as kidneys.

However, new techniques now used to match the tissue types of donors and recipients make an acceptable graft more likely, and, when used with immuno-suppressive techniques, these can allow a new kidney to move in and take over. The trouble with immuno-suppressive techniques is that the patient having them used on him is temporarily vulnerable to overwhelming attack by infection. This is why the management of such patients is so complex and costly.

Women's disorders and childbirth

In a purely biological sense, we are born for one purpose only – to reproduce our species. Nature cares above all for the continuation of life, at whatever cost to the individual who carries the major burden of reproduction. Human females, like those of most animal species, are definitely the bearers of the heaviest load. And although conceiving, bearing, giving birth to and feeding a baby are normal physiological processes, they do not always run as smoothly as they might, so women need a lot of care and support while they carry life on to the next generation. The doctor who gives these to a great degree is the gynaecologist and obstetrician. These two specialities are almost always followed by one individual, although in fact they are different. A gynaecologist is involved in the care of the diseases of women's generative organs – uterus, tubes and ovaries – while an obstetrician is involved only with the care of women in childbirth. But the two interests make an obvious pair.

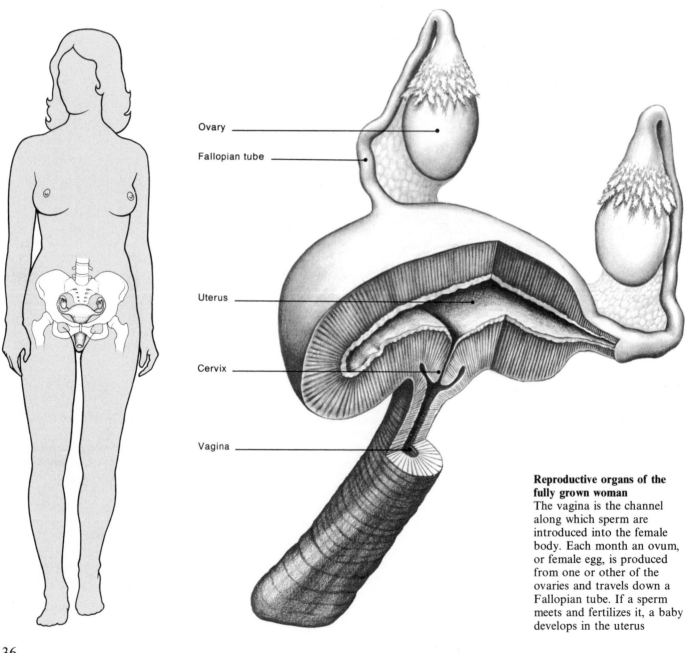

Ovary

Fallopian tube

Uterus

Cervix

Vagina

Reproductive organs of the fully grown woman
The vagina is the channel along which sperm are introduced into the female body. Each month an ovum, or female egg, is produced from one or other of the ovaries and travels down a Fallopian tube. If a sperm meets and fertilizes it, a baby develops in the uterus

Why do little girls become sexually mature so long before they are physically fit to have babies? Has nature gone wrong?

Nature seldom goes wrong. She is interested only in survival and the continuation of life, and as soon as any creature is capable of giving birth, it does so, provided that the circumstances are right.

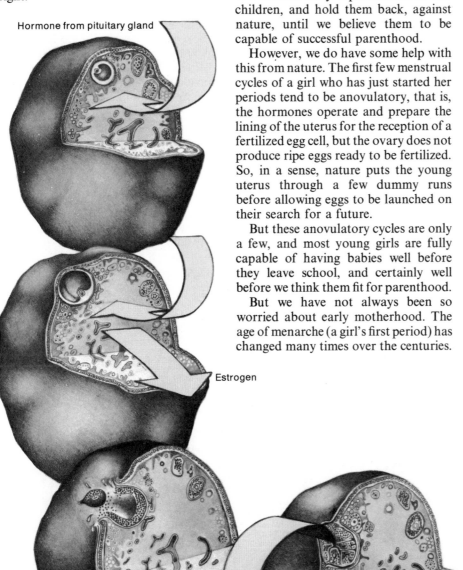

Hormone from pituitary gland

Estrogen

Estrogen
Progesterone

So it is incorrect to say that little girls are physically unfit to have babies once they reach sexual maturity, although, from our civilized point of view, they are emotionally and socially unfit to do so. We control early reproduction in our children, and hold them back, against nature, until we believe them to be capable of successful parenthood.

However, we do have some help with this from nature. The first few menstrual cycles of a girl who has just started her periods tend to be anovulatory, that is, the hormones operate and prepare the lining of the uterus for the reception of a fertilized egg cell, but the ovary does not produce ripe eggs ready to be fertilized. So, in a sense, nature puts the young uterus through a few dummy runs before allowing eggs to be launched on their search for a future.

But these anovulatory cycles are only a few, and most young girls are fully capable of having babies well before they leave school, and certainly well before we think them fit for parenthood.

But we have not always been so worried about early motherhood. The age of menarche (a girl's first period) has changed many times over the centuries.

At present it seems to be getting younger: a century or so ago the average age was reported to be 15 and now it is 12. There have, of course, always been variations on each side of the average age – some starting much younger, some much older – but the average is what matters.

Some people suggest that the reason for this current dropping in age, and it seems still to be going down, is improved nutrition and healthier life-styles. But if you go farther back in history you find that girls reached physical maturity just as young as they do today – indeed younger. Shakespeare's Juliet is a good example. She was not yet 14 when the action of the play happened, and her mother came to talk to her of marriage, remarking that '. . . younger than you . . . are made already mothers: by my count I was your mother much upon these years that you are now a maid'.

And there is evidence that motherhood in girls of 12 and 13 was not all that unusual in other parts of the world, for example in Asia, America and Africa. But although our worry about schoolgirl mothers would appear to be an artefact of our times, it is obviously something which nobody would want to encourage. Young girls who are not yet 15 years old are barely out of childhood themselves and are psychologically and economically unready to be parents.

Development of an ovum
Each of the almond-sized ovaries is guided by hormones and also produces its own.
1 Early in the monthly cycle, hormone from the pituitary gland causes several ova to begin to develop coatings, becoming structures called follicles. **2** The follicles make the hormone estrogen, which causes the uterus lining to thicken in preparation for a pregnancy. Only one follicle reaches maturity. **3** The follicle bursts, releasing the ovum into the Fallopian tube. **4** The remains of the follicle make estrogen and also progesterone, which helps to prepare the lining of the uterus for pregnancy

Women's disorders and childbirth

Why do periods vary so much from woman to woman? After all, most other body functions – bladder and bowels, for example – are fairly regular.

Bladder and bowel actions cannot be compared with periods; the first two are excretory functions, needed to rid the body of wastes, and the latter is not. The fact that blood leaves the body does not mean that it is 'bad' blood, or that unless it is discarded there is a build-up of toxins inside the body. Many women probably believe this mistaken idea because the blood of a period leaves the body from an opening close to the openings of the bladder and bowels. (In this connection, one old Scottish surgeon observed mournfully, 'Far be it from me to criticize the ways of Providence, but what was the good Lord thinking of to put the nursery between the sewers?')

So, it is not absolutely essential for total health for a woman to have a regular blood loss each month. Indeed, some experts believe that it is basically abnormal for a woman to have a period at all. They say that in a truly natural state a woman would be always either pregnant – during which time the periods are definitely suppressed – or lactating,

during which time the periods are often suppressed (though not always) and that this would continue throughout her reproductive years until the menopause, or sheer exhaustion, brought it all to an end.

But, of course, most women do menstruate often, and the variation from one to another, and even in the same woman from time to time, is immense. The textbook rule is that the periods happen every 28 days, with ovulation occurring midway, on the 14th day.

The number of women who actually conform to that exact cycle is probably comparatively small. Many have three-week cycles, many have 33-day cycles and many have quite unpredictable cycles. It is what is normal for the individual that is significant, not what is normal in a textbook.

The causes of the variation are many. First of all, the periods are under the control of the ovarian hormones – two of those complex chemical messengers which are involved with so many of our physical and emotional functions. The

ovarian hormones work in concert with the other hormones, from the thyroid, the pituitary, the adrenals, and so on, and disturbance of their function can affect the function of the ovarian hormones. This is why, for example, a woman suffering from hyperthyroidism will have scanty or absent periods.

The endocrine glands are intimately involved with the emotional state. A change in their levels can cause a change of mood, and vice versa. This is why extreme emotional experience can greatly affect periods. It is common for a woman to find her periods stop altogether for a few months when she is bereaved, or when she changes her life style – when starting college, say, and leaving home for the first time in late adolescence. Marriage and the start of a regular sex life can also suppress periods in some women.

Weight levels are also very much involved. There appears to be an ideal weight range for every woman, and if she goes below or above it her periods stop. No one has yet been able to

The monthly cycle
The ovaries, brain and pituitary gland interact in the processes that end in a period or pregnancy.
Days 1–5 During menstruation the pituitary gland, under the influence of the hypothalamus in the brain, sends a burst of follicle-stimulating hormone (FSH) to the ovaries.
Day 12 As the follicles ripen, they send out their own hormones that both prepare the uterus for a possible pregnancy and cause the pituitary to send a fresh wave of hormone to stimulate ovulation at about mid-cycle.
Day 21 The ovaries' hormones keep the uterus in readiness for a pregnancy and switch off the hormones from the pituitary. What happens next depends on whether the released ovum is fertilized or not

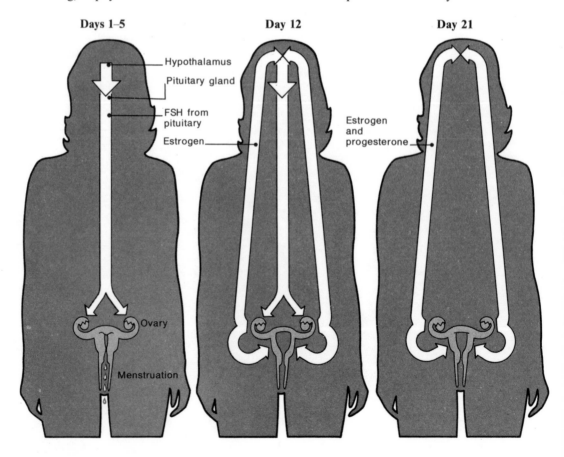

Days 1–5

Day 12

Day 21

Hypothalamus

Pituitary gland

FSH from pituitary

Estrogen

Ovary

Menstruation

Estrogen and progesterone

measure the range with any accuracy but that it is important is undoubted. The woman who goes on a strict reducing diet may well find her periods stop; the one who gains sharply has the same problem. This, incidentally, is the fact behind the old country saying 'thinning before a fattening'. Long before modern science came along and proved it, people noticed that fat women had trouble in conceiving because their ovaries and periods had been suppressed by their obesity. If they lost weight, the ovulation cycles and periods were restored and they conceived – and 'fattened' again.

Periods are also a useful diagnostic pointer in the psychiatric illness of anorexia nervosa. In this, anxious adolescent girls become compulsive dieters and lose a great deal of weight. Amenorrhoea (failure of periods) is an early response to the dieting and may drive the girl to her doctor for help. She does not know that she has anorexia nervosa, or even that her dieting habit is abnormal. But the reaction of her hormones is an indication of her abnormal state.

General health also plays a part in menstrual rhythm. Women with anaemia, for example, may find that their periods are absent or scanty; it is as though the body were conserving its low stocks of vital blood.

There is also a theory that climate and altitude play a part. Women who travel often find that their periods change rhythm, but this of course could be due not so much to the physical effects of the new habitat as the emotional effects of leaving a familiar one.

Cessation of periods is only occasionally an important symptom; of course, it is important in diagnosing pregnancy, in dealing with fertility problems, and, if it is associated with other symptoms, in suggesting the presence of disease, either physical or psychiatric. But otherwise, most women need not worry about it. Much more important and worth a medical check are heavier periods than usual, or extra blood loss, or loss at unusual times. These could indicate gynaecological disease.

I've been told that if I go on the Pill it will cure my spotty skin and greasy hair. Is this true, and if it is, why? I thought the pill was just to prevent pregnancy.

The Pill is indeed primarily a pregnancy preventer, but because it is hormonal and exerts its effect through the body's hormonal system, it can do other things as well. There are some women who have skin and hair problems because of the balance of estrogen and progesterone in their bodies, and for them the change in balance caused by using the Pill (which contains either or both hormones in varying quantities) can change the balance and, with it, the skin or hair problems.

Similarly, there are women who suffer from painful menstruation who find that their symptoms are relieved by the use of the Pill; others who suffer premenstrual tension (in which there is a depressing fluid build-up just before each period) are relieved when they take the Pill. For them the Pill may be advised for its therapeutic side effects rather than as a contraceptive, though it will still act as a contraceptive, of course.

When I got brown patches on my face my doctor made me stop using the Pill. Why?

In some sensitive women – nearly always brunette and olive-skinned – the action on the skin of the hormones in the Pill results in brownish patches forming, especially where the skin is exposed to sunlight. These are similar to the brownish markings some brunettes get in pregnancy, and are, like them, irreversible. So unless you don't mind the patches, listen to your doctor and use another contraceptive method. Or, stay out of direct sunlight at all times.

The condition, by the way, is given the medical name of chloasma.

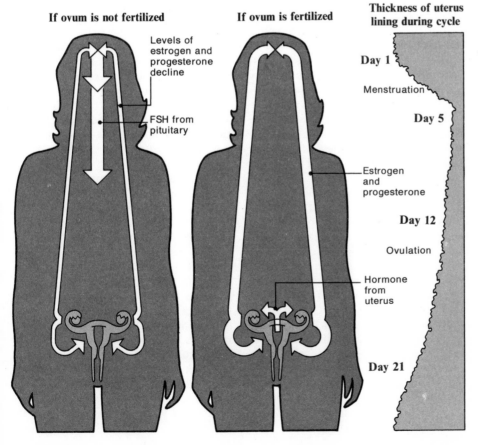

If ovum is not fertilized

Levels of estrogen and progesterone decline

FSH from pituitary

If ovum is fertilized

Estrogen and progesterone

Hormone from uterus

Thickness of uterus lining during cycle

Day 1

Menstruation

Day 5

Day 12

Ovulation

Day 21

If the ovum is not fertilized: the level of estrogen released from the ovaries falls, causing the release of FSH, which renews the cycle

If the ovum is fertilized: hormone from the uterus stimulates the ovaries to continue their hormone production, which maintains the uterus lining, and keeps the FSH production switched off

Women's disorders and childbirth

If nature's main concern is the continuation of the species, why do so many people seem to have trouble in starting a pregnancy?

Most couples think they will be able to have babies as and when they are ready. They think that they will only have to stop any contraception, continue to enjoy intercourse and then expect the birth of a baby nine months later. In fact, it has been estimated that one couple in six is involuntarily childless. It is not possible to find accurate figures as a great many couples hide their distress about their childlessness because of mistaken shame. But such shame is foolish. Sub-fertility is a common problem and considerable medical research has been made into it, so that much help can now be given to the unwillingly childless couple.

For a pregnancy to start it is necessary for a male sperm to meet a female ovum inside the woman's body, under conditions that make it possible for the fertilized egg to bury itself in the uterine wall and grow into a baby. The necessary conditions are: there must be healthy, active ovaries producing fully ripe eggs; there must be a clear passageway from ovary to uterus along which the egg can travel; there must be a healthy, fully developed uterus with a prepared lining in which the fertilized egg can embed itself; there must be a healthy vagina and cervix through which sperm can travel to meet the egg; and there must be healthy sperm deposited in the vault of the vagina, which means that the man must have fully developed, healthy testicles.

Many people believe that any and every act of intercourse will result in a pregnancy. It is true that it is possible but it is by no means always the case. A woman is usually fertile – that is, capable of conceiving – for only about two or three days in any one menstrual cycle (this is measured from the first day of one period to the first day of the next). This fertile time occurs after an egg cell has been thrown out of the ovary, and while it is travelling along the Fallopian tube on its way to the uterus. Intercourse will not result in pregnancy before ovulation (the egg shedding) because there is no egg cell for the sperm to meet, and intercourse after the egg has reached the uterus is too late, because the egg is past being fertilized.

It is possible to pinpoint the fertile days and make sure that intercourse takes place at the right time. If a woman has a really exact 28-day cycle, which is rare, then she can assume that ovulation happens on the 14th day, because ovulation always occurs 14 days before each period. Intercourse on the day preceding the 14th day itself, and one or two days after that, is most likely to lead to a pregnancy. The day before is suitable because it takes the sperm a little while to reach the part of the tube where fertilization can happen, and by the time the sperm get there, the egg is on its way to meet them.

For women with less regular cycles, the temperature test can be used. It has been noticed that at ovulation time a woman's body temperature takes a small dip and then a sharp rise. If a woman takes her temperature first thing in the morning before getting out of bed and charts it on a special chart, she will soon see the pattern of ovulation and so pinpoint the best time to have intercourse.

This method alone has helped lots of people to have the baby they so much wanted, because, when you think about it, unless a couple is sexually active enough to have intercourse more than five times a week, it is all too easy to miss the right time. This is not unusually active, of course, but many people don't make love that often, which is why they are disappointed in the parenthood stakes.

But there can be other reasons for failure to conceive. A general illness can have a definite effect. This does not mean that an ill woman cannot conceive; far from it. In the past there were many women with severe tuberculosis or malignant diseases from which they were dying who still conceived. So it must never be thought that a general illness can be regarded as contraceptive. But, at the same time, it is known that general illness may be the cause of an apparent sub-fertility. An obvious example would be a hormonal disease such as thyrotoxicosis, which has the effect of disturbing the ovaries. The various forms of anaemia may also lead to temporary sub-fertility. In these cases, treatment of the general illness will usually lead to conception.

There may be local problems in the sex organs. An infection of the vagina or cervix, causing offensive and heavy discharge may prevent sperm from making the journey to the uterus.

Lack of a special mucus made by the cervix can also affect conception. At the time of maximum fertility, there is usually an increase and a thinning out of this mucus, which helps the sperm to swim on their way to meet an ovum. Some women do not make the extra mucus needed.

Treatment and cure of any local infection in such a case may lead to conception, but treatment of the inadequate cervical mucus is not so easy. It may be due to disorder in the ovaries (which produce the hormone that encourages the cervix to produce the mucus) and that is a more complex medical problem.

There may be a blockage of the Fallopian tubes. These tubes have a very fine channel and it takes very little to close them; when this happens the ovum is prevented from reaching the uterus. It is possible for an infection called salpingitis to cause scar tissue that results in a blockage.

Doctors checking on this may inject an opaque dye into the uterus and then take an X-ray picture. This will show whether the dye can travel from the uterus and along the tubes, measuring the resistance it meets. It will also show whether or not the tubes are open. If there is a blockage it is sometimes possible to restore the clearway by an operation.

In some cases the ovary does not produce ripe eggs. This may be obvious in some women because they will not have periods. Absence of periods usually means absence of ovulation. However, the reverse is not necessarily true. It is possible for a woman to have periods even though her ovaries are not producing ripe eggs. This is because of the effects of other body hormones.

Treatment of failure to ovulate can be difficult. Much research has been done in recent years with various hormone treatments, but there were problems with them. There have been cases of women who have undergone these treatments and who have produced several ripe eggs at a time, all of which have

The beginning of a child
A pregnancy passes through these stages in the first 10 days: **1** The ovum is swept along a Fallopian tube and there meets sperm: only one sperm can penetrate it. **2** The ovum, now fertilized, divides repeatedly. **3** It becomes a globular mass of cells before reaching the uterus. **4** The globe of cells implants itself in the uterus wall. **5** In a few more days it buries itself. Here the baby grows

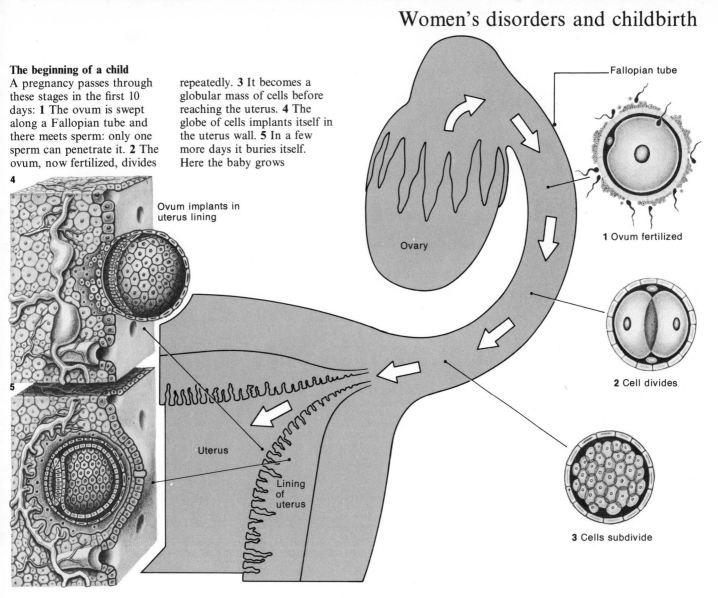

Fallopian tube

Ovary

1 Ovum fertilized

2 Cell divides

3 Cells subdivide

Ovum implants in uterus lining

Uterus

Lining of uterus

4

5

become fertilized. This has led to multiple births. Some of these unlucky women produced six or seven babies at once, none of whom lived. But doctors using these 'fertility drugs' are becoming more and more skilful and fewer multiple births happen now. A woman offered the treatment today should not be afraid of it; it has helped many childless women to become mothers.

Although the popular belief is that childlessness is always a feminine problem, as many men as women suffer from reduced fertility.

These men are perfectly potent: they are able to enjoy intercourse and orgasm (climax) and eject semen, but the sperm they produce are in some way inadequate. It may be that the man is producing a large number of sperm but they are not fully developed, or he may not be producing enough. Only one sperm is needed to make a baby, but many millions must be produced to make it possible for one sperm to complete the long journey to meet the egg.

An examination of a woman within a few hours of intercourse will reveal whether or not a man is producing healthy sperm. Some of the sperm will still be living within her body and can be seen under a microscope. This test is called a post-coital test.

If sperm are not seen, or appear to be of poor development, the cause may be one of many. The testicles must be at a temperature of around 95 degrees Fahrenheit to function properly. This is why they are positioned on the outside of the body – which is usually around 99 degrees Fahrenheit. If a man wears tight underpants which keep the testicles close to the body they are kept too warm and therefore are unable to function properly. If he gives up wearing this sort of underwear and wears the loose, boxer-type pants instead, this may be quite enough to improve his sperm production sufficiently for conception to occur within a few months.

The overweight man may also keep his testicles too warm. Fat people are hotter than thin ones because their circulation has to work harder in order to return blood to the heart. Loss of weight may be enough to correct the problem.

A great many men suffer from varicose veins which are knotted around one or both testicles. These, too, keep the temperature of the glands much too high. Surgery offers the solution for men with this problem.

In some cases, a man may be advised to bathe the testicles in cold water at regular intervals (usually twice a day) for some weeks. This may have the desired effect.

In other cases, permanent damage to the testicles has been suffered; men who

Women's disorders and childbirth

Obstacle course to fertilization

Hundreds of millions of sperm may be released in one ejaculation, yet only one can fertilize the ovum. The vagina is a hostile environment for sperm except for a short time around ovulation. If sexual intercourse takes place at that time, the vagina, uterus and Fallopian tubes actively assist the sperm. But only a few reach the ovum, and none may succeed in penetrating it

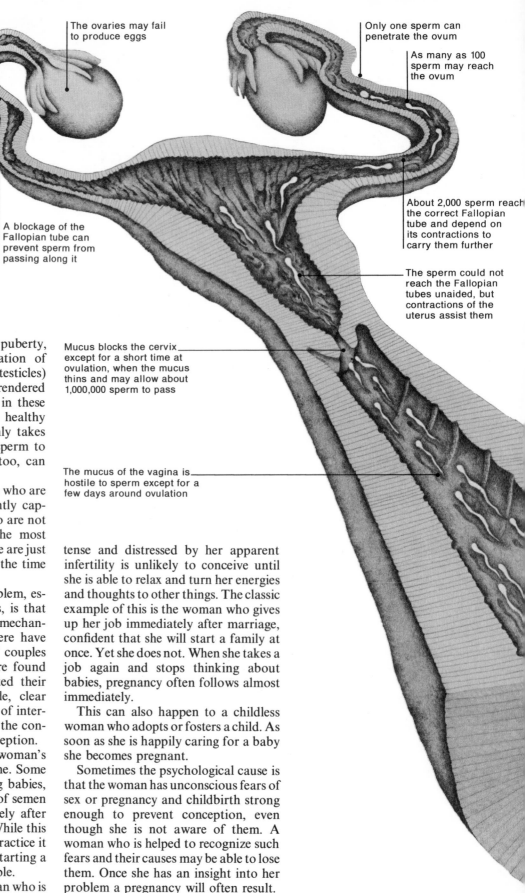

The ovaries may fail to produce eggs

A blockage of the Fallopian tube can prevent sperm from passing along it

Only one sperm can penetrate the ovum

As many as 100 sperm may reach the ovum

About 2,000 sperm reach the correct Fallopian tube and depend on its contractions to carry them further

The sperm could not reach the Fallopian tubes unaided, but contractions of the uterus assist them

Mucus blocks the cervix except for a short time at ovulation, when the mucus thins and may allow about 1,000,000 sperm to pass

The mucus of the vagina is hostile to sperm except for a few days around ovulation

have mumps after the age of puberty, and who suffer the complication of orchitis (inflammation of the testicles) affecting both glands, may be rendered sterile. This is rare and, even in these cases, it is possible that some healthy sperm can be produced. It only takes one testicle to make enough sperm to make a baby, so these men, too, can hope.

Sometimes, there are couples who are both perfectly fit and apparently capable of conceiving, and yet who are not able to start a pregnancy. The most common cause is that the couple are just not having intercourse during the time of the woman's fertility.

An even more common problem, especially in very young couples, is that they lack understanding of the mechanism of sexual intercourse. There have been many reported cases of couples seeking medical help who were found not to have fully consummated their marriages. For such a couple, clear explanation of the mechanism of intercourse may be enough to help the consummation and therefore conception.

Yet another cause may be a woman's exaggerated attention to hygiene. Some women, while actively wanting babies, are distressed by the presence of semen on their bodies and immediately after intercourse get up and wash. While this is not exactly a contraceptive practice it can certainly spoil chances of starting a pregnancy in a sub-fertile couple.

It has been noted that a woman who is

tense and distressed by her apparent infertility is unlikely to conceive until she is able to relax and turn her energies and thoughts to other things. The classic example of this is the woman who gives up her job immediately after marriage, confident that she will start a family at once. Yet she does not. When she takes a job again and stops thinking about babies, pregnancy often follows almost immediately.

This can also happen to a childless woman who adopts or fosters a child. As soon as she is happily caring for a baby she becomes pregnant.

Sometimes the psychological cause is that the woman has unconscious fears of sex or pregnancy and childbirth strong enough to prevent conception, even though she is not aware of them. A woman who is helped to recognize such fears and their causes may be able to lose them. Once she has an insight into her problem a pregnancy will often result.

Why do some pregnancies end in a miscarriage? Can they be prevented?

The correct word for a miscarriage (the loss of a pregnancy before the baby is able to survive on its own, that is, before the 28th week of the pregnancy) is abortion. Unfortunately, over recent years this word has come to mean deliberate termination of a pregnancy, and a woman who greatly wants her baby and has a miscarriage may be upset if she hears doctors or hospital staff use the word abortion to describe her condition. But she should not be distressed by the word because no medical person using it is suggesting she

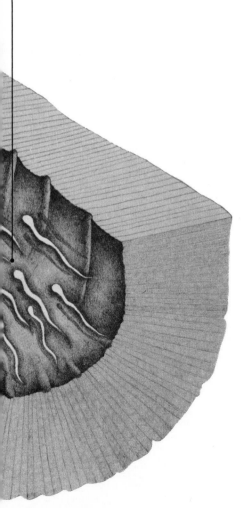

As many as 400,000,000 sperm may be ejaculated into the vagina, but many of these will be abnormal, and not capable of fertilizing the ovum

deliberately ended her pregnancy.

There are many causes of spontaneous abortion or miscarriage, only some of which are understood. It is certainly a common happening – it has been estimated that about one in every five pregnancies ends in miscarriage, and that the most common time is during the first three months.

One cause of miscarriage at around the 10th to 12th week is the 'blighted ovum'. Instead of developing normally, the cells fail to start the proper growth into a baby; the mother's body recognizes this because of differences in the hormone responses and discards the pregnancy. This, many people feel, is something to be grateful for rather than to mourn, because it is surely better to lose a pregnancy than to suffer the birth of a severely handicapped child. There is no suggestion that there is anything wrong with either parent if this happens; the growth needed to make a baby from two tiny cells is so incredible that the remarkable thing is that so many cells develop normally, rather than that a few don't.

Another cause of early miscarriage is hormonal upset. If the hormone control is not established as it should be, the pregnancy cannot survive. One of the most vulnerable times is between actual fertilization and implantation in the wall of the uterus – without the right hormonal activity implantation may fail. A miscarriage at this stage may not be noticed as such because the woman will not have missed a period and will not have known that she was pregnant. She will assume she has had a delayed and, perhaps, rather heavy period.

The next few weeks of pregnancy are also vulnerable because there are stages at which the developing placenta (the afterbirth) has to take over some of the hormone production from the mother's ovaries. These times tend to coincide with what would have been a period time, which is why some doctors advise extra rest during these few days,

Sometimes miscarriage is due to a mechanical failure. Women who consistently lose their pregnancies between the 12th and the 28th weeks of pregnancy may have an inefficient (incompetent) cervix; instead of remaining firmly

closed to protect the developing baby, it gapes a little and so the pregnancy fails. The cause of this incompetence may be a natural fault or damage due to previous childbirths, or operations of various kinds. The problem can be treated by inserting a 'purse-string' suture round the cervix (it is called Shirodkar's stitch) at about the 13th or 14th week, and then removing it when the baby is ready to be born. This is successful in about three out of four cases.

General illness in the mother can lead to miscarriage, though by no means always. There were women in concentration camps during World War II who suffered dreadful privation and illness and yet went on to give normal birth to normal babies. But it can happen that the old wives' tale that severe shock or upset can lead to miscarriage is occasionally shown to be true. If a woman's hormones are thrown out of balance by severe shock or distress then her pregnancy may suffer. But this is very rare indeed.

There is little evidence that the tales told about stretching, reaching and lifting causing miscarriage are true, although excessive or violent exercise at times when a pregnancy is vulnerable may precipitate a loss. However, it could be that the loss would have happened anyway, and the exercise only speeded things up. Generally speaking, it is not necessary to treat pregnancy in a normal healthy woman as a time to be excessively passive, or to avoid exercise.

Sexual intercourse has also been blamed by some people for miscarriage but here again, unless a doctor specifically forbids it, there is no need to be alarmed. A doctor is only likely to forbid sex if the woman has miscarried before, is suffering from pain or is bleeding. Anxiety about sex during pregnancy is based more on unnecessary guilt about sexual pleasure than on real risks.

There are many more causes of miscarriage, including disorders of the uterus itself, and no one can ever foretell in a particular woman what the outcome of her pregnancy will be. But the majority of women who have suffered miscarriage go on to have perfectly normal pregnancies and babies.

Women's disorders and childbirth

Why do I get vaginal discharge?

The normal healthy vagina is a naturally moist self-cleaning area of the body. It produces secretions which are designed to wash away unwanted foreign bodies, such as dust, which might invade the vagina – it resembles the nostrils in this – and also to maintain the right acid-alkaline balance, making sure that unwanted micro-organisms are destroyed.

The vagina also produces secretions that help in its reproductive function. To be successful, it needs to be lubricated for sexual intercourse, to allow the penis to move inside it – and the penis needs stimulation for the ejaculation of semen. So, under the prodding of sexual excitement, the vagina pours out a quantity of fairly thin lubricating liquid. This varies in quantity from time to time, and from woman to woman. Some of these secretions are re-absorbed through the vaginal walls which are usually in contact with each other (the vagina, like the gullet, is rather like an empty toothpaste tube – capable of considerable expansion when full, but usually collapsed), but if there are a great deal of secretions they escape to the surface of the vulva (the outer sex organs) and are regarded as a discharge.

There is a tendency for the vagina to produce more secretion during pregnancy and during different stages of the menstrual cycle. For example, at ovulation (the time when a ripe egg is shed ready for fertilization) the cervix at the top of the vagina produces more of its own secretion, in a thinner form. This again can escape to the surface as a discharge.

Normal sexual intercourse deposits a considerable amount of semen in the vagina. A certain amount of this is drawn up into the cervix and so on into the uterus (unless, of course, there is a barrier over the cervix, such as a diaphragm) and the rest of it will escape and be felt as a discharge.

These are all natural and healthy discharges, and most women can recognize them as such and not worry about them. However, sometimes the discharge changes in quantity and nature and then it does cause worry.

A common infection of the vagina is thrush (Candida albicans). This is a yeast-like organism which produces itching, redness and a thick curd-like discharge that dries on underwear to a yellowish-brown and can smell offensive. (Incidentally, thrush may affect other mucous membrane, for example in the mouth). There is also TV (trichomonas vaginalis), another organism that gives rise to an unpleasant frothy yellow discharge as well as itching and soreness. And there is gonorrhoea which produces a persistent yellow discharge.

Thrush can be caught by any female of any age (it has been diagnosed in babies and elderly nuns) and is not necessarily connected with sexual intercourse; TV can be picked up from infected bedding or clothing, though it is frequently passed on via sexual intercourse; and gonorrhoea is only passed on by intercourse. Each of these, once diagnosed, is treated by the use of medicines which are known to destroy the organism; penicillin for gonorrhoea, for example, and metronidazol (Flagyl) for TV.

Another cause of vaginal discharge is the condition that has been labelled (inaccurately) cervical erosion. In this the neck of the uterus (the cervix) develops a reddish, sore-looking patch which produces a lot of extra secretion. This was once thought to be due to damage to the area from rubbing – hence the name erosion – but is now known to be a pouting outwards of cells that usually lie inside the cervical canal. Why they pout like this is not always known, but it is a tiresome problem when it occurs because it can give rise to a lot of extra secretions being poured out. Also the pouting cells are susceptible to infection from thrush or TV. The treatment then is to give the medicines which combat the organism involved, and also to remove the pouting cells, by chemical cautery, electrical cautery or by cryosurgery.

Types of hysterectomy

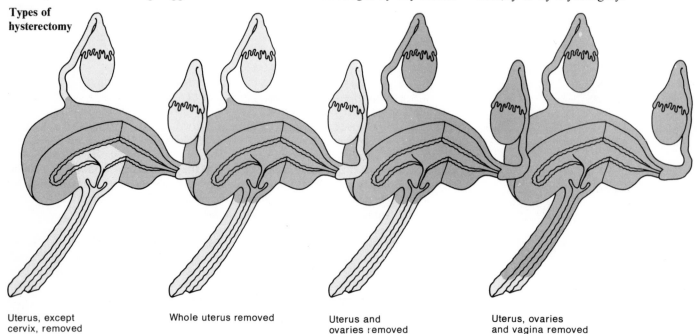

Uterus, except cervix, removed

Whole uterus removed

Uterus and ovaries removed

Uterus, ovaries and vagina removed

What is done at a hysterectomy? And how long does it take to recover from it?

Good surgeons take only what they must. Ideally they try to leave the ovaries, because these have a function apart from causing periods. The ovaries do not work quite as they did before the uterus was taken away (losing their main target organ seems to reduce their activity a little, in some cases) but it is worth keeping them for their other effects on skin, bones and general well-being.

In some cases, however, they do have to be removed, if the cause of the operation is a malignant disease which is affected by hormones. Some cancers are definitely affected by estrogen, and so loss of the organs which produce estrogen makes sense.

But a woman is always left with a functional vagina. Every effort is made to ensure that she can and does go on enjoying normal sex life after surgery. It is a myth that loss of the uterus puts paid to happy sex. It does not. Indeed, it can add to it, for once the possibility of unwanted pregnancy is gone many women find themselves so relaxed that they become much more amorous. One surgeon, observing this phenomenon, described the operation as 'Taking away the nursery and leaving the playpen'.

Some surgeons operate via the abdomen, usually making a 'bikini line' incision – that is, inside the pubic hair line. Then, after surgery, when the hair regrows, there is no scar. Others prefer the vaginal route, in which case there is no scar at all.

Surgical practices vary from one surgeon to another, but the average hospital stay for hysterectomy is between 10 and 14 days, and a convalescence of between two and four weeks is advised afterwards, with gradually increased activity over the next month. Most women should be back to normal life within three months of surgery – though sexual intercourse can restart much sooner than that. In fact, the sooner it restarts the better, for both psychological and physical reasons. The woman who delays her return to sex too long may find she has trouble in enjoying it as she used to, and she may find the vagina rather tight and uncomfortable, not because of the surgery, which does not reduce the size, but because of the delay. So, lovemaking three or four weeks after the operation is usually advised.

It is not true that hysterectomy causes greying hair, spreading figure, lined face or anything else of that sort. Some women feel so much better after it that they eat more and so put on weight, but this is not the fault of the operation. And the signs of aging happen to all of us, but may be more closely looked for by a post-operative woman who has become over-anxious.

By and large, if the operation is done for the right reasons it leaves a woman feeling better, and looking it, too.

Why do some women have to have hysterectomies?

The operation to remove the uterus and sometimes its attachments (the Fallopian tubes) has been more fashionable at some times than at others, rather like tonsillectomy. There was a time when surgeons were removing uteruses in their thousands for very slight reasons. This fashion is now, fortunately, dying out.

The operation is done nowadays mainly to remove growths, both benign and malignant. The commonest form of benign growth is a fibroid – a large outcropping of tissue in the muscular walls of the uterus. It can grow as large as a football if it is not dealt with, and can greatly increase the area of the lining of the uterus and so cause heavy bleeding at each period. This can lead to severe anaemia and much misery.

In women under the age of menopause who might want to have more babies, the surgeons try to perform a myomectomy, which means that they shell out the fibroid and leave the uterus intact. Otherwise most surgeons think that hysterectomy is the answer.

Obviously, malignant disease needs removing, both with surgery and with radiotherapy and there is a high cure rate for cancer of the cervix, if it is diagnosed early enough. The use of the Papanicolaou (cervical smear) test, in which cells from the cervix are examined for signs that they might some time in the next 10 years become cancerous, has helped to improve this cure rate greatly. It is an important and simple test and well worth having done.

Some women suffer from severe and exhausting bleeds at each period because of dysfunctional uterine bleeding. This is the label given to a range of conditions which are sometimes hard to deal with. The woman's hormone balance seems either to cause or to be unable to prevent the heavy blood loss. Sometimes the use of estrogen and progesterone treatment will control it.

However, when this treatment cannot control the heavy blood loss, then the surgeon and his patient have to weigh up the arguments for and against trying to cope with the bleeding as it is or removing the uterus altogether. The uterus, it must be remembered, is in essence a healthy organ in this situation; it just is not working as it should.

The reason why so many surgeons once performed hysterectomies so freely was that they, and also their patients, did not stop to think about why the hormone balance was so uneven. It can be due to emotional factors. An unhappy woman is more likely to have period problems than a serene and fulfilled one. And in the past, many women who had the operation, ostensibly to cure heavy periods, were actually trying to 'cure' failed marriages, or the unfilled gap of grown-up children who had left home, or distress over inevitable aging, or even sheer boredom. All of these factors can and do lead to ovarian hormone imbalance and therefore period problems.

Nowadays most doctors will try, somehow, to find a way to relieve the symptoms without radical surgery. An honest assessment of a failed marriage, or a new interest in life can restore happiness and, with it, normal periods. Many women are glad that they tried this conservative approach to the problem and so avoided surgery.

Women's disorders and childbirth

My doctor says I need a repair operation, because I have some bladder control trouble. What does he mean exactly?

The vagina runs between the bladder at the front and the rectum at the back. It is a distensible organ – it has to be so in order to accommodate the passage of a fully grown baby's head – and in some women the elasticity in the walls is damaged. It may happen in childbirth, and it may happen because of obesity. A woman carrying too much weight puts extra strain on her vaginal muscles.

Whatever the cause, the vaginal muscles no longer hold up as firmly as they did and the bladder can bulge backwards into the vaginal space, or the rectum may bulge forwards. This makes control of these organs difficult as well as causing a good deal of discomfort.

The solution used to be a pessary – a hard rubber ring pushed high into the vagina to hold the walls back. This was sometimes effective, but was quite often uncomfortable.

Today, the ideal answer is to operate on the muscular walls and tighten them by removing a triangular piece of tissue and then sewing up the space. It is rather like taking in a tuck in a too loose dress, and it works very well indeed. The control which was lost should return soon after the operations.

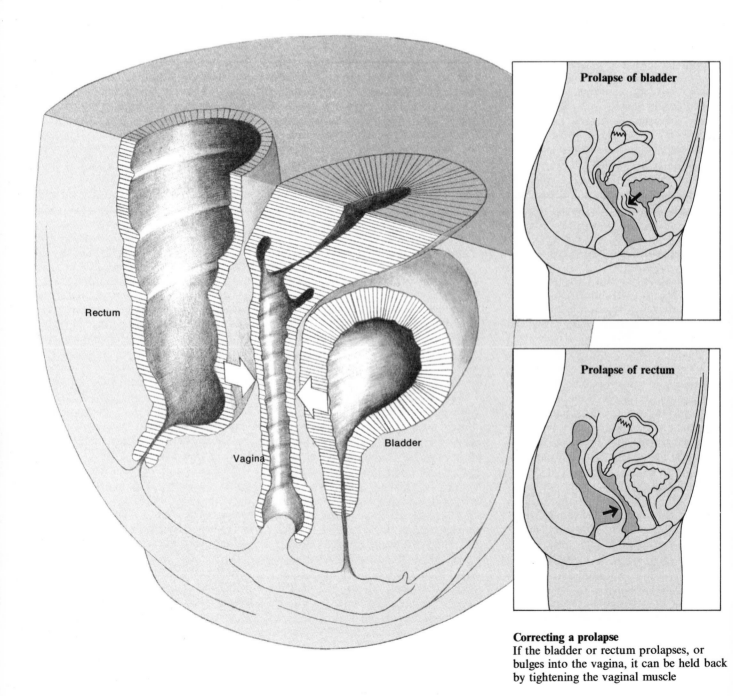

Prolapse of bladder

Prolapse of rectum

Rectum

Vagina

Bladder

Correcting a prolapse
If the bladder or rectum prolapses, or bulges into the vagina, it can be held back by tightening the vaginal muscle

What is a D and C operation and why is it done?

The letters stand for dilation and curettage, which mean simply stretching and scraping. The part that is stretched is not the front passage (the vagina) but the little opening (the cervix) of the uterus itself which lies at the top end of the vagina. It has in its centre a small channel which is usually closed, but is a little wider open in women who have had babies than in women who have not.

The first stage of the operation is to widen the channel. The surgeon, after his patient has been given a general anaesthetic, gently opens the vagina with a speculum – an instrument designed to make it easy for him to see and reach the deeper structures.

Once the surgeon can easily see the cervix he uses an instrument called a sound with which he measures the exact depth of the uterus, because each woman varies a little. It is important that the surgeon pushes his next instruments in only as far as they should go, and the sound tells him how far that is. Then he uses the dilators, a series of curved metal rods, gradually increasing in thickness. Using one after the other he gently enlarges the cervical opening.

He then uses an instrument called a curette, which is slender and long and with a loop at the far end. The loop has either a sharp or a blunt edge, although the sharp one is not all that sharp. With this the surgeon carefully scrapes the surface of the inner walls of the uterus, to remove the lining there. It does no harm to the deeper structures.

The surgeon, once he has passed his curette over the whole surface, to ensure it is all clear of lining, removes his instruments, takes away the speculum which was making the way clear for him and the patient is then almost precisely as she was before he started. She has no stitches, no injuries, no source of any pain. She has only a slightly wider open cervix and a uterus which is free of any lining. She may bleed a little for a day or two, for the uterus responds to the operation by shedding some extra blood. The only other after-effect the woman may have is that she may find her next period is an extra heavy one.

The patient who has a D and C can probably go home in a day or so, unless for any reason she needs further treatment in the hospital.

This is how the operation is done, but the reasons for doing it are more interesting. There can be several reasons, and they fall into two distinct groups, diagnostic and therapeutic.

In the first group come the operations done to investigate why a woman is bleeding heavily during periods or bleeding, even slightly, between periods. These symptoms should always be investigated. If the surgeon is able to look at some of the lining of the uterus under the microscope he can tell precisely what is causing the bleeding.

Sometimes it helps to look at the lining of the uterus in cases of childlessness; examination of these pieces of tissue can tell the surgeon how the woman's hormones are behaving.

A D and C can also be used for treatment; some doctors try it for a girl who has painful periods. It is not absolutely clear why it should prevent painful periods in the future, but it has been noticed to have this effect. Nowadays most women with this particular pain problem can gain relief from the use of hormones, given as the Pill.

A much more common use of a therapeutic D and C these days is for an abortion. Properly done, early enough in the pregnancy, it is simple, safe and effective, for the lining of the uterus contains the small developing egg and all of it can be removed, often using a hollow suction instrument – a catheter – rather than the scraping curette. If a termination is required later in the pregnancy it is not so easy and it may be necessary to perform an abdominal operation and remove the pregnancy via an incision into the body of the uterus.

Another important use of D and C is following a spontaneous abortion (a miscarriage) or after a birth, if bleeding continues. It can happen that shreds of placenta (afterbirth) remain behind after the uterus has emptied, and these tiny shreds can lead to prolonged bleeding and possibly infection. In such cases a D and C operation is necessary in order to tidy up the uterus.

Instruments for D and C
Successively larger dilators are used to widen the cervix gently and allow the curette (*far right*) to be introduced

Can the black bits in potatoes cause spina bifida in babies?

The answer is no. There was some research a while ago which suggested that the eating of potatoes with greenish skins played a part in causing these distressing neural tube defects in babies (they include not only spina bifida, where there is a defect in the structure of the spinal column, but also hydrocephalus, in which there is excess fluid build-up in the brain, and other forms of congenital and often profound mental handicap). However, later checks showed that potatoes were not the cause, but the memory of the first reports seems to have lingered on and it has left some people afraid of eating potatoes. There is no need to be.

Can diseases transmitted by pets damage the unborn baby?

Sometimes, yes. Most animal diseases do not affect us, but there are some which do; they are called the zoonoses. They include ringworm, rabies and toxocara, a particularly nasty form of parasite which, if it reaches the human body, can do a good deal of damage. In some cases there have been reports of toxocara eggs reaching an infant across the placental barrier and causing damage to eyes and other structures.

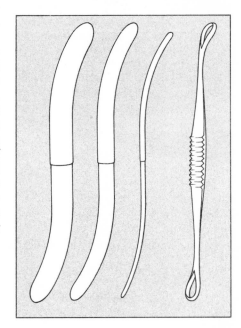

Women's disorders and childbirth

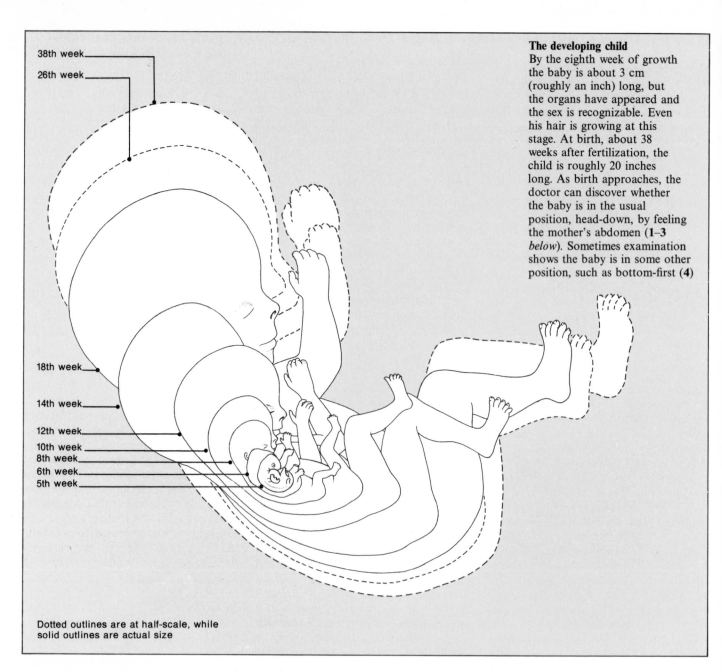

38th week

26th week

18th week

14th week

12th week

10th week

8th week

6th week

5th week

The developing child
By the eighth week of growth the baby is about 3 cm (roughly an inch) long, but the organs have appeared and the sex is recognizable. Even his hair is growing at this stage. At birth, about 38 weeks after fertilization, the child is roughly 20 inches long. As birth approaches, the doctor can discover whether the baby is in the usual position, head-down, by feeling the mother's abdomen (**1–3** *below*). Sometimes examination shows the baby is in some other position, such as bottom-first (**4**)

Dotted outlines are at half-scale, while solid outlines are actual size

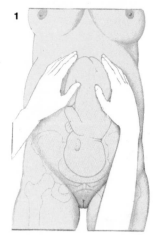

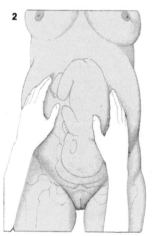

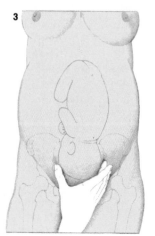

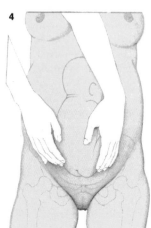

Why do some births have to be induced? Why has there been so much fuss recently about the method?

The 'traditional' method of handling childbirth is for doctors to wait until the mother's own uterus starts to contract and relax rhythmically in preparation for pushing the baby out, and to stand by, offering support and help, while the process occurs spontaneously. The drawbacks to this natural method are that there may be delay in the action of the uterus, leading to distress and even, in complicated cases, damage or death to the baby; also, there may be exhaustion for the mother and damage to her muscles resulting in later gynaecological disorders.

Doctors are trained to recognize signs of baby distress and maternal exhaustion in time to intervene. The use of forceps to facilitate a birth in such cases has been practised for close on 200 years, and surgical intervention – such as a Caesarean birth – has been used for far longer.

And in cases where the mother's body is slow to start labour by itself; or a condition like high blood pressure causes anxiety and the baby seems to be at risk of being damaged in consequence – he may be deprived of oxygen as the placenta becomes less efficient at supplying his needs – then doctors have triggered birth by various methods.

One method is to use enemas and laxatives – vigorous activity by neighbouring body structures can sometimes encourage the uterus to start its own work. This is called medical induction and is rarely used these days.

Another method is called surgical induction and involves snipping the bag of waters in which the unborn baby floats. Release of the fluid makes the baby's head push more firmly against the neck of the uterus and encourages the uterus to contract and then open out to allow the birth to proceed.

More recently, a third technique has been added by the use of hormones. Because the whole birth process is under the control of naturally occurring hormones made in the mother's body, extra doses speed up the process.

A new group of medicines for which there are considerable hopes are the prostaglandins which derive from natural body sources and which appear to play a part in normal labour. Once they have been fully identified and made easily available they will surely play a big role in the future care of mothers.

Such intervention has always been needed by a certain proportion of mothers and babies and all the methods, including the hormonal, have been in use for many years. Recently, however, there have been arguments as to whether it is right to apply active induction methods using rupture of the membranes plus hormones, usually given in an intravenous drip, for all mothers, instead of waiting to see if only some of them need it. There are doctors who support the 'traditional' method of waiting for nature, and others who prefer the modern 'active management of labour' technique. Their reasons may be based on the mother's needs or on the baby's needs, and in a few cases there may be social reasons.

With careful use of induction techniques it is possible to arrange that a baby is born at a time that is convenient to the mother or the doctor or both, and some people have suggested with great indignation that today's obstetricians induce births simply in order to ensure they get their game of golf when they want it.

This is most unlikely; obstetricians are doing their particular work because they care about it. Reaching consultant status demands a degree of devotion, a struggle to learn and gain experience and sheer dogged hard work of an order that would be unthinkable for most of us, and a man or woman who put personal considerations such as golf before work would not choose obstetrics as a career, nor would he or she achieve any degree of success in it.

However, there may be times when both doctor and patient will agree that it is wise to arrange for a birth to happen at a time when all the necessary staff are easily available and fully alert, and when all services that may be required are operating at top level. And clearly the middle of the night when personnel are tired and not able to give of their best, or Christmas Day, when ancillary staff tend to be off duty, are hardly likely to be such times. So, induction is used to by-pass such high-risk situations.

It is important to realize that even if induction is used, a labour is normal, in that the contractions enlarge the cervical opening and eventually push out the baby, with the mother's own pushing help. In other words, there is nothing all that artificial about it. But induction is a life-saving technique when used for mothers and babies at risk, and no mother should listen to the horrific tales which some people delight in telling about it, because these tales are unlikely to have any relevance to what will happen to her. And, of course, if she is anxious she can discuss it all with the clinic staff before her baby is due.

When I was in early labour the doctor said he wanted to examine my uterus but actually did a rectal examination. Why?

Because the vagina lies neatly between the rectum and the bladder, it is possible to check what is going on in the vagina by passing an exploratory finger into the rectum. This examination is often preferred because it avoids introducing any infection into the vagina, and so on into the uterus – a risk which is there however carefully the hands are washed and encased in sterile gloves. Also, many patients prefer it. In Europe it is quite a common practice for this examination to be done but it is never made by a physician in the US.

Rectal examination
A doctor can learn what is happening in the vagina by passing a finger into the rectum

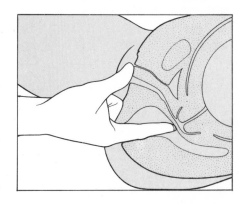

Women's disorders and childbirth

Why does giving birth cause so much pain when it is a natural experience?

The idea that 'natural' equates with 'painless' is false. A certain amount of pain in childbirth is probably inevitable, and it is certainly widespread among mammals. Is is a myth that cows and horses and simple peasant women crouching between the bean rows have an easy time of it. They do not.

But some of the pain which a civilized woman experiences may be a creation of her civilized state. She may know more about the risks and pains of childbirth than her more primitive sisters, and so become more frightened and tense (though primitive women, too, can be equally terrified, not so much by the risk of an induction drip, say, as from fear of evil spirits) and fear causes tension which causes pain. The woman pulls against the natural tendency of her muscles to move in one way and so causes some of her own misery.

This is why the use of deep relaxation techniques and modified self-hypnosis – the psycho-prophylactic method – have become so popular. They do help to remove these added causes of pain. But few women escape pain altogether, although there are many who report a degree of enjoyment of it, resulting as it does in a wanted infant.

There are some moralists who say that a mother loves her baby because she suffers pain in producing it, and for this reason, they object to the use of pain control methods. There is no evidence, however, that this is true; indeed, in some cases, mothers who have had a particularly painful experience have greater trouble in relating to the new-born infant than those who had a normal experience.

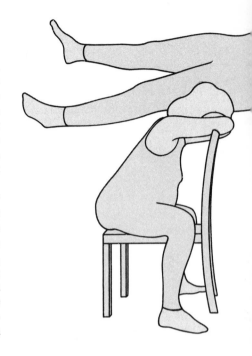

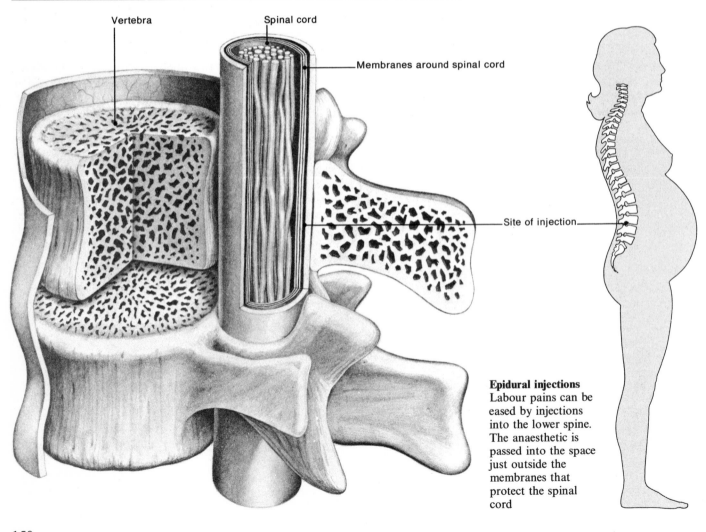

Vertebra

Spinal cord

Membranes around spinal cord

Site of injection

Epidural injections
Labour pains can be eased by injections into the lower spine. The anaesthetic is passed into the space just outside the membranes that protect the spinal cord

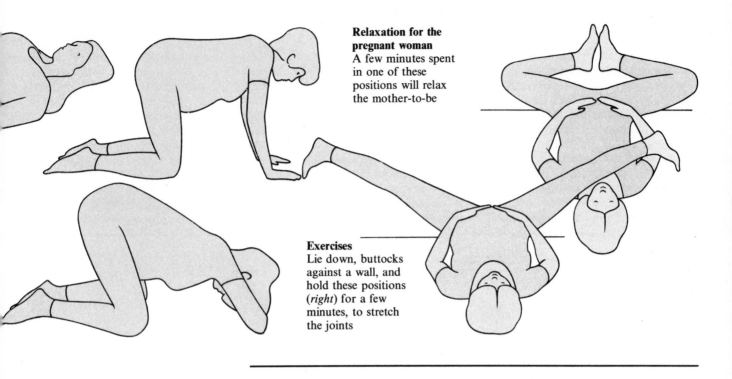

Relaxation for the pregnant woman
A few minutes spent in one of these positions will relax the mother-to-be

Exercises
Lie down, buttocks against a wall, and hold these positions (*right*) for a few minutes, to stretch the joints

Does being born hurt the baby? How much can he see and hear and feel?

The answer to this is unknown because an experience is usually handed on from one person to another via speech, and babies are born speechless. However, mothers and babies do use much 'nonverbal' language, which is called 'imprinting'.

But, there is every reason to suppose that the baby experiences a good deal as the result of his birth passage. He is squeezed, pushed and tugged by powerful external forces and his body is capable of recognizing these effects, for at birth he is well developed, with a functioning nervous system. If he can feel pain, distress, cold and heat immediately after he is born, which he demonstrably can, then obviously he can immediately before and during birth.

Theories about the effects of the birth experience on the baby are many, the latest being postulated by Dr. Frederick Le Boyer of France. He advocates a musical, low-lit gentle environment for childbirth – which is undoubtedly most agreeable for the mother and for the obstetrician, though it is hard to say what effect it has on the baby, since he still has to make that complex journey down the tight, resisting vagina, and may not notice the lights and music because he is preoccupied with other sensations.

If you ask whether being born can damage a baby, the answer has to be 'yes'. There are hazards in this, the most important journey a person makes in a whole lifetime, and they cannot be denied. Birth damage accounts for a considerable proportion of both physical and mental handicaps. Modern obstetrics are aimed at minimizing the risks, and preventing as far as possible any unnecessary damage. Hence the high-technology labour units and modern management techniques. It is a pity that some women have turned against these as 'unnatural' since they are designed to offer precisely what the mother most wants – a healthy undamaged baby born of a healthy undamaged mother. The natural way leads to a high death and damage rate, unfortunately.

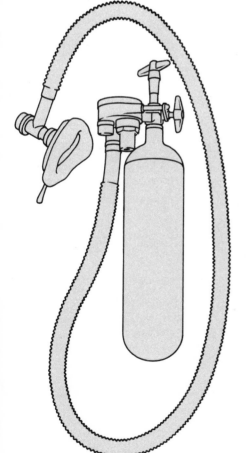

Pain relief on demand
A woman in labour can breathe pain-killing gas from this cylinder whenever she chooses

Women's disorders and childbirth

How does the mother's body know the right time to start labour? Why doesn't she push the baby out too soon?

How pregnancies are controlled is still partly a mystery. It is known that hormones are greatly involved with the placenta, the organ which acts as go-between for mother and baby and whose hormone output changes as it ages.

The weight of the baby inside the uterus seems to trigger a change in hormone production and have an effect. This is probably why multiple pregnancies tend to end prematurely, when the combined weight of the babies is that of a single full-term baby.

The baby's body itself may be involved, producing trigger hormones when it is sufficiently mature which then affect the mother's body.

One thing is sure; it is exceedingly rare for a sudden shock or dramatic experience to trigger immediate labour. Emotions, of course, have an effect on pregnancy and labour, but it is not such a violent or dramatic one as is sometimes suggested in the movies.

Why do babies have gaps in their skulls when they are born?

This is one of the mechanisms that make it possible for the baby to go on developing safely inside the uterus for a longer period while its brain grows. The skull bones are designed to glide over each other during the birth process and this makes it possible for quite a large head to be born safely. If the skull were as rigid at birth as it later becomes, it would fracture and damage the underlying brain as the pressures were put on it during the process of birth.

Before birth
A large gap still remains between the bones of the baby's skull (*right*)

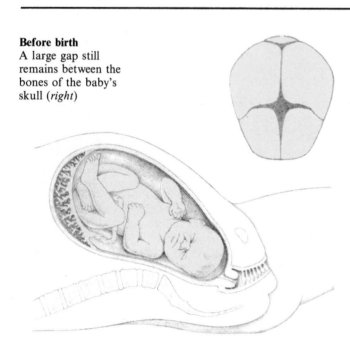

First stage
As the baby's head is squeezed through the cervix, the skull bones close up

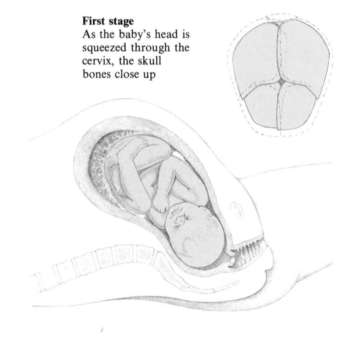

Second stage
'Crowning' is the emergence of the head as the baby is pushed out of the vagina

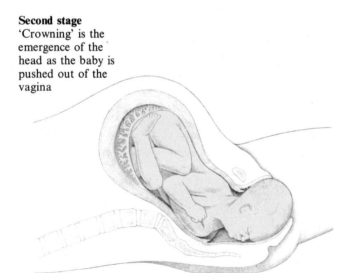

Afterbirth
Finally the placenta and umbilical cord, the link to the mother, are expelled

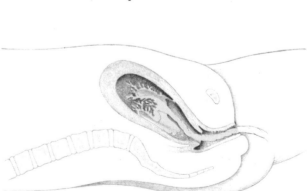

Obviously babies don't breathe inside their mothers, or they would drown. How is it they can breathe as soon as they are born?

When a baby is born fully conscious, that is, not depressed by anaesthetic drugs given to his mother, he takes his first gasp, probably as a reflex action following the cooling of his skin, as he hits the outside air. This first gasp is extremely powerful and can inflate his hitherto collapsed lungs. Once that has happened, comparatively weak breathing movements are enough to keep the oxygen flowing. It takes about 40 minutes for the baby's breathing to become totally easy and without effort.

Another effect of this sudden expansion of the lungs is alteration of the pressure of the blood inside the heart. This pressure change has the effect of closing a little passageway which the blood has used throughout intra-uterine life and which enabled it to bypass the lungs, and so forces the blood to go through the lungs. The baby's own body then takes on the job of supplying oxygen to his tissues – the job which the mother's placenta used to do for him.

Fetal blood flow
Circulation in the uterus takes routes (*dotted*) that close at birth. One is through the umbilical cord. Another bypasses the lungs, which are not yet functioning

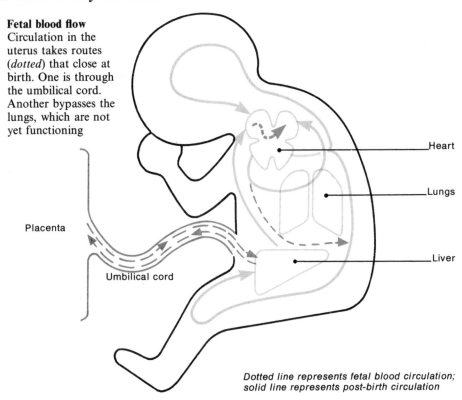

Placenta
Umbilical cord
Heart
Lungs
Liver

Dotted line represents fetal blood circulation; solid line represents post-birth circulation

Why are babies so helpless compared to new-born animals?

The most significant thing about the human species is its big brain. It is that which sets us apart from our animal relatives. A big brain demands a big skull to hold it, and a big skull is difficult to give birth to, unless the mother has a large pelvis.

Over the millennia we have evolved a pattern of gestation and birth that allows a baby to develop as far as is possible within the body, then allows it to pass as safely as possible through the narrow birth passage, followed by a system of care that allows it to complete its development to full self-reliance.

Our babies are still pretty immature when we produce them, but not as immature as all that. They can suck – a complex and vital action for survival; they can hold on (put your finger in your baby's palm and feel the power of his grip – he can support his own weight with it) and respond to many stimuli. The reflex actions of the new-born baby are, in their own way, as complex as the new-born foal's walking ability.

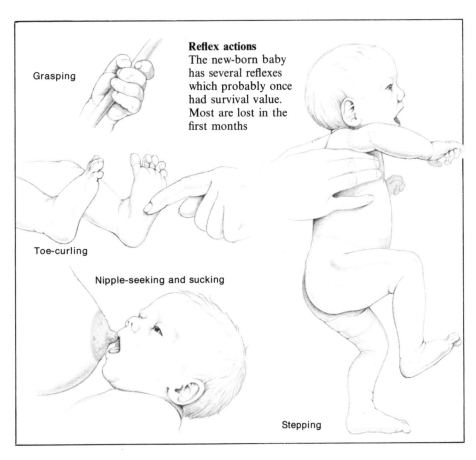

Grasping

Reflex actions
The new-born baby has several reflexes which probably once had survival value. Most are lost in the first months

Toe-curling

Nipple-seeking and sucking

Stepping

Women's disorders and childbirth

Why does a new mother not make food for her baby until three days have passed? Does the new baby not need food?

Although true milk may not appear in the mother's breasts until the third day after delivery, other food called colostrum has been made in the breasts throughout most of the pregnancy. It is a thick, yellowish, highly nutritious food, rich in antibodies to protect the baby against illness, and it is best to put the baby to the breast from birth, to receive colostrum at regular intervals. He may not take much of it at first, but what he takes he needs. Also his suckling will encourage the milk to come in sooner because suckling stimulates the gland tissue of the breast to produce more. This is why the more a baby feeds the more there is for him to be fed on.

Does breast-feeding ruin a woman's figure?

It may well change it. The human breast goes through a number of changes in a normal lifetime, and the changes from virgin to pregnant and then lactating are among them. It is a bit unreasonable to assume that a figure is 'ruined' just because it has changed from one state to another. It is not realistic for a woman still to expect to have the breasts of a 17-year-old when she is 37 and has had two or three children.

In fact a lot of women do manage to maintain the shapeliness of their breasts by watching their diets (excess fat spoils more breasts than pregnancies and feedings) and the use of supportive bras. The no-bra look may offer liberation but it also allows the breasts to sag, which is probably natural. Look at the pictures of African tribeswomen to see how adult breasts are probably meant to look.

It is really pointless to avoid feeding for fear of losing breast shape or size. It is the changes of pregnancy that alter the shape of the breasts, rather than the effects of milk-making and giving. Some women are constitutionally designed to become flatter and more pendulous after a birth than others – it's more luck than judgement.

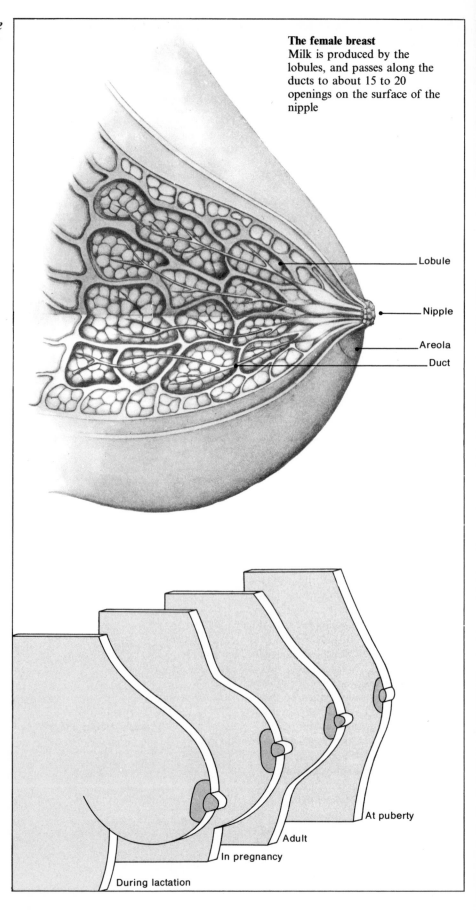

The female breast
Milk is produced by the lobules, and passes along the ducts to about 15 to 20 openings on the surface of the nipple

Lobule

Nipple

Areola

Duct

At puberty

Adult

In pregnancy

During lactation

Why do some mothers fail when they try to breast-feed? Does this mean their babies would die if we didn't have artificial feeding methods?

There can be many reasons for feeding problems, both physical and psychological. Some women have nipples which are difficult for the baby to grasp. Some have excess fat tissue and this gets in the way of the baby's nose and mouth when he is put to the breast. Some women experience a delay in producing enough milk and so the baby is unsatisfied and will not suckle because he is frustrated. This means that the breasts are not stimulated and that less and less milk is made, which is a vicious circle.

Feeding can also be affected by a mother's psychological state. She may have a deep-down dislike of the idea of breast-feeding, or regard her breasts as sexual objects to share with her partner rather than feeding objects to share with her baby. The possible hang-ups about breast-feeding are many and attempts to nag or coax or shame a mother out of them only make them worse, usually because they are ill understood by the mother herself.

In a purely natural, that is, primitive state, babies of such mothers probably would die – which is what survival of the fittest is all about. But we have artificial methods which, properly used, are safe and effective, so today these babies live and grow healthily, and their mothers are happy.

Breast feeding
The baby's vigorous sucking of the nipple stimulates the flow of milk

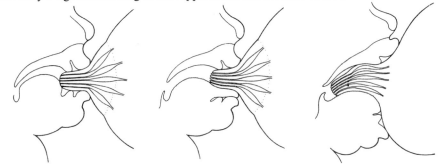

Removing the baby's mouth from the nipple

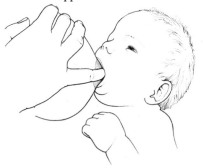

Why do women's nipples keep on changing from smooth and flat to pointed and wrinkled?

A nipple, like the clitoris (the sexually responsive area in a woman's vulva – the surface sex organs) and the male penis, is made of erectile tissue. It can take in a lot of blood which fills the spaces in it, and holds on to it so that it becomes hard and erect.

There are several stimuli apart from a baby ready to feed which make the relaxed nipple erect – cold air, for example. Another is sexual excitement and this is closely linked with the feeding experience. The pleasure a woman feels from nipple stimulation triggers the pituitary gland, which in turn encourages the erection of the nipple and other signs of sexual arousal. It is a loop action – getting a stimulus gives pleasure which seeks more stimulus which increases the pleasure. This is why a breast-feeding mother gets physical satisfaction out of feeding her baby. It is similar to the pleasure she gets from lovemaking, and it is meant to be. Some women are embarrassed by it, and try to hide it, which is a pity.

If I have an operation to enlarge my breasts will it stop me from breast-feeding any babies I have later on?

It depends on the operation that is done. A careful implant should not interfere with breast gland tissue and it is the glands which make the breast milk. A good cosmetic surgeon operating on a young woman is always aware of the need to maintain the breasts' function while changing their appearance.

Operations to reduce breasts can also be done with a view to preserving breast-feeding ability later on.

The areola in pregnancy
The areola, the zone around the nipple, is pink in a light-skinned woman who has not borne children. During pregnancy, it becomes darker and the glands beneath it swell, giving it a bumpy appearance. After the breast-feeding period the areola lightens but always keeps a brown colour

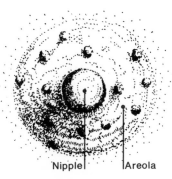

Nipple | Areola

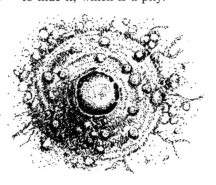

Babies and children

Most of the illnesses which affect adults can also affect children; so the specialist doctors who look after adults can also look after their children. A gastro-enterologist, an ophthalmologist, an endocrinologist has as much to offer to children as anyone else. However, children are rather more than just miniature adults. The problems they have are special: because childhood is a time of rapid growth and development, this must affect any illnesses they have. So, the speciality of paediatrics has developed – the care of the ills of children. In one sense, a paediatrician is a Jack of all trades, since he does not confine his expertise to any one body system. He applies it to an age group. But he is expert in the needs of that age group, and in many families enjoys the status of a friend.

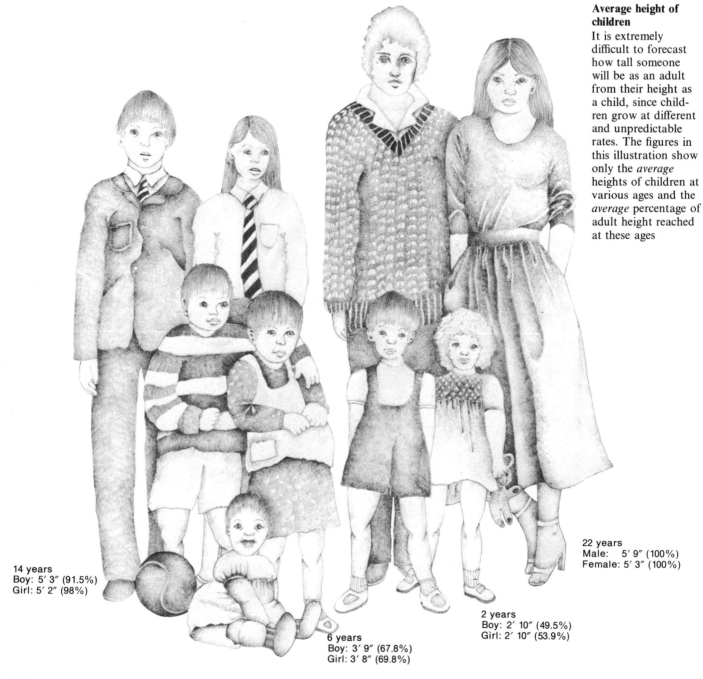

Average height of children
It is extremely difficult to forecast how tall someone will be as an adult from their height as a child, since children grow at different and unpredictable rates. The figures in this illustration show only the *average* heights of children at various ages and the *average* percentage of adult height reached at these ages

14 years
Boy: 5′ 3″ (91.5%)
Girl: 5′ 2″ (98%)

6 years
Boy: 3′ 9″ (67.8%)
Girl: 3′ 8″ (69.8%)

2 years
Boy: 2′ 10″ (49.5%)
Girl: 2′ 10″ (53.9%)

22 years
Male: 5′ 9″ (100%)
Female: 5′ 3″ (100%)

Can you foretell a child's eventual height and appearance when he is a baby?

A baby changes a great deal as he develops and many of his later characteristics will not show at all when he is an infant. No baby is born with a large curving nose – nearly every baby's nose looks like a dab of putty. Similarly, a square-cut chin, high cheek bones or a broad brow may be built into the baby for the future, but it will not show for many years yet.

Eye colour will change, and so will hair; eyes are always blue at birth (announcing eye colour in a new-born baby has always struck me as somewhat absurd for this reason) and slowly develop their permanent colour over the first months of life, just as hair colour changes, especially in light-haired children who become darker.

Height depends on two factors; the baby's genes, and the sort of environment and feeding which he receives. Many of the shortish older people around in the world were born to be six foot, but were not fed sufficiently to get them much beyond five foot or so.

During World War I the British authorities were appalled to discover just how wizened and underdeveloped the men conscripted from the slums were, and a new policy regarding the nutrition and care of the poor was born as a result. Today we feed our children with greater care than we were fed ourselves (though sometimes we tend to overfeed them, which is another form of malnutrition) so that most of them will achieve their full growth potential.

One rule of thumb that can be used is that 'like produces like'. So, two tall parents will have mostly tall children, and two short parents will have mostly short ones. If a tall man marries an average-sized woman, their children will probably be shorter than he is; if a short man marries an average-sized woman, their children will probably be taller than he is.

The sex differential should be taken into account, of course; there is supposed to be a six-inch difference between the sexes (the average European and American male is five feet eight inches, the average female five feet two inches). However, as we all know, few of us are average, and most of us seem to choose partners close to us in height. So, a man of five foot eight inches may well have a five-foot-seven-inch wife, which counts as tall for statistical purposes, and their children will probably be rather taller than average as a result.

Growth is rapid in the first two years of life, but slows down around the second birthday, so another popular rule of thumb is that a child of two is half his adult height. Not his adult weight, however; he will weigh only one eighth of that. One experimenter measured his two-year-old child, and found that all his body proportions – height, girth, leg length and so on – were half that of his own. But his son weighed 28 pounds while he weighed 210 pounds. Height can be accurately predicted from an X-ray analysis of the wrist bones of a child. This is important for certain careers, for example, acceptance at a ballet school.

My new-born babies are twins. How alike will they be?

It depends on what kind of twins they are. If they developed from a single egg – these are called monozygotic or monovular twins – they will be of the same sex, and identical in appearance, unless they grow up apart, in which case appearance will be modified. We all get a good deal of our appearance from our environmental experiences.

If the twins developed from two separate eggs – dizygotic or binovular – they are fraternal twins, and no more similar than any other pair of brothers and sisters. They may be of the same sex, or different.

It is fraternal twinning that runs in families, incidentally – as a tendency for women to release two eggs from the ovary at the same time, both of which are fertilized. Fertility drugs can also cause twinning, stimulating the ovaries to release extra eggs, and these twins again are fraternal.

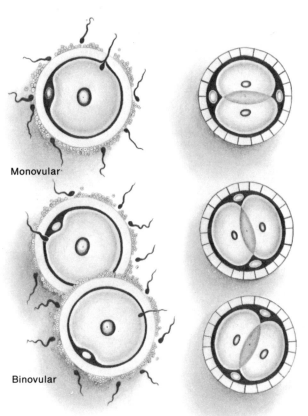

Monovular

Binovular

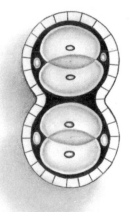

Conception of twins
Twins may be caused either by a single fertilized egg dividing (monovular), or by two separate eggs being fertilized at the same time (binovular). Monovular twins will be identical in both appearance and gender, while binovular twins will be no more alike than ordinary brothers or sisters who were conceived at different times

Babies and children

Why do doctors fuss so much about breast-feeding? After all, bottle-fed babies do just as well, and make life easier for a mother.

The feeding of babies has always been subject to fashion. There was a time in the early part of the century when bottle-feeding was regarded as more 'scientific' and therefore better. Then there came a revulsion against modernity, and a new and now widespread interest in Nature and Ecology, and this made breast-feeding fashionable again among some sections of the population.

Inevitably, this means that individual mothers may be confused and worried, especially if they have anxieties about breast-feeding, for any reason. Not all women want to breast-feed, perhaps because of misplaced prudery, or because of fear of damage to the breast which they value more for its sexual characteristics than as feeding equipment, or because of a husband who resents sharing his wife with his own infant. Whatever the reason for her unwillingness to breast-feed, such a mother may be made uneasy by hectoring on the subject.

The physiological facts are that there is a great deal of evidence that breast-fed babies are healthier and have fewer feeding problems than bottle-fed ones. This is because human milk is the ideal food for the human infant. It contains the precise nutrients that the baby needs, in the precise mix, and also offers antibodies – disease-fighting materials – from the mother. The milk comes to the baby uncontaminated by any infecting organisms, is always at the right temperature and is always available at the drop of a hat, or certainly the unbuttoning of a shirt. Breast-fed babies rarely suffer from allergy (many bottle-fed babies react unfavourably to cow's milk), rarely get obese (a common problem in the bottle-fed), and hardly ever suffer from gastro-enteritis (a condition that in severe cases can be fatal and which is a risk in bottle-feeding).

So, there are many strong reasons to encourage it. However, there is also a psychological aspect to be taken into account. The bond between mother and baby must be strong if the baby is to thrive. Babies need more than mere food and physical care. Love is an essential nutrient. And if a mother breast-feeds against her will, and feels resentment of the baby as a result, it will not benefit him.

So, in some cases bottle-feeding is acceptable, if not ideal. As long as scrupulous care is taken to sterilize all feeding utensils, and the milk mix is carefully worked out for the individual baby, he will grow and thrive well.

Good paediatricians know this, and though they will regret a refusal to breast-feed, they should be able to help a mother and her baby do well without making her feel she has failed in some sort of way as a mother.

Why do babies have so much trouble with wind?

There is no real evidence that they do. For many years mothers who have been unable to find any other reason for a baby's fretfulness have said he was suffering from wind in his belly which caused pain, but this is rarely, if ever, the case. A baby will swallow a good deal of air while sucking, especially if he has an inexperienced mother who does not know how to help him to get his jaws firmly round the nipple. This air will fill the stomach, and may make the child stop sucking before he has had enough food. He will then sleep as usual but some time during his sleep will either burp the wind up again, or it will pass on through into his gut, leaving him hungry again. So, he will cry for more food. Also, when he burps, he may bring up some of his milk with the air, and this, too, adds to his hunger.

For this reason, mothers have learned to sit a baby upright half-way through a feed to burp up swallowed air, and then top him up with more milk. It doesn't really make much difference to the baby if she doesn't – he will happily wake and demand feeding after two hours and not care. But his mother, who would rather he slept for four hours, will care. So she can do it if she wants to, but it is not essential to do so.

Some babies do suffer a form of colic in which they seem to experience discomfort from spasms of the gut, but again there is no evidence that air in the gut has anything to do with it. It is more often due to an anxious mother in whom tension has built up during the long day, or it is possibly due to boredom. By the age of three months or so a baby is ready to add something more interesting than feeding and sleeping to his life. The discomfort tends to clear up by itself after a few exhausting weeks, by which time the mother has probably found out why her baby is crying, and has removed the cause.

Extra milk
The supply of a mother's milk may be uneven in the first weeks following the birth, and this may mean that she has some milk left in her breasts at the end of a feed. They should be emptied either by gently squeezing the breast as shown, or by the use of a simple hand pump

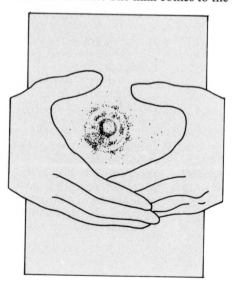
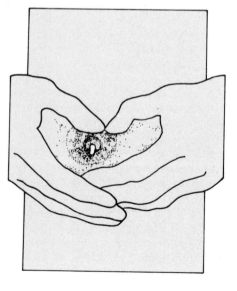

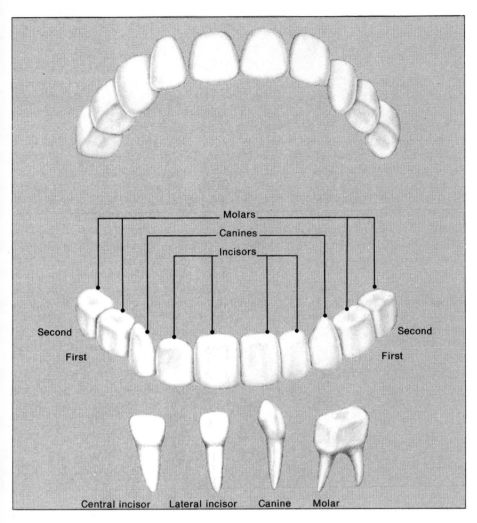

Molars
Canines
Incisors

Second
First

Second
First

Central incisor   Lateral incisor   Canine   Molar

Milk teeth

The milk teeth usually begin to grow between six and 10 months after birth, when the central and lateral incisors appear. These are followed during the second year by the first molars and the canines. The second molars are the last to appear, sometime during the third year. Usually the lower teeth appear before the upper set, and girls begin, and end, teething before boys do

Why does teething cause a baby so much misery? Can anything be done to prevent it?

This is another myth, similar to the 'wind' one. In fact, teething is not inevitably painful. The only thing we actually know that results from teething is teeth. Most babies start showing their milk teeth at around the age of seven or eight months, and will go on doing so until the age of around two-and-a-half years. They also produce new teeth from the age of six or so until the age of 13 plus, but no one ever says a six-year-old is suffering from 'teething' problems. Only babies are so diagnosed.

The reason is that during the first two or so years of life a baby is exposed to many infections, and develops symptoms as a result. Also, he is having to learn how to fit into a complex adult world with all its (to him) absurd rules and regulations. This makes him frequently angry and unhappy. The result of both experiences is often fretfulness, sleeplessness, fever, nausea and vomiting – it is hard in the very young to sort out physical from emotional difficulties. To have something convenient to blame for such episodes helps adults – and teeth are a handy scapegoat.

The only symptoms which can be directly ascribed to pain from teeth are dribbling, and a red patch on the cheek over the affected side. If a mild painkiller removes the symptoms, then the reason was a sharp tooth. But it is really comparatively rare. All other unexpected ills – vomiting, wheezing, coughs and colds, fevers – need to be treated seriously and not dismissed as 'mere teething'. Too often, because of this false idea, babies have been allowed to get quite ill instead of being taken much earlier to a doctor.

Why do children have two sets of teeth? What is the use of milk teeth?

We really are rather deprived in terms of teeth, in having only two sets. Many other animals can produce set after set, as each one wears out – for example, the shark. Other animals have teeth that go on growing in length all their lives, because they wear them down with eating – for example, the horse.

The milk teeth, the first set, which are shed between the ages of six and eight years or so, start appearing at around the age of seven to eight months, though there is great variation in the normal range. They are small, and this is probably why the permanent teeth are held back; the jaw has to grow, and permanent teeth, which must be large enough to fill it and strong enough to last a lifetime, or as much as possible of it, could not fit a young mouth.

Their value is the same as that of permanent teeth – to enable a child to chew his food. They also help to shape the growing jaw; if they are absent the second dentition is affected because the jaw has remained so small that the permanent teeth may come through crowded and crooked. This is why the care of milk teeth is as important as later tooth care. They must be regularly brushed and, if necessary, filled to preserve them. It is also the reason why it is so important to limit a child's intake of sugary foods. These can stick to the teeth and make a perfect medium for organisms, and this leads to dental caries – decay. To say 'it doesn't matter – they're only the milk teeth' – is tantamount to saying that the later teeth don't matter either.

Babies and children

Why do children get so many illnesses?
It seems like one thing after another in the first
years – chickenpox, measles, colds and coughs.

We are all of us always under attack by the micro-organisms that share this world with us (and which were undoubtedly here before we were). Our bodies have developed effective immune systems to repel these attacks. When we are invaded by an organism, special cells make antibodies (substances which have a specific killing effect against the invading organism). We also produce other fight-back mechanisms, including white cells which gobble up the organisms, and the liver which destroys the poisons which the organisms make.

We need to be exposed to a specific organism only once to be equipped with a lifelong supply of antibody against it. Chickenpox, measles, whooping cough and the other childish illnesses are cases in point. Once you have had these, you won't get them again because the invading organisms will be routed at once.

New-born and breast-fed babies have a supply of antibodies collected from their mothers and this confers protection for the first few weeks or months, but not for a lifetime. The child has to manufacture his own antibodies when he encounters the various organisms.

That is why children get the illnesses – measles and so on – which adults do not: the adults have already had them.

Coughs and colds are slightly different. These can be caused by a wide range of different organisms, often viruses, which do not have the specific effect of those that cause, say, measles. There are probably hundreds if not thousands of different organisms which cause the symptoms of a cold. This means that although we may have antibodies to one virus, we will not to another, so we get cold after cold all through our lives. But we get them more often in childhood because we have not yet built up any antibodies at all. As people grow older they build up an armoury and get fewer such infections as a result.

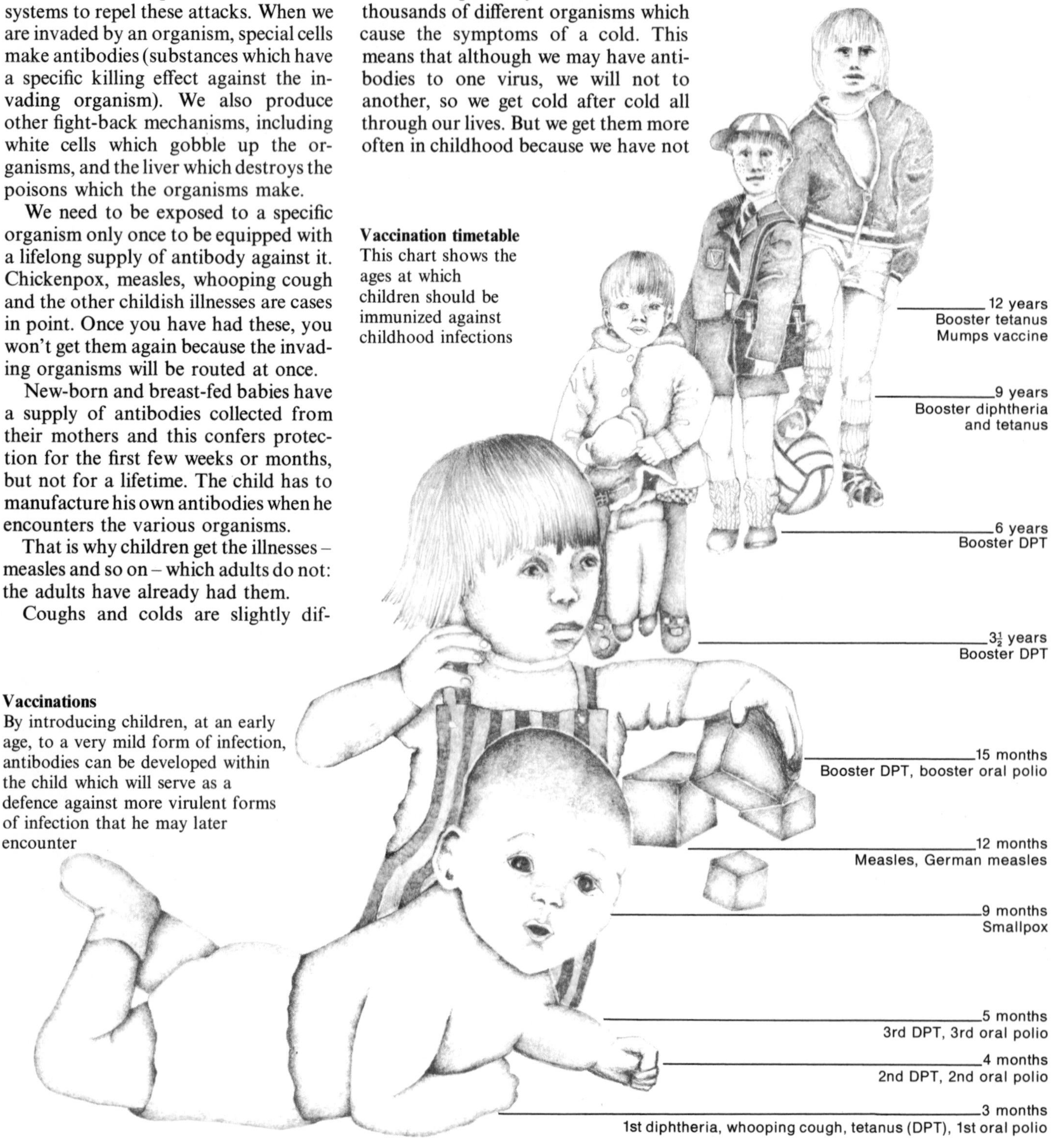

Vaccinations
By introducing children, at an early age, to a very mild form of infection, antibodies can be developed within the child which will serve as a defence against more virulent forms of infection that he may later encounter

Vaccination timetable
This chart shows the ages at which children should be immunized against childhood infections

12 years
Booster tetanus
Mumps vaccine

9 years
Booster diphtheria
and tetanus

6 years
Booster DPT

$3\frac{1}{2}$ years
Booster DPT

15 months
Booster DPT, booster oral polio

12 months
Measles, German measles

9 months
Smallpox

5 months
3rd DPT, 3rd oral polio

4 months
2nd DPT, 2nd oral polio

3 months
1st diphtheria, whooping cough, tetanus (DPT), 1st oral polio

How do immunizations work? Are they really safe for babies? We hear so many stories of babies who have been brain damaged by them.

In simple terms, an immunization is a deliberate triggering of the immune response, but by using a dose of the organisms which is too small and too weak to cause a full-blown disease. It takes very little to get the antibodies going, and immunization techniques are based on this.

As for the danger – the hard facts are that millions of humans have died over the centuries from diseases such as smallpox, diphtheria, polio, tetanus, and typhoid which we no longer suffer, or very rarely. This is because of widespread immunization programmes which have prevented epidemics.

More recently, the development of a vaccine to protect us against measles has saved many lives, for this is a potentially very dangerous illness indeed, and a vaccine which prevents rubella (German measles) also helps to protect unborn babies who may suffer damage if their mothers catch it while pregnant.

The vaccine that has caused a certain amount of anguish is the one given to prevent whooping cough. This disease, too, can be severe, even fatal in some cases, and protection is well worth seeking. Sadly, a small number of children have reacted unfavourably to it and sustained brain damage, but this does not mean that all immunization programmes are likely to have this effect. Millions of children have been safely protected, and it would be tragic if the diseases were allowed again to get a hold over us, for fear of a risk that is, in truth, a very small one.

Children at risk of bad reactions to whooping cough vaccine can sometimes be identified. A child with a history of allergy or asthma or eczema (both of which can have an allergic base) or one who is not in the best of health at the time, should not have the vaccine, but be occasionally reassessed for suitability.

Travel sickness
An infant who has a tendency to be travel-sick is always safer if he is kept lying on his front to prevent the risk of his inhaling vomit

Why do babies sometimes have fits when they have high temperatures? Does this mean they will develop epilepsy later on?

No, it does not, provided that the convulsions are proved to be due to high fever. The brain of a small child is less stable than that of an adult and more easily irritated by fever. A sharp rise in temperature of the sort that commonly happens in an infection in a child, stimulates the brain which triggers the nerves supplying the muscles and causes the alarming rigidity and twitching. There is also temporary unconsciousness and the baby may froth at the mouth and breathe stertorously – an alarming sight indeed.

A convulsion (the word means the same as fit) is always followed by sleep. Never leave a child in a convulsion, because although it is never fatal, if a child vomits during a convulsion he may choke. So he needs someone with him to make sure that this does not happen (keep the child turned to the side so that any potentially choking material can run out of his mouth).

An epileptic fit may look the same, and a doctor may have to perform tests, such as an EEG to make a firm diagnosis. But once a parent has been assured that a fit was merely fever-induced, she need not fear that the nature of the fits will change into epilepsy. These are two separate conditions.

Incidentally, a tendency to feverish convulsions may run in a family.

Why do children get travel-sick?

The organ of balance, which is the ear, is disturbed when unusual motion is experienced and this sets up a chain of reflexes that spread into the brain and reach the vomiting centre. This is why the travel-sick person throws up.

The condition is, therefore, partly physical in nature, but there is a strong psychological effect. A person who fears and expects to be travel-sick may start to vomit even before a ship moves. So, a child who has parents who expect him to be sick in the car will usually oblige.

A calm uninterest in whether the child vomits or not will help to reduce the amount of sickness. Being equipped with receptacles, deodorizers and clean-up tissues helps parents to relax, and therefore helps the child to be less sick than he might. Many children as they grow up and become less susceptible to their parents', and other adults', behaviour and expectations, lose the tendency for car-sickness. It is rare in adults, though sea-sickness is a common problem at all ages.

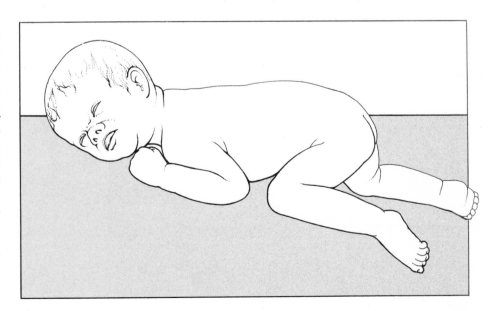

Babies and children

My little boy of 10 is so nice, friendly, easy-going, polite. But my 13-year-old nephew, who used to be the same, is so repellent – stubborn, noisy and difficult. Are adolescent miseries inevitable?

Adolescent change is inevitable and it would be dreadful if it weren't. No one would want to rear an adult who was in behaviour, attitude and outlook a 10-year-old.

Some children and their parents are able to weather the changes with the minimum of fuss. They have their disagreements, but the parents are able to remember how it felt to be adolescent and respond with sympathy and firmness, and they don't bully or nag or complain unduly.

Other parents, however, are less skilful and themselves foment many of the family hassles that arise. They seem almost to set out to make life tough for the developing personality – they complain they are having terrible trouble with their child when, in fact, he is having much worse trouble with them.

Also, the personality of the child comes into it. Some are particularly sensitive, touchy, fast to rise to a taunt, secretive and withdrawn by nature. Others are docile, outgoing, easy-to-get-on-with people. Allowing for these individual personality differences is an essential part of parenting this age group.

With a lot of good will, common sense, and an understanding of when to keep your mouth shut and when to put your foot down, parents can make the change-over quite pleasant. But it is never easy, for either side.

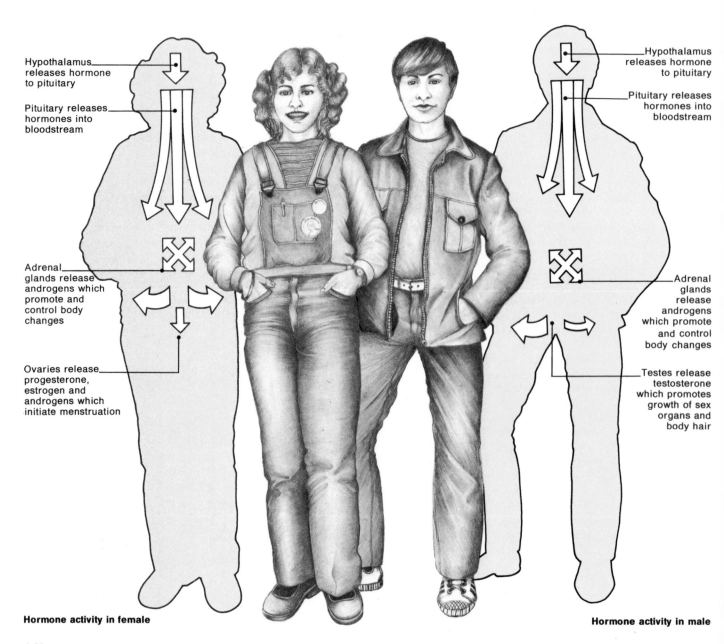

Hypothalamus releases hormone to pituitary

Pituitary releases hormones into bloodstream

Adrenal glands release androgens which promote and control body changes

Ovaries release progesterone, estrogen and androgens which initiate menstruation

Hypothalamus releases hormone to pituitary

Pituitary releases hormones into bloodstream

Adrenal glands release androgens which promote and control body changes

Testes release testosterone which promotes growth of sex organs and body hair

Hormone activity in female

Hormone activity in male

I have noticed that sometimes one of my four-year-old son's sex organs disappears. It comes down again, especially when he is in the bath, but I am afraid he is not growing up right.

It is very common indeed for this to happen to a boy's testicles. As long as the testicle can come down easily you have no need to worry. In time – when he reaches puberty – it will start to grow and won't be able to slip up inside its little tube quite so easily. The reason testicles do this is that they first develop inside the body where they are safe and protected, and only later come down at around the time of birth. In some young boys they do move around a lot.

Hormone activity of adolescence
The onset of adolescence is triggered by hormonal action within the body. Under the influence of the hypothalamus, the pituitary releases hormones, which act on the adrenal glands, testes and ovaries, and cause them to release other hormones which promote the physical changes of adolescence

Physical changes in adolescence
During adolescence the body undergoes physical changes which mark the step from child to adult. There is no set pattern for these changes, which can be confusing and awkward for the adolescent, and the age at which the changes begin may vary greatly from one child to another

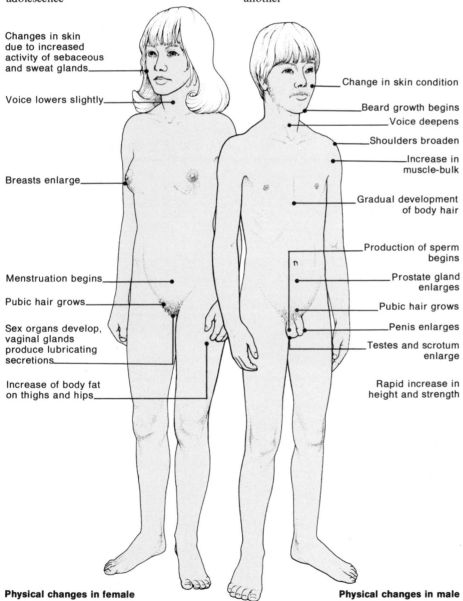

Changes in skin due to increased activity of sebaceous and sweat glands

Voice lowers slightly

Breasts enlarge

Menstruation begins

Pubic hair grows

Sex organs develop, vaginal glands produce lubricating secretions

Increase of body fat on thighs and hips

Change in skin condition

Beard growth begins

Voice deepens

Shoulders broaden

Increase in muscle-bulk

Gradual development of body hair

Production of sperm begins

Prostate gland enlarges

Pubic hair grows

Penis enlarges

Testes and scrotum enlarge

Rapid increase in height and strength

Physical changes in female

Physical changes in male

Why do some babies have a belly button that sticks out, and some have one that is turned in?

The belly button, or navel (umbilicus is the proper term) is the stump of the cord that connected the baby to his mother before birth. The way the cord is cut and tied may affect the size of the resulting scar – some are rather larger than others.

The other factor that matters is the depth of fat over the belly wall. A baby with a lot of fat will have a dimpled navel, as the fat rises all round it. One with a skinny build will have a bump.

In a few cases, there may be a hernia – a loop of the underlying gut pushes up into the scar tissue because this is a weakened area. Such a hernia is not dangerous, but it may be considered unsightly. A pressure bandage to push the loop of gut back often cures the problem, if it is used until the belly muscles have tautened enough to control the hernia themselves. In a very few cases, a simple operation is needed.

My son is 14 and is a fine healthy boy, but he's told me he's very worried because his breasts are growing just like a girl's. He won't show me and he refuses to go swimming. I do notice it through his shirt sometimes. He won't go to the doctor, and I'm getting extremely worried about him.

There is no need for either of you to worry. This is called 'gynaecomastia' which means literally 'feminine breasts' but it does not mean that your boy is changing sex, or failing to develop as he should. It is something that happens to a great many boys (more than half, in fact) as they go into puberty – the stage at which their bodies change from those of children to those of men – and in the vast majority of cases it disappears within three years. Some men, however, are always a little more fleshy over the chest than others: of course allow your boy to cover himself, because he's entitled to his privacy, and suggest to him that he tells his friends that he has a sensitive skin and has to wear a tee-shirt when he swims in case of sunburn.

Sexual disorders

Sex therapists are the newest of all the specialists. There was a time when no one talked much at all about sex, and certainly never to complain about the quality of the erotic experience. Today, however, expectations of all kinds of happiness run high among the richer peoples of the world – and this includes expectations of sexual happiness, in a climate where contraception is increasingly reliable. The pioneer workers in this field were the American researchers Masters and Johnson; their studies produced new ideas and techniques which can be used to improve considerably the sexual satisfaction of couples; sex therapy is the application of these ideas and techniques.

Forms of contraceptive

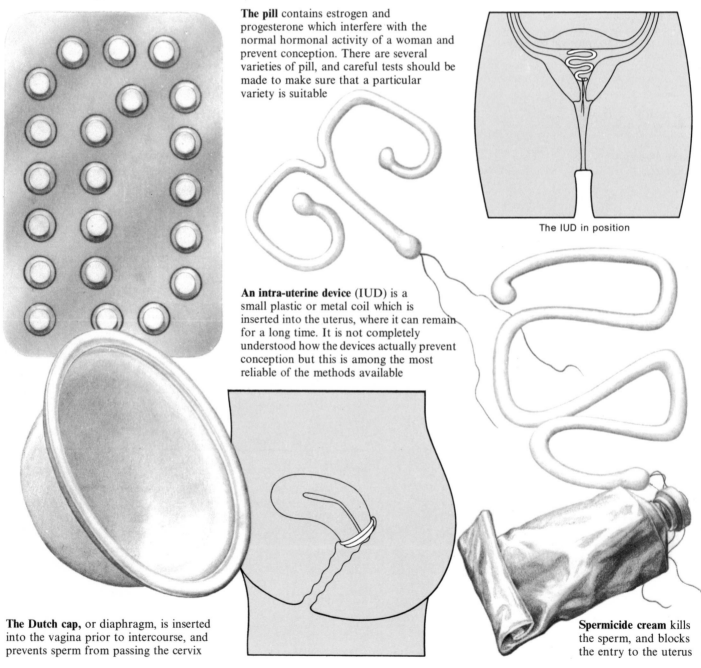

The pill contains estrogen and progesterone which interfere with the normal hormonal activity of a woman and prevent conception. There are several varieties of pill, and careful tests should be made to make sure that a particular variety is suitable

The IUD in position

An intra-uterine device (IUD) is a small plastic or metal coil which is inserted into the uterus, where it can remain for a long time. It is not completely understood how the devices actually prevent conception but this is among the most reliable of the methods available

The Dutch cap, or diaphragm, is inserted into the vagina prior to intercourse, and prevents sperm from passing the cervix

Spermicide cream kills the sperm, and blocks the entry to the uterus

What is the best method of contraception nowadays? There have been so many scares about the different ways.

We really are very lucky. Our great grandmothers had really only one choice. No babies? No sex. We, however, have an embarrassment of choice; the Pill, various barriers, chemicals, sterilization, rhythm. Different people have different needs but with so many possible methods, few are unable to find one that suits them.

A method has to be judged on three basic factors; its contraceptive safety, its health safety and its personal accept-

ability. One that is less contraceptively safe than another, but more safe in health terms for a particular individual, will make it more personally acceptable. For example, a woman aged 35 who is overweight and a cigarette smoker faces health hazards if she uses the Pill. So, she (and her doctor) will feel happier with an IUD (intra-uterine device) or the cap or diaphragm, although that is less contraceptively sure. If she is bothered by the need to remember to use her cap

and fears she cannot trust herself to be reliable, then she may find the IUD the most personally acceptable. If she dislikes them both, and her partner is happy to use the condom then that might be the most personally acceptable method. The permutations have to be worked out for each individual couple.

The chart here may help you decide, but it is always wise to discuss the matter with your doctor or at an International Planned Parenthood Centre.

Contraceptive safety	Health safety	Pro	Con
Pill 98% +	Some women at risk of thrombosis: the over-30s, the overweight, smokers, those with high blood pressure or a family history of blood vessel disease. If more than one of these is present, the risk rises	Simple to use. Makes some women feel extra well. Controls painful periods. May control acne. Protects against benign breast disease	Makes some women headachey/depressed, lose sex drive (may be psychological effects, not hormonal). Occasionally causes weight gain. Other drugs, attacks of diarrhoea or vomiting, may alter the Pill's effect
I.U.D. 97%–98%	.001% have perforations. Under 1% of users have sepsis	Simplest of all – no need to think about it, once fitted	May cause heavy, crampy periods at first. May be pushed out altogether
Cap/Diaphragm Below 90% if used alone. 96% – 98% if used with chemical	May be allergic response in sensitive subjects. Cystitis sufferers may find their condition aggravated	Linked only with intercourse. Does not interfere with normal body processes	Demands preparation for every act of intercourse. Needs regular washing and care
Condom 94% if used alone. 98% if used with chemical	May be allergic response in sensitive subjects	Male method. Absolves woman of responsibility and control	Male method. Deprives woman of responsibility and control
Chemicals 60%–90%	May be allergic response in sensitive subjects	Linked only with intercourse. Gives added lubrication	May be messy. Often unreliable and should not be used alone
Sterilization (males) 100% after tests (females) 98%–99.8%	May be depression in unprepared people	Permanent. Removes all fear of pregnancy for always	Permanent. Difficult to reverse if you change your mind and want another child
Rhythm 60%–90%	Nil	Suits Catholics who cannot use mechanical methods, and naturalists	Very unreliable. Demands considerable control of sex drive
Withdrawal 60%–90%	Nil	Cheap. Needs no doctor's advice – so is very personal	Very unreliable. May leave woman unsatisfied

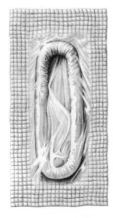

A condom prevents sperm from entering the vagina

Sterilization is a surgical operation, which results in permanent loss of fertility. In the male operation the vas deferens tubes, along which the sperm travel from the testes, are cut. In the female operation the Fallopian tubes are cut

Condom

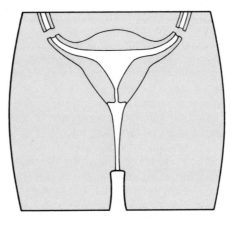

Female sterilization

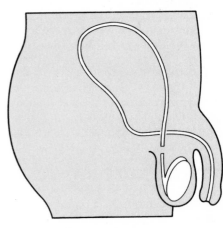

Male sterilization

Sexual disorders

Why do some women lose their sex drive?

The most obvious cause is the fractured marriage. It can happen that there are deep emotional and psychological rifts between the partners that have never been consciously admitted. When this happens, a disturbance in sexual feeling can be a symptom of underlying unhappiness, and needs to be recognized for what it is.

The physical causes are often, though not always, linked with emotional/psychological ones. Sex drive, like so many body functions, is under the control of the hormones.

These derive from a number of different glands but the ones most involved in sexual feeling are the hypothalamus and pituitary, situated deep in the brain, and the sex organs, which in women are the ovaries.

The hypothalamus, acting via the pituitary, sends out a little spurt of stimulating hormone, which affects the ovaries, and they in turn produce two important hormones, estrogen and progesterone. These are involved with periods, egg production, conception, pregnancy and birth, and also sex drive.

Generally, it is believed to be estrogen which makes a woman feel in the mood for sex; but women vary enormously in the way they respond to their own estrogen levels. Some women are eager for sex on quite low estrogen blood levels; others need to have much higher ones before they feel any flicker of interest. And some women are more responsive to a high progesterone level than to a high estrogen one. There are many factors involved in this whole subject of the chemistry of sex that still remain mysteries to the researchers.

So, what triggers the production of hormones, and thus creates the levels that lead to a desire for sexual intercourse?

The triggers are both physical and psychological. Simple mechanical stimulation of areas of the body that are responsive to sexual touch – they have been labelled the 'erogenous zones' and they include the lips and tongue, the breasts, especially the nipples, and the surface sex organs, especially the clitoris – can be enough to make the hypothalamus send out its initiating spurt of hormone. This is why foreplay, the kissing, cuddling and caressing that precede intercourse, are so important to a woman.

But the hypothalamus often needs an additional nudge to make it start off hormone production, and this comes from the brain cortex – the thinking part. The sight of an attractive man, the thought of sexual contact, sounds, sights and smells that have previously been linked with enjoyable sex, all these can make a woman think of lovemaking, and set her hormones into action.

And, very importantly, the operation of hormones affects other hormones in the body because each stimulates the others. The hypothalamus responds not only to touching of erogenous zones and conscious thoughts about sex, but also to blood levels of hormones. So, after it has started off sexual feeling the hypothalamus goes on triggering more because it responds to the changes it has itself created. Sexual appetite increases the more it is fed, and decreases the less it is fed. Which is why sex therapists say so often 'If you don't want to lose it – use it.'

Clearly, any disorder of the hypothalamus, the pituitary and the ovaries which results in changes in the ability to create the necessary hormone levels can affect the way a woman feels. Disorder of the hypothalamus and pituitary is fairly rare but disorder of the ovaries is much more common. The most common is the menopause.

When women reach the end of their reproductive years, the ovaries falter and slowly lose their ability to release new eggs to be made into babies; they also produce their hormones in differing ways. In some women this results in a loss of drive – but by no means in all women. Many of them find that the changes of the menopause result in hormone levels that make them much more eager for sex. This is because a woman's natural male hormone, androgen, (all women have some) is less constrained by estrogen, and androgen is a potent sexual stimulator.

There are other times in a woman's life when a normal change in the way the ovaries operate can affect her sex drive. Pregnancy is an obvious one: some women feel greatly increased sex drive during pregnancy, others lose all interest.

Similarly, some women find in the early months after a birth that their drive is greatly diminished. Indeed, this is so common that some researchers wonder whether this might not be a biological reaction. They suggest that perhaps nature has equipped new mothers with a form of built-in contraceptive; by making them unresponsive it protects them from getting pregnant again too soon. Such a loss of sex drive in the first months, or even the whole year, after a birth, is common. Other researchers, however, see it as a symptom of post-birth depression.

Not only the dramatic changes of conception, pregnancy and birth alter a woman's responses; so can the regular monthly ebbing and flowing of hormone balance that is marked by the periods. Some women suffer an imbalance of their hormones in the week before their period is due that results in a build-up of body fluid, weight gain, headaches, irritability, loss of concentration and loss of sex drive.

The use of the Pill method of contraception which acts by changing hormone balances, may lead to a loss of drive. Gynaecologists help each woman to find a brand of Pill which suits her and does not cause this side effect.

All these might be called the 'normal disorders' of the ovaries in that they are certainly not diseases; the ovaries are simply not running as smoothly as they might.

The next obvious cause of lack of sexual drive is illness.

In certain diseases involving the uterus the operation of hysterectomy (removal of the uterus) is sometimes advised, and if this operation includes the ovaries it can lead to a sex-drive problem. If the ovaries are removed, the hormone levels are profoundly affected. However nowadays, when the ovaries are removed, most doctors will replace the missing hormones in pill form, and after an initial readjustment period the woman should be able to regain her old responses.

Other illnesses that can sometimes result in changes in sex drive include diabetes (itself an illness involving hormones) various forms of anaemia and, most important, the mental illness of depression. This is not simply the change of mood which the word means to most of us, but the actual illness called clinical depression. The full causes of this distressing and widespread illness are not yet fully known, but many doctors believe it involves brain chemistry and hormones.

Another common disease of our times which also contributes considerably to loss of sex drive is obesity. Not only because the fat woman feels less attractive and therefore less interested in sex, but because being overweight undoubtedly affects hormone levels.

It depresses the action of certain of the hormone-producing glands. A recent finding is that women with a great deal of peripheral fat – that is, fat distributed on the outer parts of the body – actually produce different amounts of estrogen, the fat deposits providing the raw material for the hormones' manufacture and storage.

Marked changes in body weight certainly lead to marked changes in hormones and it is well known that a woman who seems infertile when she is heavy may become pregnant as soon as she has lost enough of her excess fat. But she must not lose too much, for overloss of weight and over-dieting can lead to a halt in the periods, because again the hormones have been put out of balance. One of the symptoms of anorexia nervosa (the self-starving illness) is the loss of periods and loss of sex drive.

These are all physical causes but, of course, emotional and psychological factors come into play as well. The hormone loss of the menopause may not itself be profound enough to make a woman totally lose her sex drive, but if because she is aging she feels old, unattractive and unsexy, then that, added to the underlying hormone problem, can be enough to quench her sexual interest.

The girl who has a new baby to care for may have a slight hormonal imbalance which is not on its own enough to upset her sexual drive, but when anxiety about the baby, the new responsibilities, or a jealous husband who resents the infant's demands is added to the hormonal imbalance, the result is a switching off of her sexual feelings.

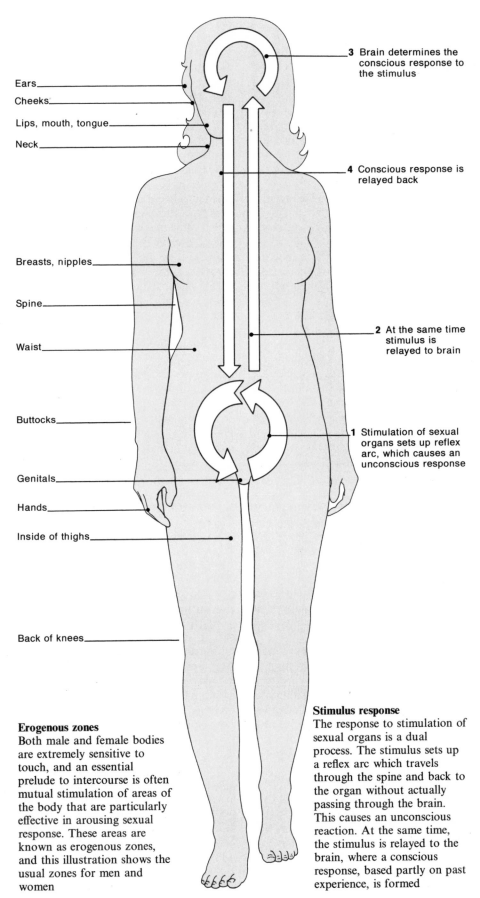

3 Brain determines the conscious response to the stimulus

Ears

Cheeks

Lips, mouth, tongue

Neck

4 Conscious response is relayed back

Breasts, nipples

Spine

Waist

2 At the same time stimulus is relayed to brain

Buttocks

Genitals

1 Stimulation of sexual organs sets up reflex arc, which causes an unconscious response

Hands

Inside of thighs

Back of knees

Erogenous zones
Both male and female bodies are extremely sensitive to touch, and an essential prelude to intercourse is often mutual stimulation of areas of the body that are particularly effective in arousing sexual response. These areas are known as erogenous zones, and this illustration shows the usual zones for men and women

Stimulus response
The response to stimulation of sexual organs is a dual process. The stimulus sets up a reflex arc which travels through the spine and back to the organ without actually passing through the brain. This causes an unconscious reaction. At the same time, the stimulus is relayed to the brain, where a conscious response, based partly on past experience, is formed

Sexual disorders

What is frigidity? Why does it happen?

Sexual arousal leading to a willingness to take part in and enjoy intercourse culminating in orgasm is part of a complex series of sensations and responses. Women who, for some reason, lose their responses are sometimes said to be frigid, but it is a bad word, because it seems to imply a judgement of a whole person, rather than a description of the actual problem, which is failure of a physiological mechanism. This is why most modern doctors prefer to use the terms sexual dysfunction or orgasmic incompetence.

The range of this problem is wide. One woman will complain that she feels nothing at all in sexual terms; no arousal, and sometimes actual revulsion, possibly accompanied by a muscular spasm of the muscles of the vagina that makes penetration by the penis impossible. This is called vaginismus.

Another will say that she can be aroused and will enjoy preliminary sex play – stimulation of breasts and clitoris (the peak of sensitive tissue at the front of woman's surface sex organs) – but loses all feeling when intercourse starts.

Another will say she enjoys foreplay and intercourse but that she can never reach orgasm, the climactic pleasurable muscular response that arousal should lead to.

Yet others are orgasmic if they receive manual stimulation of the clitoris, but not in intercourse.

The causes are similar to those already listed; a woman who has once enjoyed normal complete response and then loses it is in much the same situation as one who has never had it – except that she is better able to recover. Anyone who has once been able to enjoy sex can do so again; the woman who has never enjoyed sex usually needs more help, and over a longer period of time.

The help that can be given ranges from emotional counselling – discussion of personal attitudes and needs in a particular relationship – to the behavioural approach pioneered by such sex researchers as Masters and Johnson. With the help of counselling, many people are taught to recognize and respond to their basic sensations. The physiological fact is that no healthy adult is incapable of sexual response; but the psychological aspects are so important and so integral a part of sexual drive that they can overwhelm an otherwise normal physiological state.

How frequent should sex be for a normal couple?

Once again, there can be no norm. One couple will regularly have intercourse every night and every morning, another only once a month or less. As long as both are content with this, then it is normal and healthy for them. Attempts to set 'proper' levels and make rules about sexual behaviour tend to damage the spontaneity of responses, and may lead to sexual problems such as failure of erection or failure of arousal for a woman.

Having said that, it can be added that research by various experts suggests that the average frequency appears to be two to four times a week.

Why don't we find all members of the opposite sex attractive as animals do?

Sexual attraction, at a purely physiological level, depends first of all on the appearance and behaviour of the potential partner. If a member of the opposite sex looks as though he or she is interested in, available for, and ready to engage in sexual intercourse this can be arousing.

Smell comes into it also, even though we do not always realize it. The human body, like all animal bodies, produces powerful scents called pheromones which, though they may not be recognized at conscious level, profoundly affect behaviour. A woman who is at her fertile phase – who has just ovulated – produces a different odour from one who is menstruating, and this difference can make her seem more attractive to a man who unconsciously recognizes it.

There are other body odours, some coming from the sexual areas and some from other parts of the body such as the armpits, which also throw out special sexually attractive smells. In modern life we tend to be afraid of the power of these, and deodorize ourselves heavily – which seems a pity, to say the least. Not all the 'unpleasant' body odours that the advertisers have trained us to fear are all that unpleasant.

Apart from these physiological triggers to sexual attraction, there are the far more important psychological ones. A potential sexual partner will be judged on a wide range of factors, including likeness or dissimilarity to parents. A girl who had a close, warm and happy relationship with her father will find men who look, sound or behave like him attractive, just as a man who related well to his mother will be attracted to girls like her. This is so well known that it even makes the subject of popular song lyrics: 'I want a girl just like the girl who married dear old Dad...'

Also, fashion comes into it. Men and women are exposed constantly to images of the 'ideal' sex partner and tend to respond to them. At present, the ideal female is thin, so skinny girls are regarded as beauties and are much sought after by males. Also, they feel themselves to be sexually desirable, since they fit into the current beauty pattern, and so send out 'I-am-attractive' messages. At the turn of the century, such girls would have been passed over in favour of the fashionable beauties of that era, who were voluptuous – women whom we would today regard as fat and therefore undesirable.

Men are as affected by fashion as women, of course. Today we admire the thin, boyish-looking, pallid males who were once passed over in favour of meaty, heavily muscled men. No doubt the fashion in looks, for both sexes, will change again during the present century: it always has, and always will.

Incidentally, many animal species are just as choosy about their sexual partners as we are. Pandas and gorillas are good examples of this.

Why do some men become impotent?

This, again, is a bad word to use because it seems to suggest that the whole man is useless rather than that he is having a sexual difficulty.

The causes of male sexual dysfunction are similar to the female's, except that hormonal disorder is less common since men have a less complex hormone balance. With a few fairly rare exceptions, most men who suffer from failure of erection (a penile erection being the obvious sign of male sexual arousal) have a psychological problem. Masters and Johnson's research has shown that men are capable of initiating and enjoying intercourse culminating in orgasm well into old age, though there is a loss of drive in most older men.

The causes may be rooted in a man's view of himself (if he feels a failure in his work or other aspects of his life, he will not be able to display his normal sexuality) or in his relationships (if his partner responds to him with coolness or rejection, his self esteem and therefore his sexual responses will be damaged) or occasionally in physical disorder. Some drugs, notably alcohol, interfere with the physiology of sexual arousal. Shakespeare referred to the way alcohol makes a man 'stand to, and not stand to . . .' and British men joke sardonically about 'Brewer's droop'. The medicines that are particularly likely to have a side effect on sex drive are some of the ones that are used to treat high blood pressure, and some of those used to treat depression or anxiety, namely the anti-depressants and the tranquillizers.

General chronic illness such as anaemia can affect sex drive, as can an acute illness such as an attack of influenza. Some conditions are more likely than others to do so; one example is diabetes, and others are multiple sclerosis and Parkinson's disease. However, treatment of the underlying problem and psychological help can often maintain a high degree of function for men with such illnesses.

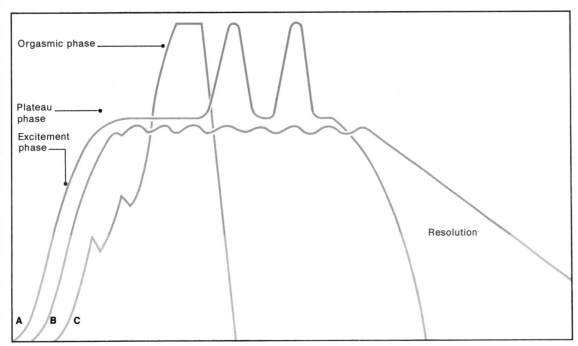

Sexual intercourse
The duration of sexual intercourse is marked by three distinct phases. The excitement phase, at the start of intercourse leads to the plateau phase, which (if it is sustained) leads to the orgasmic phase in both men and women. Women can respond to intercourse in three ways. (**A**) is a gradual rise through the excitement and plateau phase to a multiple orgasm. (**B**) is a gradual rise to a sustained plateau phase without orgasm, while (**C**) is a rapid rise through excitement and plateau to a single orgasm

Orgasmic phase

Plateau phase

Excitement phase

Resolution

A B C

How long should intercourse last?

If this refers to the age of the participants, then the answer is 'as long as you like'. There is no reason why people of advanced age should not enjoy sex, and many geriatricians (specialists in the ills of the old) recommend an active sex life as a way of maintaining general health.

If the question relates to the individual episodes of sexual intercourse the answer has to be 'as long as the participants choose'. Some people make a rapid transit from arousal to orgasm – just a few minutes – and they are content with that.

Other people can keep themselves aroused for hours at a time. In the East, in some religious cults, male adherents were taught a practice called *karezza* in which they could persist in intercourse for inordinately long periods while avoiding orgasm. This, while it gave a great deal of satisfaction to the woman, offering her multiple orgasms, resulted in minimal pleasure for the man. However, since the practice was regarded as a religious duty, perhaps that didn't matter too much.

For most couples, the length of time devoted to sex play and intercourse is related to the amount of time which is available. If they have only 10 minutes, then 10 minutes is enough. If they can spare an hour, they will go on for an hour. There is no absolute norm, happily for all of us.

Sexual disorders

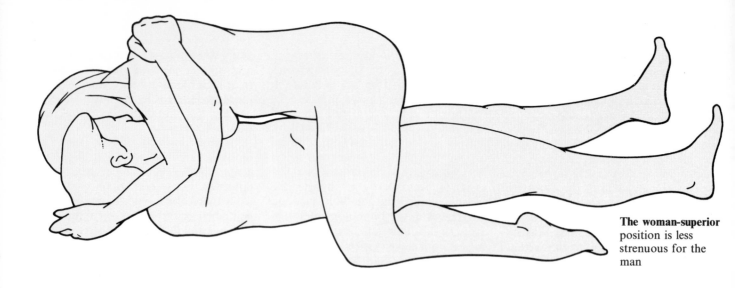

The woman-superior position is less strenuous for the man

Can a person have a sex life again after having had a heart attack?

That depends on the degree of damage caused by the heart attack. If a person remains very ill, suffering breathlessness and angina at the least exertion, his or her ability to respond to sex will be severely limited.

But most people who have recovered from a coronary thrombosis attack and who have been told by their doctors that they may return to normal living may also return to normal sex. Unfortunately, many do not do this because they are often too shy to ask the doctor about it, and simply assume that they may not. But it is not only usually safe, but also a healthy way to recover from an attack and to prevent a future one. Graded exercise is part of the recovery programme for many heart attack patients, and sex is excellent exercise.

To make a return to sex comfortable and reassuring after a heart attack, the couple should start with gentle arousal, go on to stimulating to orgasm manually – masturbating – then on to 'lazy' intercourse, with the healthy partner making all the necessary movements (the woman-superior position if the man is the patient) and finally back to their previous active ways. If there is any point at which the effort is too much it will be signalled by a twinge of pain that will stop the patient anyway.

It should be noted that this answer to the question should be used only as a general guide. Before returning to a normal sex life, each person, of course, should discuss his or her individual case with his or her own doctor.

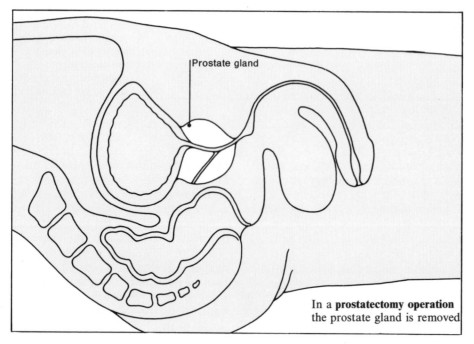

Prostate gland

In a prostatectomy operation the prostate gland is removed

Is a man's sex life damaged by the operation of prostatectomy?

Most men who have had this operation can and do return to a normal sex life, although there may be a little nervousness at first, which is inevitable after any surgical procedure involving the sex organs. Some men have the problem of retrograde ejaculation after the operation – they have erections and orgasms but the semen goes into the bladder instead of out through the penis. But even men with this problem can and do enjoy sex.

In common with nearly all aspects of sexual response, it is what a person expects to happen that governs what does. If a man who has had an operation believes all will be well afterwards, then it almost certainly will. If he has doubts, his sexual responses will falter.

Is it safe to have sex when you're pregnant?

Usually, yes. The times for the woman at which there may be a risk to the pregnancy, if there is deeply penetrating intercourse with orgasm, are the first few weeks (during which time she may not even know she is pregnant anyway) and the last few days, when the experience might trigger labour. However, this can be an agreeable way to induce a birth, in a healthy full-term pregnancy.

Only if an obstetrician expressly forbids intercourse – which is rare – need a couple abstain. This is just as well, because many women find their sex drive increases when they are pregnant both because of their altered hormone balance and the excitement of expecting a baby.

Sex during pregnancy
Providing that due care is taken, sexual intercourse can be enjoyed even at an advanced stage of pregnancy. As this illustration shows, the uterus and vagina are not in direct alignment, and even quite deep penetration by the penis will not come close to the fetus, which is well protected in the uterus

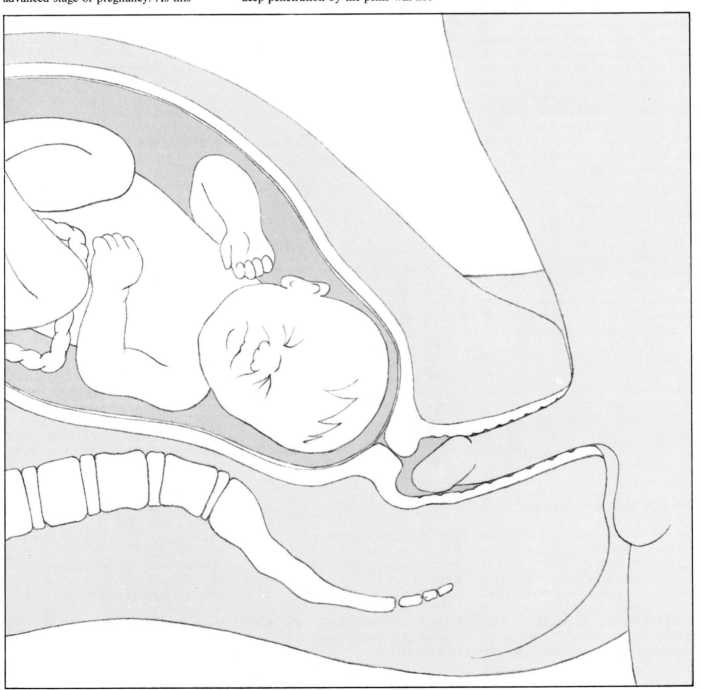

Sexual disorders

Why do some foods and drinks make people more sexy?

There are very, very few true aphrodisiacs – substances which trigger and increase sexual desire. Those that do include certain hormone preparations, and some highly irritant materials which have a stimulating effect on sex organs. The best-known of the latter is Spanish Fly (cantharides), an irritant poison said to have been used by Casanova. These preparations are risky, since even small doses can lead to death.

Certain foods have been labelled as aphrodisiac because of lingering beliefs in sympathetic magic. This system says, *inter alia*, that something that looks like another thing can have an effect on it. For example, a food which looked like an erect penis or a vulva was believed to have a direct action on these organs. So, long phallic-shaped foods are said to be male stimulants – celery is an obvious example – and enclosed foods are thought to help women – and the obvious example here is the oyster.

But there is nothing in either of these (or any others) that contains even a hint of an actively sexually stimulating substance. The same is true of rhino's horn, the phallic-shaped material that is sometimes still powdered down and fed to sexually tired men. However, if anyone believes that these substances will have an effect, then they will. It is a psychological effect.

Alcohol is rather different. It does not contain a sexually stimulating substance, but it does have an effect on the brain and its controls. Inhibitions may be discarded and underlying sexual drive allowed free play. This is why giving an unwilling girl a few drinks has always been part of the seducer's stock in trade. But of course the dose must be carefully controlled. Too much alcohol can damp down sexual response altogether.

Phallic-shaped foods have long been held to act as male stimulants. Sadly the results usually belie the promise

Do men have a menopause?

No. The word means literally 'end of the periods' – and men do not have periods.

However, they do have a form of mid-life climacteric – a change that in some ways mimics the female experience. They may become aware of their aging and become depressed by it. They may become anxious about their sexual prowess, and become either sexually more active, even promiscuous, or lose their drive altogether. Anxiety about work, growing children and future activity are just some of the things which could lead to depressive illness.

The only possible treatment is to deal with the anxieties as they arise, coming to terms with the inevitability of change as life goes on.

Why won't some doctors give women hormones at the menopause, when it is the loss of hormones that causes the symptoms?

The only symptoms that have been definitely proved to be due to the hormone changes of the menopause are hot flushes, in which the woman suddenly gets red and sweats heavily, and changes in the mucous membrane of the vulva and vagina, leading to dryness and soreness. These can be relieved by the right sort of hormone treatment and few doctors will refuse this.

However, in recent years there has been a campaign to make women, and their doctors, see the menopause as a deficiency disorder characterized by a huge list of symptoms, including depression, irritability, headaches, loss of skin tone, poor hair condition, loss of sex drive and many, many others.

It was argued that the giving of estrogen prevented or reversed all the problems, ensured strong bones (some women develop thinning of the bones in old age, which can occasionally be prevented by estrogen) and generally made a woman feminine forever.

Other doctors resisted this vigorously, making the point that many of the symptoms of the menopause are due to anxiety and stress about being middle aged and that they are often linked with personal anxieties over the quality of a marital relationship, and the loss of children as they become adult and leave the parental home. In the opinion of these doctors, to give estrogen would not cure the problem and, in some women, it might create other, more worrying problems. The lining of the uterus is susceptible to estrogen because it is the target organ for the hormone, and in some cases early cancerous disease has developed after the use of estrogen treatments. For this reason, many doctors will not prescribe estrogen therapy. Also, estrogen therapy may be linked with gall bladder disease, and some circulatory disorders. This, too, discouraged some doctors.

The controversy will no doubt go on for a long time. There are so many factors involved that there cannot be an easy answer.

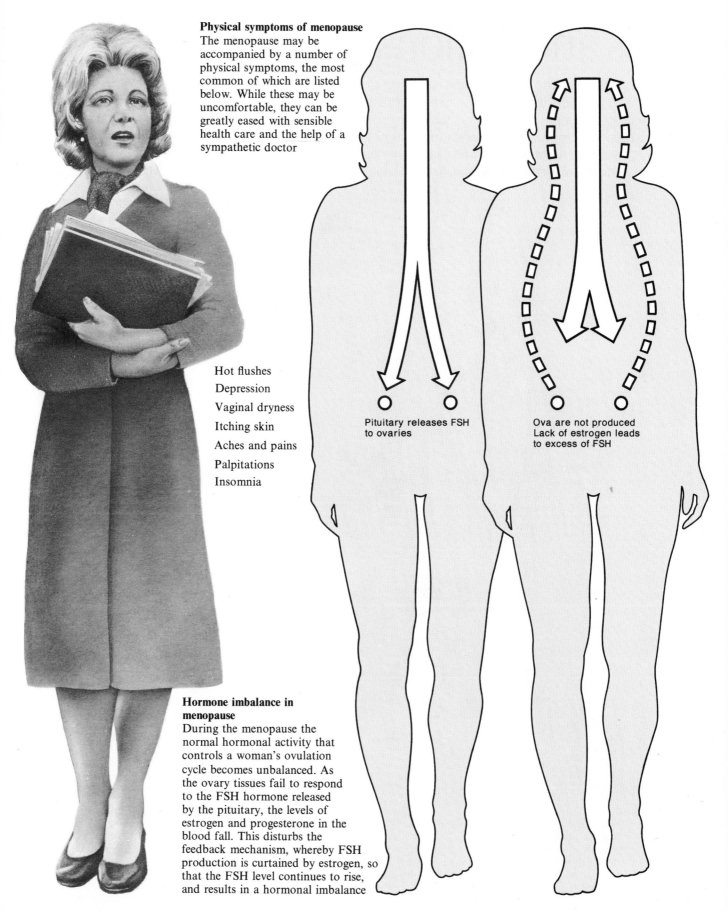

Physical symptoms of menopause
The menopause may be accompanied by a number of physical symptoms, the most common of which are listed below. While these may be uncomfortable, they can be greatly eased with sensible health care and the help of a sympathetic doctor

Hot flushes
Depression
Vaginal dryness
Itching skin
Aches and pains
Palpitations
Insomnia

Pituitary releases FSH to ovaries

Ova are not produced
Lack of estrogen leads to excess of FSH

Hormone imbalance in menopause
During the menopause the normal hormonal activity that controls a woman's ovulation cycle becomes unbalanced. As the ovary tissues fail to respond to the FSH hormone released by the pituitary, the levels of estrogen and progesterone in the blood fall. This disturbs the feedback mechanism, whereby FSH production is curtained by estrogen, so that the FSH level continues to rise, and results in a hormonal imbalance

Pills and potions

The human being who was the first to have the courage – or perhaps it should be called foolhardiness – to swallow a particular berry, leaf or root to relieve a painful symptom is one to whom we should all be grateful. He was the forerunner of the pharmaceutical industry which has brought us a great deal of benefit, although it has also brought some problems. The more powerful and potentially useful a drug, the more potentially dangerous it is. However, considerable efforts are made to protect the users of medicines, and doctors are as aware of the risks as they are of the uses.

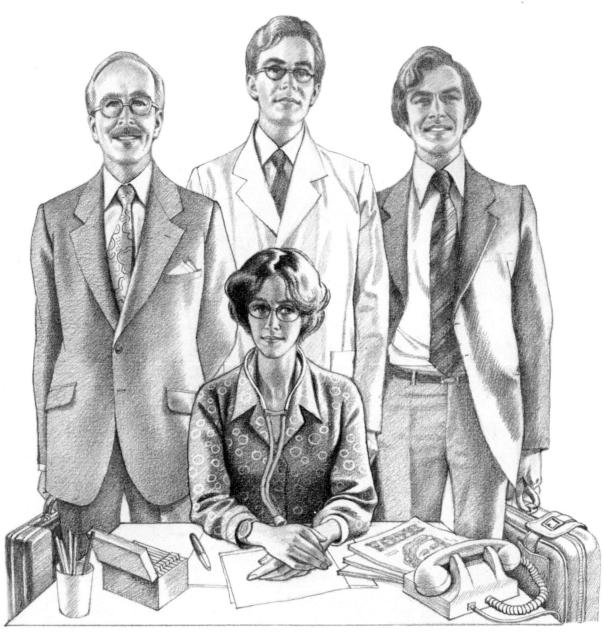

The people behind the prescriptions
Every drug that your doctor prescribes is the result of a vast effort by the manufacturers. Their research scientists screen new substances for their possible therapeutic effects and modify existing drugs for new applications. New products are tested for safety and effectiveness in trials that are closely scrutinized by government safety officers. Drugs are marketed by the maker's representatives, who deal with family doctors, hospitals and pharmacists, and also supply information on the medicines' dosages, benefits and possible side effects

How can I be sure that the medicines my doctor gives me are really safe? There are so many different ones these days . . . surely no doctor can really know all there is to know about all of them?

This is indeed one of the biggest problems facing doctors today. In the past, when it was a case of prescribing the pink medicine or the white medicine and it didn't much matter which since neither was much use for anything, there were few problems. But today, when every doctor can prescribe very powerful medicines with just a flick of his pen, the situation is much more complicated.

The first line of protection which patients, and doctors, have is the stringent controls on the manufacture, testing and distribution of medicines. These controls operate in all major countries, though there are parts of the world where there is a black market in medicines, which is exploited by cynical profit-makers and which causes a great deal of damage. But those of us who live in 'civilized' countries are fairly well protected.

The second line of defence has to be the personality and attitude of an individual doctor. Some doctors have a special interest in pharmacology and make sure they are up to date in all developments. Clearly they will prescribe knowledgeably.

Others are less aware, but are slow to prescribe new drugs and are suspicious of the blandishments of the many pharmaceutical companies which spend a great deal of money advertising and promoting new medicines. These doctors write as few prescriptions as possible, and then usually only for medicines they understand.

Others lack knowledge and are prepared to listen to the advertising and the sales representatives without question. They prescribe freely.

The doctor likely to do us the least harm is in the first or second of these categories. The last kind is one to be worried about.

How can you tell whether your doctor is prescribing wisely? You could try asking him his views on new medicines. And also ask him what the medicine is, what it is supposed to do, and whether it is likely to have any unwanted side effects. If he is a careful prescriber he will be willing to answer.

It also helps if you control your own urge to be 'given something'. Many patients put considerable subtle pressure on their doctors to prescribe, when the doctor would be much happier not to do so. And even though the doctor is technically 'in charge' it sometimes can be difficult for him not to allow a patient to put pressure on him to prescribe medicines which he is not really comfortable about.

Why do some medicines have to be used as suppositories— put into the body through the anus?

For any medicine to be effective it has to be carried to its target. One way it can enter the bloodstream is via the mucous membrane. The medicine dissolves if it is solid, or is diluted if it is liquid, and its molecules get through the membrane and through the blood vessel walls and are carried on their way.

The mouth is lined with mucous membrane, and many medicines are given by mouth to be absorbed directly from there. An example is glyceryl trinitrate, which is used to relieve attacks of angina pectoris (heart pain), tablets of which are dissolved under the tongue or in the cheek. And, of course, there are glucose tablets which athletes suck to lift their blood sugar level and with it their energy.

Swallowed medicines also enter the bloodstream through the mucous membrane lining the stomach and the gut. However, the stomach has a very specialized lining and also produces some powerful digestive substances, including pure hydrochloric acid. These substances can alter and damage the medicine and make it useless. Also, some medicines are unpleasant to take, and some patients tend to vomit easily. For example, giving medicine by mouth to relieve a migraine attack which is accompanied by vomiting would be a waste of time.

So, another mucous membrane area must be used, and the most available is the rectum. Medicines suspended in a slow-melting material such as paraffin wax can be shaped into pledgets called suppositories and when these are pushed into the anus and left there to dissolve, they release the medicine through the membrane walls.

This route is sometimes used not only because it is useful, but because it is culturally acceptable. In France, Belgium, Italy and other European countries the majority of remedies are presented in this form; people expect it and prefer it that way.

Incidentally, in women the vaginal route can also be used for medicines, but generally it is not, except for those medicines which are meant to treat gynaecological problems, for example progesterone-containing vaginal pessaries are used to treat the symptoms of pre-menstrual syndrome.

If you have to take different kinds of medicine, do they act in the same manner as if you take them separately? Or do they get in each other's way?

Some medicines can share the human body at the same time and have no effect at all on each other. Others may interact to create a combined effect that is greater than each alone could have caused; this is called synergism. Others may cancel each other out or act against each other; this is called antagonism.

Sometimes such effects can be dangerous. If a person who is suffering from a tendency to thrombosis (blood clotting) is given the anti-blood-clotting medicine, warfarin, and is also given the anti-rheumatism medicine, phenylbutazone, both of which work via the blood in the same way, the phenylbutazone can interfere with the warfarin. The result is sometimes quite severe bleeding in various parts of the body.

Sometimes medicines increase each other's effects – alcohol and mood-altering treatments for example. A person taking tranquillizers who also takes wine may become inebriated, and that can be lethal if he or she is working with machinery or driving.

Pills and potions

How do medicines know which part of the body to work in? For example, a cough medicine affects your lungs and a laxative affects your bowels.

Medicines do not in fact 'know' anything. When they are taken into the body they are carried by the bloodstream to the whole of the body. Swallowed medicine which is meant to help you cough up thick mucus from your lungs, for example, reaches your big toes as well as your chest. But because big toes do not contain mucous membrane, they don't respond to it.

However, other parts of the body do respond. A medicine which is meant to help you cough up clogging mucus in your air passages acts by stimulating the glands in the mucous membrane to produce more fluid. This softens the thick stuff, and so loosens it and makes it easier to get rid of. But the medicine also acts on the mucous membrane glands everywhere else, including the bowel, so an expectorant cough medicine can exert a laxative effect, by adding fluid to the bowel contents.

There are other kinds of cough medicines apart from expectorants; there are the sort that stop you from coughing, and they are used to cure irritating dry coughs rather than the catarrhal ones. They act directly on the cough reflex centre in the brain and also affect all involuntary muscle to a certain extent, which means that they act on the muscles of the gut walls. They slow the muscles down, which is why some cough treatments – codeine is an example – cause constipation.

Some medicines have their specific effects because they act only on certain target tissues. For example, iodine is always taken up by thyroid tissue, digitalis by heart tissue and fluoride by bony tissue, especially teeth.

Why mustn't I eat things like cheese and pickled herrings when I take the pills my doctor gave me for depression?

It is not only medicines that can interact on each other – some foods can. The medicine you are taking is one of the group called monoamine oxidase inhibitors (MAOI). They can be most helpful in lifting the misery of depression, but one of their side effects is to suppress a body enzyme which is needed to break down certain substances found in food, and to render them fully acceptable to the body. When this enzyme is prevented from doing its work the chemicals from these foods can build up and cause raised blood pressure, severe headaches and some eye complaints and other unpleasant symptoms. It is foods which contain the substance tyramine which are a problem, and they include certain cheeses, pickled herrings, Chianti-type wine and extracts prepared from meat or yeast, and, oddly enough, broad beans.

Rather than prescribe MAOI medicines, doctors are now tending to use the more recently developed antidepressants called the tricyclic compounds which are less likely to cause the side effects.

Why do some medicines have to be taken before meals, and some after meals?

Obviously, if there is food in the stomach, this will strongly affect the rate at which the medicine sharing the stomach will be absorbed. Consider alcohol again. Taken on an empty stomach it reaches the brain very rapidly indeed; on a full one it does not.

Some medicines should be absorbed quickly to be useful, so users are advised to take them before meals.

Other medicines may be rather irritant to the stomach lining and so are more likely to upset an empty stomach, or the rate of absorption needed may be slower. So for them an after-meals regimen is best.

Why do injections have to be used when they hurt? Couldn't the medicines be swallowed just as easily?

Because mucous membrane produces substances of its own, swallowing medicines may not be the ideal way for certain of them to enter the body. Insulin, which diabetic people need, is a case in point. If it goes into the mouth and stomach it is destroyed by the secretions there; the only way it can be used by the body is if it enters directly from depots in the subcutaneous fat or muscle. That is why insulin has to be injected.

Another reason for using injections is speed; it takes far longer for a medicine to reach the whole system via a mucous membrane route than if it is injected directly into the blood itself.

Can drugs get into your body any other way apart from through your mouth and your anus?

They can get in through the skin; creams and lotions containing medicines can be smeared on and will be gradually absorbed through the skin layers and reach the bloodstream. This method used to be applied for babies suffering from marasmus, profound malnutrition due to severe illness or starvation. They would be rubbed all over with cod liver oil in an attempt to get the essential vitamins it carries into their systems.

Inhalation is another method of entry; the membranes lining the breathing passages can allow medicines through them just as can those in the mouth or gut. The obvious example is ether or chloroform or other anaesthetic gases.

The last available method is via intravenous injection, in which the medicine is passed through the skin directly into the subcutaneous fat or the underlying muscle, from which it can be absorbed, or directly into a blood vessel.

What is the difference between a medicine and a drug?

There is no difference. All medicines are drugs in that they affect the way the body works. Aspirin is a drug. So is heroin. So are tea and coffee and cola drinks and cocoa (they contain, among other things, the stimulant caffeine); and, of course, alcohol is a drug.

Unfortunately, many people have come to use the word 'drug' to mean something exceedingly powerful that may do harm and 'medicine' to mean something that always does good. They are wrong. Calling something a medicine does not make it safer or more effective than calling it a drug: and calling something a drug does not make it potentially evil. But medicine is probably a better word because it alarms people less than the emotive word 'drug'.

A point that must be made is that any medicine that has any really useful effect is potentially damaging. A medicine that is incapable of doing any harm at all is unlikely in the extreme to be capable of doing any good either. In the past, most medicines were fairly harmless, and therefore had hardly any effect on the people who used them. Modern medicines, however, are often extremely effective and must therefore be used with great caution because they can have marked side effects.

There is one property of all medicines, whether they are chemically powerful or not, and this property is extremely useful, and a little odd. It is called the placebo effect.

In simple terms it means that any substance a person takes in the belief that it is a medicine can exert an observable effect. People with headaches, when given sugar pills and told they were strong pain-killers, reported relief from their pain. Asthmatic children, given harmless inhalations and then told that they were an irritant, promptly went into asthma attacks – and recovered just as fast when given the self-same inhalation and told that it was a treatment. People who respond like this – and about 75 per cent of us do so fairly strongly, and the remaining 25 per cent to a certain degree – are not 'neurotics' or 'malingerers'; they are affected by the powerful psychological trigger of faith. The power of the mind over the body is immense, and the placebo (the word comes from the Latin root *placere* meaning 'to please') proves this.

Incidentally, the placebo effect is as important to the doctor as to the patient; many doctors feel they have done a better job for their patients if they have given them a prescription for something even when they know perfectly well that the medicine they have given is really not much use at all for the patients' particular conditions.

Why can you only take pain-killers every four hours? What would happen if you took them more often?

When medicines are taken into the body they do not remain unchanged. They are broken down into their basic chemicals and then disposed of. Most of the breaking-down process happens in the liver, and the waste products are removed in urine, extracted by the kidneys, and to a lesser extent by the bowels as some wastes are removed in stools.

The liver is a vast and exceedingly active organ, and has the vital task of detoxifying many of the dangerous substances we put into ourselves. If the liver is unable to cope with its job then the toxins build up and the result is illness of varying degrees.

For example, a man who takes too much alcohol will overload his liver so severely that it just cannot detoxify the alcohol fast enough (and alcohol is a poison) and the breakdown products build up and contribute to the disagreeable symptoms of hangover – head pain, eye symptoms, dehydration, nausea and all the rest of it.

Excess use of medicines can also overload the liver. It has been found that about four hours' delay is needed for a dose of pain-killer to be safely dealt with and still maintain its pain-killing effect. So, the recommended way to use these medicines is at this interval. It can be shortened to three hours if the pain is severe, but this is not recommended if you value your liver's good health.

Why is it that a medicine which is safe used in one part of the body, say as eye drops, is dangerous if it reaches another part, say, if it's swallowed?

Although a medicine can be absorbed through the skin and structures such as eyes and ears, much less of it reaches the bloodstream from these routes than through mucous membrane. So, a treatment which is safe on skin, eyes or ears could be poisonous if swallowed, because all of it would reach the blood.

Also, eye drops, ear drops and skin treatments tend to be used in small amounts. One drop at a time is the norm for eyes, for example. But, if the whole bottleful were swallowed then the dose would be very high indeed and could be poisonous. This is why certain drops and ointments and lotions are labelled 'Poison – do not take by mouth'.

Why do the effects of some medicines 'wear off'? The first time I took a sleeping pill I was knocked out, but after a week of taking them I didn't feel particularly sleepy when I swallowed one.

This is habituation. When body cells are first exposed to a substance they respond briskly, but if more and more of the substance appears they get used to it, and accept it and no longer respond as much as they did.

There are some other substances that are particularly likely to have this effect. The barbiturates, the sleeping pills that were once widely used, are a classic example; others are the opiates, morphine, heroin and so on. And, of course, alcohol is the same. The more you drink the more you need to produce an effect.

Sometimes habituation goes a step further and becomes a need: people who used to take one sleeping pill become psychologically dependent on the effect, and start to take more and more of the medicine to get the same result. This can be a severe problem to deal with, and doctors are now chary of prescribing any medicine known to have a tendency to cause habituation.

Pills and potions

How do slimming pills work? And why don't doctors like giving them?
After all, being overweight is supposed to be unhealthy,
so why not encourage a treatment that helps to prevent it?

Some medicines which act on the brain, causing alertness and arousal, have a side effect of depressing appetite. Amphetamine is an example. In the past, doctors would give overweight patients these medicines in order to help them to stop eating. Unfortunately, the patients learned to enjoy the side effects of alertness and tension and to fear the 'let down' sensation when they stopped the pills. So they continued to take them and, in time, found that they lost the effect of hunger control. They went on taking the medicines and also went on and on eating.

The medicines, therefore, not only failed to do the job they were being given for: they also caused the patient to develop a dependence. This is why few responsible doctors today will prescribe these medicines except in special circumstances, and then only for very limited periods.

In the UK attempts were made to ban the medicines altogether, because too many adolescents were obtaining them and using them as artificial stimulants. In one provincial town doctors joined together and agreed never to prescribe amphetamines, so local pharmacists no longer stocked them and the incidence of abuse among the town's young dropped sharply. Similar attempts are being made to ban barbiturates which are also popular with experimenting adolescents.

If antibiotics kill germs and so many different ones have been devised, why do people still get colds in the head which can't be treated by them?

A cold, like many other infections, is caused not by bacteria but by viruses, which are much smaller creatures and of a different structure. So far, no antiviral medicines as effective as the antibiotic medicines have been devised. Attempts have been made to isolate the body's natural virus-fighting substance, interferon, to be used against viral infection, but not, so far, with a great deal of success.

Sometimes it can be useful to give antibiotics to people with colds, if they are suffering from a secondary infection from bacteria. For example, people may get a viral cold, and on top of it a severe bacterial sinusitis. Then penicillin or a similar medicine can be given for the sinusitis, although it will not affect the underlying cold.

Agents of disease
Many infectious diseases are caused by viruses, tiny structures only about a hundred-thousandth of an inch across. They are parasites, able to live and reproduce only in larger organisms, such as bacteria (some of which also cause disease), or the body cells of humans

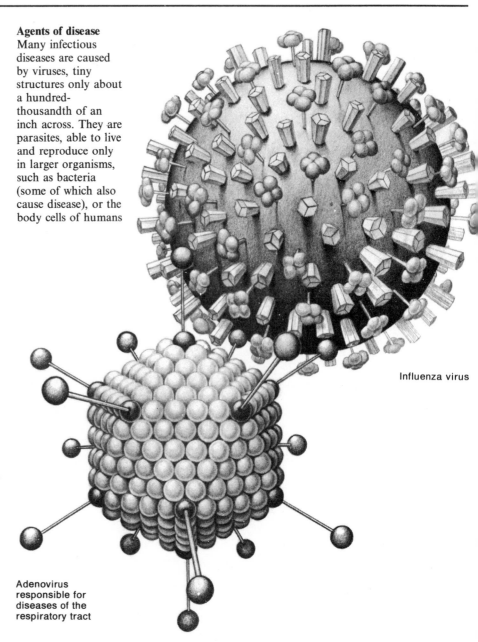

Influenza virus

Adenovirus responsible for diseases of the respiratory tract

Why do some people get rashes if they take penicillin?

They are the people who have an allergy to the antibiotic. Their natural defence systems react against it as if it were a dangerous germ invader. Hence the rash, and in some cases, swelling, wheeziness, even collapse.

If all antibiotic medicines kill germs, why are there so many different kinds? Why can't penicillin, for example, be used for all infections?

Penicillin was the first of the modern antibiotic medicines to be developed, although there had been precursors, notably the sulphonamide medicines, which exerted a bacteria-killing action. But penicillin was the first that promised a blanket effect on all bacteria.

However, it was found fairly soon that bacteria vary in their structure and their ability to resist penicillin, and different antibiotics had to be developed for different strains of bacteria. For example, the tubercle bacillus resisted penicillin without difficulty but was knocked out by streptomycin (and also by other medicines, called para-amino salicylic acid, PAS, and isonicotinic acid hydrazide, INAH) and that spelled the end of the tuberculosis plague that not so long ago had decimated whole populations.

It was also found, as time went on, that bacteria that had once succumbed to an antibiotic medicine began to learn how to resist it. The use of inadequate doses for too short periods of time contributed to this, and so more and more antibiotic medicines had to be devised.

We have now reached the stage where doctors are far less willing to prescribe these 'wonder-medicines', as they were originally labelled, for mild infections. It is often better for the patient to allow the infection to run its course and be resolved by the body's own mechanisms.

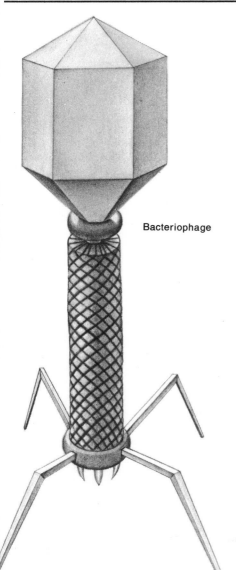

How viruses take over bacteria
The bacteriophage reproduces by injecting its own body contents into a bacterium, forcing it to make thousands of new viruses

Bacteriophage

Why is it that things you use on parts of the body, like hair dyes, are said to cause cancer in other parts of the body?

Because medicines can be absorbed via the skin, and so reach the bloodstream that way, it is obvious that other noxious substances can do the same. There is a theory, as yet unproved, that some hair dyes, in common with certain other chemical dyes, can stimulate changes in body cells that may lead to cancer, and they do this by entering the scalp. But it is worth repeating that this remains as yet an unproven theory, though considerable research work is going on at present.

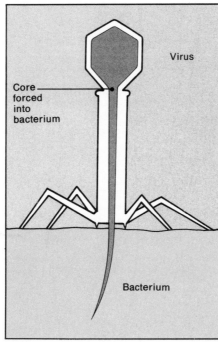

Virus

Core forced into bacterium

Bacterium

Why do some medicines have to be taken three times a day, and some only once a day?

Each medicine has its own life expectancy in the body. Some medicines are passed through the bloodstream faster than others, and some are broken down into their basic chemical parts more quickly than others. The rate depends not only on the structure of each medicine, but also on the user. In some people medicines act swiftly and are excreted swiftly; in others it takes much longer. And the rate can vary in the same person from time to time, depending on many factors. Alcohol shows this very obviously; one person will be made tipsy by one small glass of sherry, while another can swallow half a bottle of whisky and appear unmoved. And the man who can drink that half-bottle of whisky after a large meal when he's in tip-top condition and be unaffected may be bowled over by one small glass taken on an empty stomach when he's tired.

Attempts are made by medicine manufacturers to work out the way to give a medicine so that its level in the bloodstream will remain at the necessary point. Some medicines are retained in tissues (especially in fat) for a long time, so a daily dose is enough. In some cases the interval can be longer; monthly injections of Vitamin B12 can control the problem of pernicious anaemia.

Other medicines, however, are more rapidly absorbed and need more frequent administration. Antibiotics often need to be given every four to six hours to ensure high enough levels in the blood to fight the infection.

179

Anaesthetics and painkillers

In just over a hundred years, surgery has progressed from what was little more than bloodletting to open heart and brain surgery, kidney transplants, major reconstructive surgery of limbs and faces, and the most delicate of neurosurgery. None of this would have been possible without the development of safe swift anaesthesia. The skill of the anaesthetists makes the heroic efforts of the great surgeons possible. And it is the skill of the makers of analgesic drugs as well as of anaesthetics that has made childbirth a less harrowing experience for women, and less hazardous for babies.

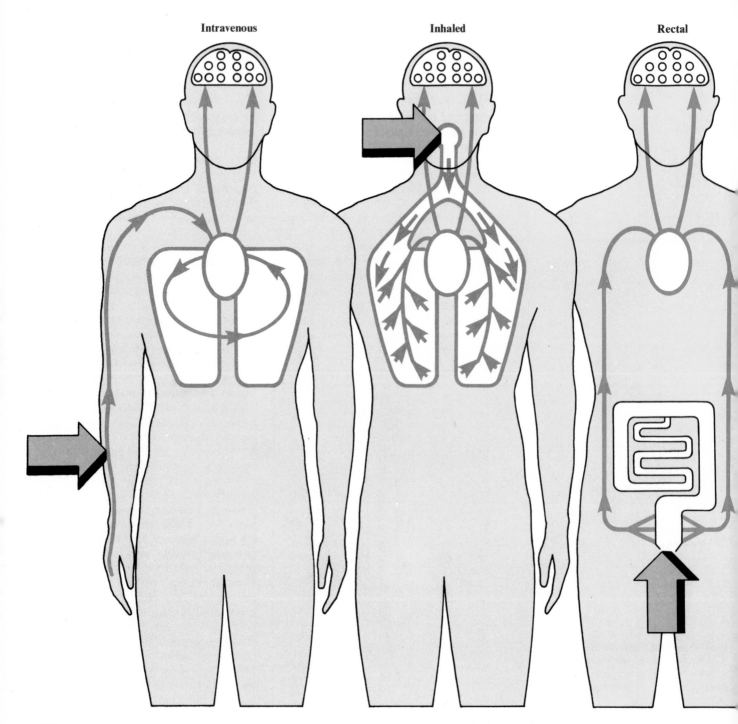

Intravenous

Inhaled

Rectal

If it is possible to anaesthetize different parts of the body with injections, why is it necessary to make people unconscious for operations?

The control of pain is not the only thing that is needed before it is possible for a surgeon to operate on a living human body. Avoiding pain may seem the most important thing to the person having the operation but, for the surgeon, there is also the problem of the control of bleeding, and the power of the muscles which he has to manipulate as he does his work.

A local anaesthetic, that is, an injection either into the tissues of a particular part of the body, or into the nerve that supplies that part of the body, only limits the pain sensation. It will not affect the blood supply nor the tone of the muscles which remain firm and often quite tense. Surgeons who regularly have to pull apart a couple of the muscles of the abdominal wall or the upper thigh, for example, can tell you just how powerful these muscles are. It takes a great effort to do it, and surgeons need to be physically strong, as well as dextrous, for this reason.

To make this muscle power more controllable, drugs can be used by the anaesthetist. He can give a muscle relaxant, which makes the muscles go floppy, robbing them of all power to move. The muscle relaxant works so well, in fact, that the patient cannot even breathe for himself, because that task uses muscles, and therefore he has to have artificial respiration. (The drugs used are often derived from the famous South American arrow-poison, curare, which killed people by totally paralyzing their breathing muscles.)

The patient also needs different gases in order to breathe – extra oxygen, for example, to ensure that an adequate oxygen supply gets to the outlying parts of the body, including the operation area. And drugs to control blood pressure are also necessary, again partly because of the importance of controlling the blood supply to the operation site, and also to ensure a satisfactory blood supply to the brain.

The experience of being given a muscle relaxant and artificial respiration would be exceedingly unpleasant for a conscious patient – probably worse than the experience of pain. So it is better for most of us to sleep our way sweetly through operations while the surgeon does what he has to do without the added difficulty of having to deal with strong, unrelaxed muscles.

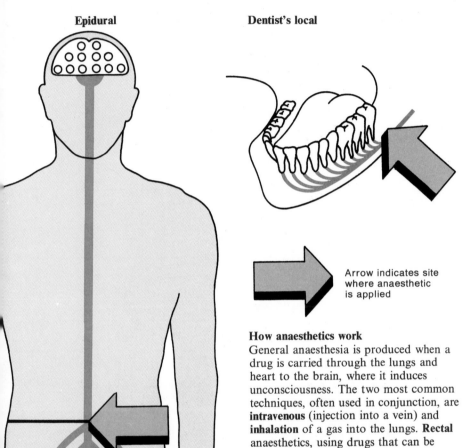

Epidural

Dentist's local

Arrow indicates site where anaesthetic is applied

How anaesthetics work

General anaesthesia is produced when a drug is carried through the lungs and heart to the brain, where it induces unconsciousness. The two most common techniques, often used in conjunction, are **intravenous** (injection into a vein) and **inhalation** of a gas into the lungs. **Rectal** anaesthetics, using drugs that can be absorbed into the bloodstream via the rectum, are slower to take effect than the intravenous or inhaled types, but appear less alarming to children.

Local anaesthetics are injected around the nerve to prevent pain signals being carried from the site of operation to the brain. An **epidural**, injected into the spinal canal, deadens all feeling from the point of injection down, and is frequently given to women in labour to enable them to take part consciously, without pain. A **dentist's local** injected into the gum or at the back of the mouth deadens pain from the nerves of the teeth being treated on that particular side

Anaesthetics and painkillers

Is it true that sometimes patients can understand and hear what is going on when doctors think that they are unconscious from an anaesthetic? I am scared this will happen to me.

When anaesthetists first started using the powerful muscle relaxants that are so much a feature of modern anaesthesia, it did happen on a very few occasions that they underestimated the amount of consciousness-blanking drug they needed to match the amount of muscle relaxant. The patients actually regained consciousness while they were still unable to move, and were still having their artificial respiration. There is no evidence that anyone ever felt any pain – but certainly a few people did hear and understand what was going on, as they were prepared for a return to bed, by being given an antidote to the muscle relaxant while they were powerless to signal to their attendants that they knew what was happening.

But, of course, the patients told the doctors afterwards, and due notice was taken. Anaesthetists learned from this how to assess the exact amount of drugs which each patient needed. There is no need to fear such an experience happening to anybody now. The problem has been solved.

Why do people having anaesthetics have to have tubes in their noses? After all, you can breathe when you're unconscious in sleep or when you've fainted.

It is the muscle relaxant and not the anaesthetic that makes the tube necessary. The muscles that you use for breathing – the diaphragm and the intercostals between the ribs – go on working during quite deep unconsciousness, but a muscle relaxant knocks them out even if you are awake. The tube is used as part of the artificial respiration which such drugs demand. Oxygen and other vital gases are fed to the lungs through it.

People having anaesthetics aren't allowed to eat or drink for a long time beforehand because it's dangerous. So what happens if it's an emergency and an urgent anaesthetic is vital but the person has just eaten?

A full stomach can be an embarrassment during a general anaesthetic because the body, when disturbed, as it is by such an experience, tends to empty the stomach by inducing vomiting. And apart from the mess, this could be dangerous because an unconscious patient may inhale the stomach contents, and suffocate. This is the reason for pre-operative fasting.

In emergencies where the stomach is full, either the anaesthetist will make special efforts to watch out for vomiting and will deal with it as it arises (as long as someone expert is there with the patient, there is no risk of suffocation) or, and this is usual because it is simpler, a stomach tube is passed to empty the stomach of its contents. This is not a pleasant experience, admittedly, but it is definitely protective for the patient.

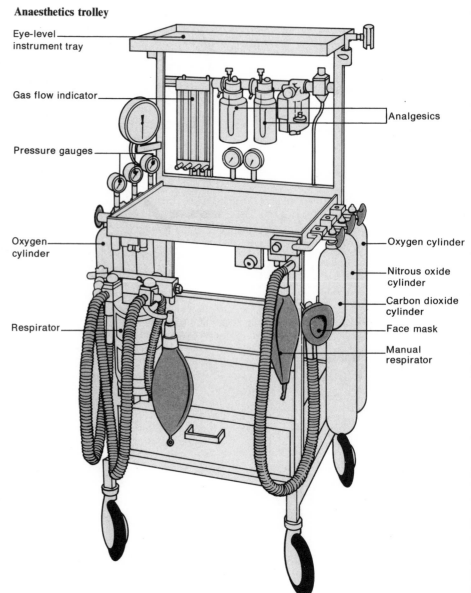

Anaesthetics trolley

Eye-level instrument tray

Gas flow indicator

Pressure gauges

Oxygen cylinder

Respirator

Analgesics

Oxygen cylinder

Nitrous oxide cylinder

Carbon dioxide cylinder

Face mask

Manual respirator

Why are people sick after having general anaesthetics? My mother felt dreadfully ill for days when she had her hysterectomy 15 years ago, and said it was worse than the pain of the operation. I'm worried because I'm having the same operation next month.

A small dose of anaesthetic can make a patient unconscious, but also leave him excitable and active. In the past, anaesthetists sometimes had to give larger quantities of the anaesthetic to control the excitability, and sometimes larger ones still to relax the muscles.

Because these drugs are so powerful, they are also potentially poisonous, and the body works hard at getting rid of them. They are broken down mainly in the liver and excreted in urine, stools and breath (that is why, in the old days,

people who had had an anaesthetic smelled so awful) and, in many cases, they caused the patient to vomit copiously, as part of the body's attempts to get rid of the poison.

But anaesthetic skills have come a long way in the last 15 years. Now, with the armoury of different drugs that can be used, it is no longer necessary to give such large doses of anaesthetic. Just enough to blank out awareness is used, and then a muscle relaxant to control restlessness.

As soon as the operation is complete, an antidote to the relaxant is given, to cancel out its effects, and there is no long-drawn-out breaking-down of the drug in the liver, and so no vomiting. The small amount of anaesthetic is rapidly excreted, so today most patients are awake, alert and quite free of any nausea within a short time of the operation. It's a much less unpleasant experience than it used to be.

Why are doctors so unwilling to give women in labour more anaesthetics and pain-killers than they do? Some labours go on for 24 hours or more; no one would be expected to have to put up with such pain during an operation, or for so long.

First of all, one point must be made clear – although a labour may last 24 hours or more from start to birth (though most are much shorter) by no means all of it is so dreadfully painful. The later stages when the contractions of the uterus are strong and frequent can be distressing and, of course, the effort to push the baby out can cause pain. But that stage lasts a comparatively short time – an hour or so usually – though it may be up to three or four hours. So, this is the only time that really

needs much pain control.

The reason why doctors and midwives are sparing with anaesthetics and analgesics during this stage is not anti-woman sadism, nor medical laziness, as has been suggested in some feminist circles. Actually, it is easier to deal with a completely anaesthetized person than a miserably complaining and distressed one.

The reason is because of the baby. He, too, is part of the deal, getting as he does all his nutrition and, most

importantly, his oxygen from his mother's blood supply. Not until he is born can he rely on his own breathing to supply his oxygen needs. So anything which affects the mother's oxygen supply also affects his. And some analgesic and anaesthetic drugs do affect this supply.

Also, the baby gets any drugs his mother gets, again through her blood supply. And he is much more susceptible to the dosage than she is because his body is so much smaller. So, the doctors have to compute as carefully as possible the dose that will give the mother adequate pain relief without knocking out the baby.

The dose must be right or the baby may be born anaesthetized, and that causes more than one problem, as anyone will know who has ever tried to resuscitate a baby born unconscious.

It is because of this problem that psychological pain control techniques have become so popular in recent years. If a woman can learn, by relaxation and self-hypnosis techniques, to handle her discomfort without drugs, her baby is much better off.

This is not to say, of course, tnat all babies born to anaesthetized mothers are damaged. But it seems foolish, to say the least, to make it harder for a baby to be born easily and safely by giving too much drug to his mother.

The needle and accessories

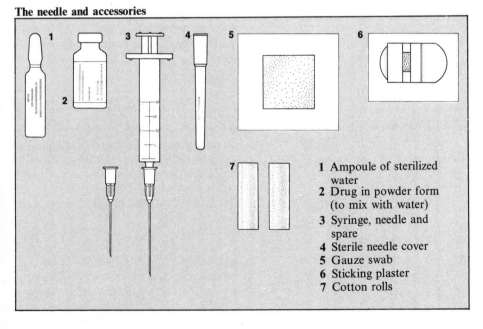

1 Ampoule of sterilized water
2 Drug in powder form (to mix with water)
3 Syringe, needle and spare
4 Sterile needle cover
5 Gauze swab
6 Sticking plaster
7 Cotton rolls

Anaesthetics and painkillers

Why does swallowing an aspirin, which goes into your stomach, relieve pain in your head and elsewhere?

The pain pathways described on page 19 show how the stimulus that comes from the knee, say, travels along the nervous pathways up to the brain, where the pain is registered and awareness of it passed on to the conscious mind.

Any interruption of the messages anywhere along that line can result in the pain message not reaching awareness.

In hypnosis, it happens high up on the line at the point where the brain sends the conscious mind the message.

In local anaesthesia, when a drug is injected right into the nerve where the pain is starting out – in this example, in the knee – the interruption comes very low down on the line.

In general anaesthesia, the message is interrupted in the brain, below the level of the conscious mind – fairly high up on the line.

Analgesics – pain-killers – can also operate anywhere along the line. But, they have to reach the line. The easiest way for them to do this is via the system that is always in contact with every part of the body, namely, the bloodstream. So, putting a pain-killer in the stomach allows it to be dissolved and subsequently absorbed into the bloodstream through the stomach and gut, and then to be swept around the body.

Some pain-killers act at the site where the stimulus is first applied, by reducing the inflammation and so decreasing the intensity of the pain signals sent to the brain. They may also reduce overall body temperature – for example, during fever.

The most common example of a medicine of this sort is aspirin. There are several others, but this is one of the most effective, with paracetamol coming a close second. But people who have gastric ulcers, or who are taking drugs to reduce blood clotting, may be advised not to use aspirin.

Other analgesics act directly, not on the actual site of the pain but on the pain centres in the brain, where the messages are received and prepared for passing on to the conscious mind. There are special receptor cells in this part of the brain on to which the drug molecules 'lock' because they fit them so exactly. They then prevent the pain messages from being registered.

A common popular example of this sort of pain-killer is codeine, which derives from opium. It is an excellent pain-killer, but can have some unfortunate side effects, just as can all the opium-derived drugs. It depresses the cough reflex, for example, which is dangerous in people with clogged lungs – you need to cough to keep your breathing tubes clear. It also slows down the action of the muscles of the gut, and can cause constipation. And it can be rather depressing, making the person who is using it feel very low. So it is the medicine of choice only in certain conditions.

All anaesthetics and narcotic drugs have analgesic effects, but the term analgesia is usually confined to milder drugs that do not cause stupor.

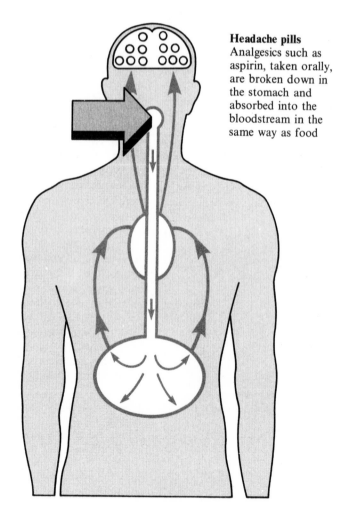

Headache pills
Analgesics such as aspirin, taken orally, are broken down in the stomach and absorbed into the bloodstream in the same way as food

---

I'm having an operation for hernia soon, and I am so afraid that I shall never wake up again after the anaesthetic. Does this happen often?

No – certainly not as a result of the anaesthetic. With modern techniques we are all safer under the care of an anaesthetist than we are crossing the average busy street – the latter activity has a much higher death rate. Anaesthetists really are the great experts at drug control and life-support-system control.

However, there is still the question of why a person is being given an anaesthetic. If he has been involved in a terrible car crash and needs surgery to repair the damage, he could possibly die during the operation, but this will

Why are so many of the drugs that ease pain – morphia and heroin, for example – so likely to cause addiction?

The drugs which are most addictive are nearly always derived from opium. Both morphine and heroin come from this Eastern poppy, as does codeine.

There are some drugs to which people become habituated; that is, they develop a psychological dependence on them. An example is cannabis indica (marijuana, pot, grass, and so on). But people do not become addicted to these drugs in the sense that their brain cells have become dependent on them in order to function. But with opiates, addiction does happen.

The extraordinary fact about the opiates is that the human brain actually contains special cells which fit them exactly. When the drug enters the body, it locks on to these cells.

But why on earth should humans have developed such cells in their brains long before the opium poppy was used to make into drugs? It seems unlikely, to say the least, that a remote Providence should design mankind ready to be exploited by drug runners.

The obvious answer has to be that the body produces a substance of its own which is meant to lock into these brain receptors and to which the opiates are similar. Once the existence of the receptor cells was discovered, researchers set out to find such a substance, and find it they did.

They discovered that when a nerve is affected by a pain stimulus, nearby cells respond by making special pain-killing substances. These go to the brain, together with the pain message, and lock on to the receptor cells, and so reduce the pain effect – built-in, natural opiate, in other words. The researchers labelled these substances endorphins, 'the morphine from inside'.

The discovery of the receptor cells showed something else as well – that they are located close to the brain areas where pleasure is registered. When the pain-killing molecules lock on to them, they not only reduce pain; they can create a profound euphoria – high spirits and a sense of joy.

This can happen in the natural way. Any sportsman will tell you that a game in which he has pushed himself to the limit of pain-endurance can result in high excitement and joy, and not only because of the psychological effects of winning or losing. It is a direct effect of the physical experience.

A similar euphoria is felt by joggers, when they push themselves to the point of pain – and this could account for the activity's current popularity.

Once someone has discovered that he is the sort of person who gets a 'high' from pain, he may have problems. Some people have great success, of course, and become great sportsmen or stuntmen or soldiers and so get the pain stimuli which trigger their euphoria in a legitimate way. Others do not, and the theory now is that some masochists (those people who find pleasure in experiencing pain) are driven to seek painful experiences by the demands of their brain receptor cells for endorphin.

It is also a commonly held theory that people who become addicted to opiate drugs are suffering from a constitutional shortage of these endorphins. Their bodies do not provide them, so they seek them from outside, and become addicted to the source of their pleasure. In other words, addiction, rather than being based on the need to escape from poverty, or arising from a search for excitement by jaded people, is a deficiency disease which is constantly struggling to correct itself.

It is an attractive theory, but unfortunately it does not entirely explain the pattern of drug abuse. Opiate addiction is much more common among the deprived, the poor and the underprivileged who throng the slum streets of big cities. They can't all be born with this particular deficiency, can they?

Why can some people be hypnotized and not feel any pain?

not be because of the surgery or the anaesthetic. It will be because of the car crash.

Similarly, if a person has a really severe and dangerous illness – say, a heart so damaged by disease that he needs a transplant – and he dies during an operation to try to reverse the effects of the disease, then it is not the surgery or anaesthetic that has killed him, it is the disease.

The chances of your dying during an operation for a hernia are far less than your chances of winning a fortune at Las Vegas.

Pain is felt in the brain. So any technique that interferes with the brain's perception of pain can stop a person feeling it.

One stage of the awareness of pain is during the transmission of the message – that is, the message that has come from the part of the body where the pain stimulus is applied – from the receiving area in the brain to the conscious mind. It is this stage which doctors think is affected by hypnosis. They admit that they are not absolutely sure about this, but it seems to be the most likely order of events.

Because the conscious mind is so active and so rich in imagination, a great deal of what goes on in it can affect the way the rest of the brain and the body works.

We all know how it is possible to make your heart beat faster with rage, or your knees shake with sexual excitement, or your eyes fill with tragic tears just by thinking about the right thing – an argument with the boss, a night in bed with a gorgeous, sexy person, your own funeral. In the same way, inducing the state known as an hypnotic trance (and no one yet knows exactly what that is) and feeding suggestions into the conscious mind can make a person feel different emotions – or cause the brain to fail to respond to pain.

It can also work the other way, incidentally. Some people under hypnosis can be made to scream with pain by being made to believe they are being burned or injured in some way.

Surgery

There was a time when every surgeon was a general surgeon. He would operate on any part of the human body, and do so with great success. Today, however, more and more specialities have evolved with surgeons devoting themselves to learning all they can about one circumscribed area. This ensures a greater development of expertise, with obvious benefits for the patient. If you need complex eye surgery, it is obvious that you will be better off in the hands of someone who spends all his time operating on eyes. This does not mean, however, that there is no longer any need for a surgeon who can deal with many kinds of different operations. All over the world general surgeons perform very competently. Most abdominal surgery is handled by general surgeons, but they also work on arms and legs, heads and hands and feet with great skill and very satisfying results.

Hospital bedside apparatus

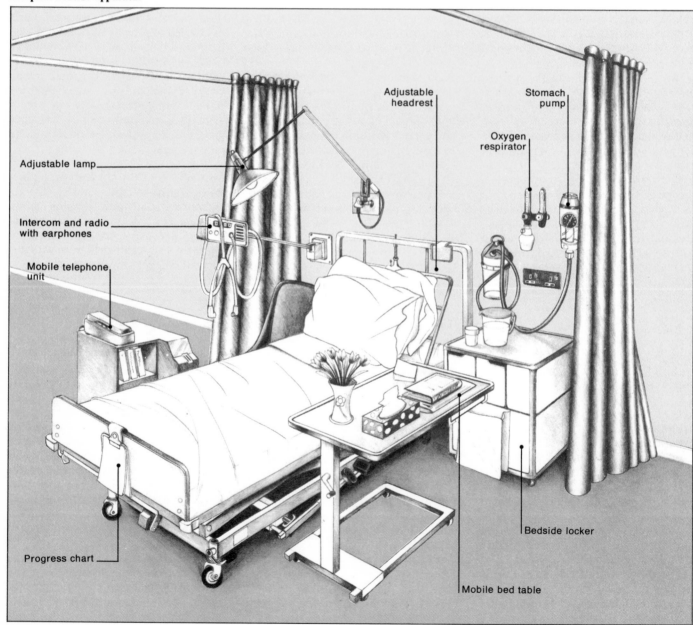

Adjustable lamp

Intercom and radio with earphones

Mobile telephone unit

Progress chart

Adjustable headrest

Oxygen respirator

Stomach pump

Bedside locker

Mobile bed table

Why do doctors and nurses make people get out of bed so soon after they have had operations? It hurts to move around so much.

And it can hurt even more if they don't move around. Many of the post-operation miseries which people suffered in the past were due, it is now known, not to the operations but to prolonged bedrest. The human body was never designed to be inactive for long periods. It slows down, becomes sluggish and can develop all sorts of disorders as a direct result of bedrest.

For example, a bedfast person tends to breathe shallowly, especially if he or she has had an abdominal operation (it is less comfortable to take a deep breath when there is a potentially painful wound on your abdominal wall) and this can lead to congestion of the lungs – pneumonia. Most people think pneumonia is due to germs, but it can also be due to the lack of proper use of the lungs.

Another effect of bedrest is the slowing down of the circulation. It becomes harder for blood to return to the heart from the lower limbs, especially when the calves are pressed against the bed as they are when you lie on your back. The blood moves more and more slowly in the deep veins of the legs, and the results can be the formation of a clot – a thrombus. Eventually, this clot can be swept into the general circulation, and if it reaches the heart or lungs or brain the effect can be a catastrophe – the blood supply to these vital organs is interrupted and the result can be severe damage, even death.

Also, muscles become soggy and lazy when they are not used. This leads not only to that dismal sense of weakness and wobbling when at last you do get up, but can also affect the muscles of the intestinal wall as well. The result is constipation which, although it doesn't really make you ill, can be uncomfortable and depressing.

Prolonged bedrest can also cause pressure sores – large painful areas of damaged skin caused by the pressure and friction of the bedclothes.

Depression, too, is a common effect of lying in bed for long periods and it can make a patient feel much more ill than his operation warrants.

And, most important of all, the general sluggishness of the bedfast patient can lead to a slowing down of the healing process. The operation wound may take longer to unite firmly, and may even, in some cases, break down once the person does get up and about. The newly stitched incision is much stronger and more able to withstand strain in a person who is moving about than a half-healed wound that has not adapted to the normal and inevitable effects of activity.

So, taking it all round, the sooner that people of all ages are coaxed out of bed after an operation, no matter how major it has been, the better. And if a patient has a condition that really makes walking about the hospital corridors impossible, vigorous physiotherapy is essential.

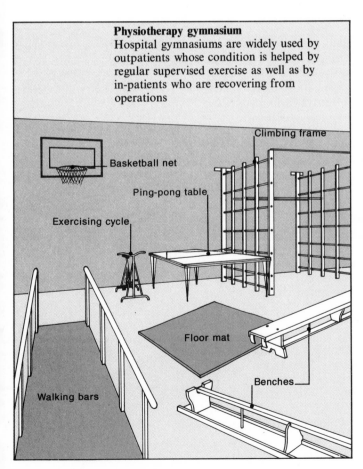

Physiotherapy gymnasium
Hospital gymnasiums are widely used by outpatients whose condition is helped by regular supervised exercise as well as by in-patients who are recovering from operations

Climbing frame
Basketball net
Ping-pong table
Exercising cycle
Floor mat
Benches
Walking bars

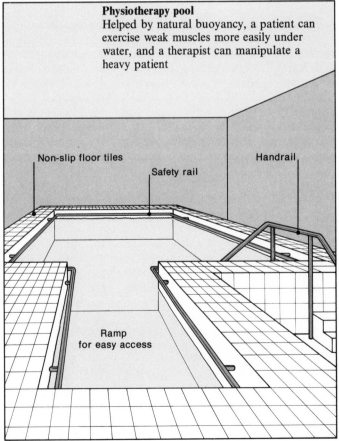

Physiotherapy pool
Helped by natural buoyancy, a patient can exercise weak muscles more easily under water, and a therapist can manipulate a heavy patient

Non-slip floor tiles
Safety rail
Handrail
Ramp
for easy access

Surgery

Why do some stitches have to be taken out after an operation?

A surprising number of different substances can be used to suture (sew up) human tissue. Horsehair, silk, nylon, cotton thread, silver or steel wire, catgut (which is nothing at all to do with cats; in fact it is made from the walls of sheep's intestines) and even strips of human tissue.

For example, repairs of some sorts of hernia – weaknesses in the muscle wall of the abdomen through which loops of intestine can push and be dangerously pinched – are often made by taking a strip of tough fascia (the covering of a muscle) from the patient's own thigh, and using it to sew up the gap. The result is a firm natural bond that is permanent – there is no need to take the strip out again.

There is also no need to remove catgut stitches because they, too, are made of organic, that is, natural material. Our bodies can absorb the strands of specially treated sheep muscle in the same way as they can absorb the lamb chops or kebabs that we eat. Stitches made of catgut are always used for deep ties in an operation. Often, when a blood vessel has to be cut and the end secured, catgut is the obvious choice, just as it is for the sewing of a deep layer of the abdomen, such as the peritoneum, the membrane which surrounds the abdominal contents.

Surface stitches, however, can be easily removed, so tougher materials can be used, and here nylon, silk, horsehair (a bit old fashioned now, but still popular with some experienced surgeons) or metal buttons holding wires come into their own. And surgeons who want to produce the most delicate scars do not stitch their wounds at all. They use a form of closure that brings the edges of the incision firmly together without actually touching them. The result is an almost invisible hairline mark.

When you have to have more than one operation in the same area does the surgeon re-open the first incision or make a new one?

A repaired surgical incision is not like a zip fastener; it cannot be reopened. Once it has healed, it is just like any other part of your skin, except that there is scar tissue there. If new surgery is needed before healing has taken place – if, for example, the surgeon has to re-operate within a day or so of the first operation – then he may remove the stitches from his original incision and operate through it. Otherwise he has to make a new cut. Usually surgeons take great care not to leave disfiguring scars, so any follow-up operations on scarred skin may be made as near as possible to the first cut to give reasonable access to the operating area, but not so close that the resulting scar will be wide and ugly.

Why did I get so much painful wind after I had my appendix out? Was it because of air trapped inside me during the operation?

No, air is not trapped in the bowels during surgery. The problem is caused by the same thing that affects the bladder emptying after surgery. Handling of the intestines in any way is an insult that results in their refusal to operate normally for a while. And this can be a problem because during an average day we all have between seven to 10 litres of gas in our intestines (some of it swallowed air, some of it resulting from the breakdown of food in digestion). Much of this air is absorbed through the gut wall, to enter the bloodstream and ultimately be disposed of, and about half a litre is passed out through the anus. But an intestine which is not producing its usual waves of expulsive action (peristalsis) does not get rid of its gas, and it balloons the gut, pressing on adjoining structures, including the operation site. All this can be extremely painful. The gut does, in time, get to work again, and the relief when the gas is at last pushed out is almost enough to make up for the discomfort that led to it.

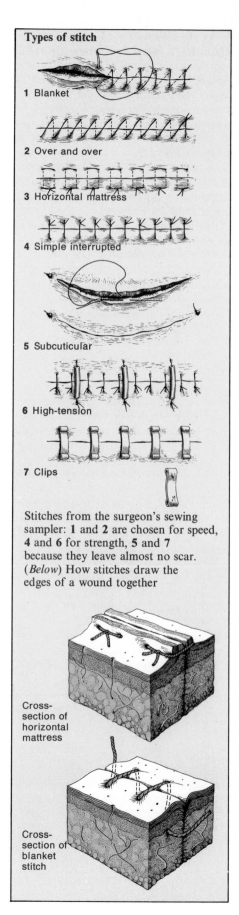

Types of stitch

1 Blanket

2 Over and over

3 Horizontal mattress

4 Simple interrupted

5 Subcuticular

6 High-tension

7 Clips

Stitches from the surgeon's sewing sampler: **1** and **2** are chosen for speed, **4** and **6** for strength, **5** and **7** because they leave almost no scar. (*Below*) How stitches draw the edges of a wound together

Cross-section of horizontal mattress

Cross-section of blanket stitch

Why do some people who have operations have IV (intravenous) lines put up? Does it mean they are in more danger than those who don't?

At one time the sight of a bottle dripping its contents through a tube into a patient's arm made everyone uneasy. It meant that the patient was at a low ebb, and his body fluids and chemicals, such as sodium and potassium, were dangerously out of balance, or that he was in need of extra blood. Now, however, surgeons and anaesthetists often use drips as a preventive method to ensure that a patient is kept in good balance from the start, instead of waiting until there is trouble as they once used to do.

The rate of flow of blood plasma or drug into the patient's vein is controlled either by a small tap near the mouth of the drip bottle (*left*), or by automatic monitoring (*right*)

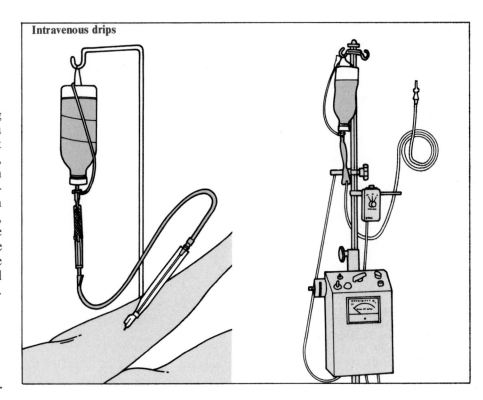

Intravenous drips

Why do some surgeons and not others insist on shaving the bodies of women who are about to have operations?

This has become a debatable issue in recent years. It used to be taken for granted by all surgeons and nurses that the only way to ensure clean skin which would heal safely after surgery was to remove every vestige of hair. So, both men and women were assiduously shaved as part of the pre-operative ritual. And women about to give birth were similarly shaved, since it was taken equally for granted that this was essential to prevent infection.

But then some feminists began to point out, sensibly enough, that women who gave birth before a doctor got to them, or who were at home under the care of unfussy midwives who didn't worry about shaving, got no more infections than women who had been denuded. And these women were spared the uncomfortable regrowth period. So the feminists suggested that shaving was just a meaningless anti-woman ritual.

Some obstetricians began to omit the shaving and found it made little difference to infection rates in child-bearing. And some surgeons, too, agreed that shaving seemed to have little effect on the germ population of the skin and they agreed sometimes to operate on

hairy skin. It really all depends on the sort of operation being done, the surgeon's willingness to cope, and the degree of risk of infection. For example, a brain operation is a high risk because infection of the brain can lead to severe difficulties. Similarly, infection of bone can create long-term and worrying problems. So, for such cases, shaving of the area to be dealt with makes good surgical sense. But for some abdominal operations, for example, an appendectomy, the shaving of the pubic and belly hair is not all that important and can often be omitted.

Why do you have trouble emptying your bladder after some operations?

The nerve supply to the bladder is closely linked with the nerve supplies to other nearby organs, such as the uterus and the bowel. And when these organs are handled during an operation, even as gently as a good surgeon does it, they are disturbed and react by stopping work, as it were. The messages from the brain just don't get through as they should. Also, of course, the effect of

fluid loss during the operation, added to fluid deprivation before it, means there is less urine to be disposed of. Usually, however, the bladder should be in full working order again within 12 hours of an operation, and if it is not, and the usual nursing tricks have no effect (running a tap where the patient can hear it, and whistling at a high-pitched note tend to have the effect of stimu-

lating the brain to intensify its messages to the bladder), putting in a tube called a catheter to drain the urine may be needed. This is less of a problem nowadays because surgical patients are encouraged to be active and out of bed, and this restores normal function more quickly. Also, it is easier to empty your bladder in the normal posture in a lavatory than perched on a bedpan.

Surgery

I've never been inside an ambulance but they fascinate me. What equipment do they carry?

A considerable amount. Apart from the obvious things such as the stretcher and blankets, there is resuscitation apparatus, splints, bandages, tourniquets and other items needed for emergency treatment at the site of an accident. And there are some mundane but very important items as well such as bedpans and urinals.

Equipment used in an ambulance
1–4 The type of stretcher used depends on the accessibility and injuries of the patient. **5** Bandages, slings, plasters, rubber gloves, and a knife for car seat belts. **6** General kit of small items. **7** Inflatable splint to cushion the limb and hold it straight. **8** Portable stomach pump. **9** Small manual respirator. **10** Oxygen cylinder and mask. **11** Flask of water. **12** Bedpan and urine bottle. **13** Spotlight. **14** Handyman kit with pliers, rope and saw

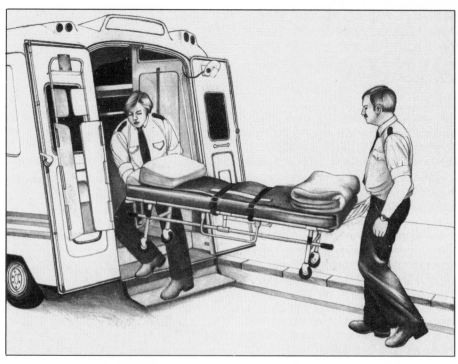

Stretchers   Medical equipment   General apparatus

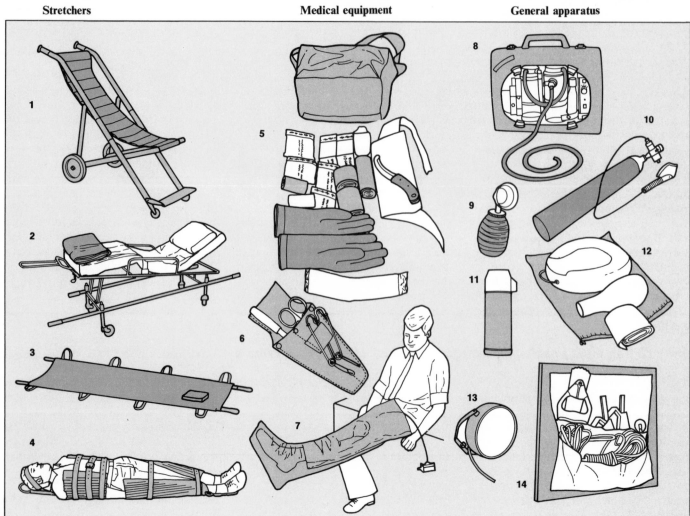

Why is it possible to remove such large parts of the body, and leave a person well? Does this mean we have a lot of useless parts?

No part of the body is useless. Whatever we have we have for a purpose, although sometimes that purpose has been lost. For example, the human appendix is not used as much today as it was in our remote evolutionary past when we ate far more cellulose (heavy vegetable matter) than we do today. The appendix played a part in digesting such material, and today we don't need it. Hence its apparent uselessness, and hence the ease with which it can be removed.

We are also, like a great many other living organisms, designed on a double system. With a few notable and important exceptions, cutting us down the middle would leave us with two matching halves. One eye, one ear, one breast, one kidney and so on, although of course we have only one heart, one stomach, one gastric system and one liver.

Each of the doubled-up organs—kidneys, lungs, ovaries and testes, eyes, ears, breasts—can take over the whole work load that usually both carry. This is why removal of one such organ leaves a person functioning well.

However, when it comes to single organs—stomach, gut, liver, heart—the situation is different. They are vital to life and health. But, with the exception of the heart, these organs can be diminished in size and still operate well. Surgeons can remove chunks of liver and several feet of gut and a sizeable portion, if not all, of the stomach, and we adapt and go on living well.

Some organs are irreplaceable, of course. Removal of the uterus usually means loss of the ability to bear children. But so remarkable is the drive to reproduce life that there have been (very rare) cases of women who have had a hysterectomy who have still conceived and carried a pregnancy 'loose' in the abdomen, with the placenta attached to another organ, such as the mesentery (the structure that holds loops of bowel in place).

Of course, much modern surgery is aimed not at removing but at repairing or improving. So there is no need to fear the loss of essential tissue.

Duplicated organs of the body
In some cases when an organ is removed its duplicate in the other half of the body can take over its function and cope with the extra work load. This is possible when someone loses the use of an eye, an ear, a lung, a breast, a kidney, an ovary (in the case of a woman), or a testicle (in the case of a man)

Spare-part surgery
Bionic men and women remain fictional concepts for the time being: spare-part surgery cannot yet provide replacements that are superior to nature's originals. However, a wide range of artificial parts is now available. They are often made from materials such as non-corrosive metal or plastic, which are not liable to be rejected by the body's defence system – as occasionally happens with the living tissue used in transplants

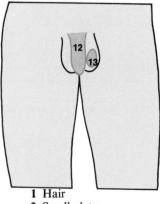

1 Hair
2 Small plate
3 Drain for excess brain fluid
4 False eye
5 False teeth
6 Artificial jaw
7 Artificial larynx
8 Heart pacemaker
9 Heart valves
10 Artificial arm
11 Main blood vessel
12 Artificial penis
13 Artificial testicle
14 Artificial leg
15 Metal plate
16 Knee joint
17 Knuckle joint
18 Hip joint
19 Bladder stimulator
20 Elbow joint
21 Artificial breast
22 Shoulder joint

Tests and checks

Even a hundred years ago, diagnosis was a very hit-or-miss affair. A doctor looked at his patient from the outside and could use only what he could see, smell or touch to identify what might be going on inside. Some doctors made shining reputations for themselves because they were particularly expert at identifying diseases with only these few signs and symptoms to guide them. They were regarded as great exponents of the art of diagnosis.

Nowadays, however, we demand science as well as art, and it is available. A large number of new techniques have been developed which have made it possible to see inside the human body, to hear its activities and to identify its chemical processes. Doctors can now inspect almost anywhere within the body where disease may be present.

Self-help breast examination
A regular monthly routine (for example, at the end of each period, when the breasts are softest) helps to detect any change. The most frequent problems – cysts, fatty and other tumours, lumps and blocked milk ducts – are all easiest to treat if they can be found at an early stage, when they are small

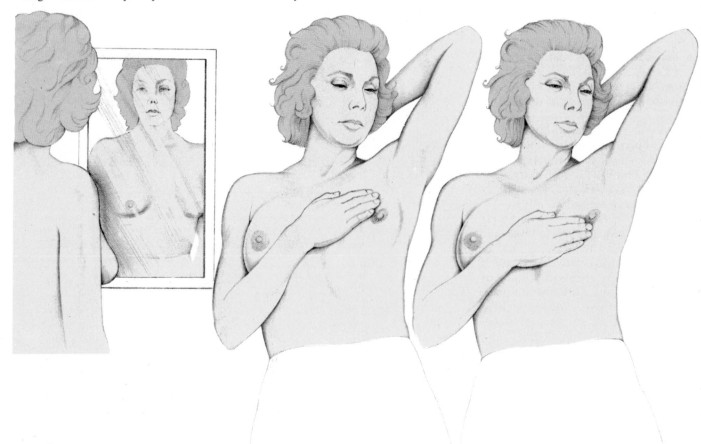

Check the appearance of your breasts in a mirror, first with your arms by your sides, and then raising them above your head. Look for changes in the texture of the skin – puckering or dimpling – and in their shape. Get to know your breasts – they are usually slightly different from each other in their shape and in their position. Examine the nipple for any unusual discharge, including bleeding

Lie down comfortably and examine your left breast with your right hand, using the flat of the fingers. Get to know their normal texture so that you can feel anything unusual. With your left arm behind your head, start by examining the upper, inner quarter. Work inwards towards the nipple from the ribs and chest area

Keep your arm behind your head while you examine the lower, inner quarter in the same way. Feel the area all round the nipple

I have to go into hospital to have a test on my lungs called a bronchoscopy. Why does this mean I have to have a general anaesthetic, when it's just a test?

For centuries doctors used to long to be able to look around inside the human body, and watch it at work. Slowly, they developed techniques which made it possible to introduce tubes with lights and mirrors on them into available body orifices, which would enable them to get a distant view – rather in the way a submariner looks through a periscope.

Nowadays, the equipment has become much more sophisticated and fibre optics have been developed which make it possible to see around corners without mirrors. So, more and more parts of the inside of the body can be looked at by a doctor from the outside.

In your case, it is the air passages that must be examined and it can be somewhat upsetting to have even the finest of fibre optics pushed into your lungs. So, a general anaesthetic is used, to make the whole procedure more pleasant for the patient.

The examination is called a bronchoscopy just as there are similar examinations called a cystoscopy (the bladder), a gastroscopy (the stomach), a proctoscopy or sigmoidoscopy (the rectum) and a laparoscopy (the belly – this technique is often used today to look at the ovaries and/or the Fallopian tubes).

I asked my doctor how I could be sure that regular checks for breast lumps were really accurate, and he sent me for a heat scan. Is this the same as an X-ray?

No. Although X-rays can be used to examine the breasts for suspicious lumps, many doctors dislike using them. This is because the too lavish use of X-rays has been known to actually lead to disease.

A safer test involves measuring the heat thrown out by different parts of the breasts. It is known that diseased areas can show up on a heat scan as a 'hot spot'. This can be a very reassuring test to have done. It is called a thermograph.

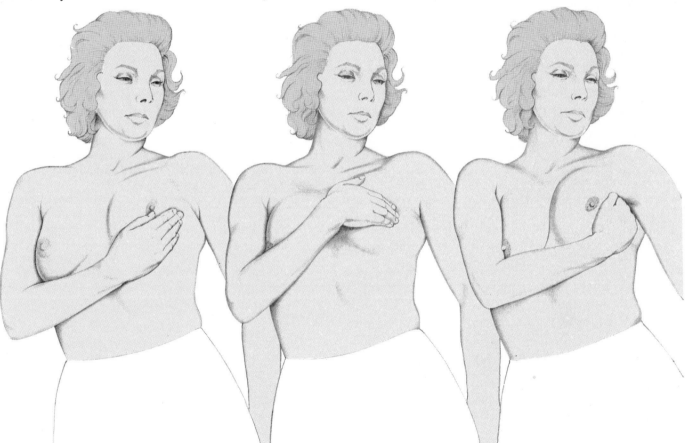

Put your arm down by your side before you examine the lower, outer quarter. Work inwards towards the nipple from the ribs, well outside the breast area

Feel over the upper, outer quarter of the breast in the same way. Check across the top of the breast to the armpit to cover the extra section of breast tissue there

Finally, feel inside the armpit itself for any lumps.

Reverse the procedure for the right breast, beginning again with the upper, inner quarter, with your right arm placed behind your head

Tests and checks

What are the blood tests that doctors do? What can they show?

Blood is a most remarkable fluid. For a start, it is not precisely a fluid, containing as it does a large number of solid bodies – the cells. There are three main types: red cells carry oxygen about the body, in the substance haemoglobin with which they are filled; white cells, which in fact are colourless, have the job of combating infection, among other things (they have other tasks but these are not all fully understood); and the platelets which act as protectors by causing the blood to clot and so plug damaged areas in blood vessel walls.

The fluid part of blood is called plasma, and it has a bewildering array of substances dissolved in it – sugar, salt, proteins, lipids (fats), hormones and various other materials which are carried from one part of the body to the other, as they are needed.

So, clearly, blood is a very important body tissue, and study of it can reveal a great deal of information about what is going on inside the body. First of all, the number of cells can be counted. Not individually – one cubic millimetre of blood, which is about the size of a large pin-head, contains five million red cells; the whole body supply of five litres has about 25 million million. The counting method used is to take a thin smear of cells in a tiny measured area. This is then multiplied to give the estimated total.

A shortage of red blood cells suggests anaemia, and the degree of anaemia is measured by estimating the amount of haemoglobin there is in the blood. Most of the tests which are commonly used measure the degree of redness of the blood against an agreed standard scale, and the answer is expressed in a percentage, or as grammes per cubic centimetre of blood.

It is also possible to measure the actual volume of individual cells (the MCV or mean cell volume), and the ratio of cells to plasma (the PCV or packed cell volume), and the amount of haemoglobin inside each cell (the MCHC or mean corpuscular haemoglobin concentration). These are complicated measurements but they give valuable and detailed information to a doctor who is investigating a patient's anaemia.

Another test involving red cells is the ESR (erythrocyte sedimentation rate – erythrocyte means red cell). It has been found that in inflammatory conditions the rate at which red cells in a specimen of blood sink to the bottom of the test tube, leaving the clear fluid of the plasma above, is accelerated. So a high ESR shows that there is inflammation somewhere that needs investigation.

White cells, too, can be counted and also checked for their shape and maturity. There is more than one kind of white cell, and since they are made in bone marrow, and also in special glands in the body, the state of the white cells indicates the state of these other structures, as well as giving warning as to whether or not infection is present.

Platelet tests usually involve measuring the amount of time needed for a specimen of blood to clot – the so-called 'bleeding time'.

Plasma tests are many and range from checking the levels of various proteins to measuring the amount of glucose, hormones, cholesterol (fats) and other substances that are carried in the flood of plasma from body cell to body cell.

Then there are tests to show the presence of disease – the Paul-Bunnell (Mono-spot in the US) test for glandular fever, the Wasserman test which reveals syphilis or the Coombs' test which shows whether there are dangerous antibodies present, for example, after a mismatched blood transfusion.

And there are tests designed to prevent disorder. One example is the Rhesus test which is done on pregnant women. If a mother has Rhesus negative blood, and she carries a second baby who has inherited Rhesus positive blood from his father, her blood may react against the baby's and destroy it. In the past this used to kill many babies. Today, early testing can reveal those women who need special protective immunization, and they go on to have healthy, normal infants. Also tests on the blood which is taken from donors to match it with the blood of an anaemic person who needs it, prevent the damage, and even death, that can result if incompatible bloods are mixed.

What are urine tests, and what do they show?

Because urine carries the waste materials out of the body, it also carries a great deal of information about how the body is producing those wastes. Not only can kidney and bladder function be measured but also endocrine and metabolic and circulatory function.

The tests that are done depend on what the doctors are looking for, and what their examination of a patient and his symptoms makes them suspect is wrong. But there is one basic test that is always done.

This routine covers the colour (darkening shows a concentration that may be due to severe fever, heart disease, diarrhoea and vomiting; pallor may show the presence of nephritis – kidney inflammation – or diabetes; bloodiness may be due to kidney damage or bladder disease); the quantity (too little urine in 24 hours may mean dehydration, too much may mean diabetes); specific gravity (a low one may suggest nephritis or diabetes, a high one concentration of urine, as in dehydration or heart disease, and also the presence of pus or blood cells, as in a kidney or bladder infection); the amount of sugar (in diabetes extra sugar is excreted) and the presence of protein (which suggests kidney disorder).

Why did my doctor ask for an early morning specimen of urine? Is it different at that time of day?

Most people do not pass urine during the night, although the kidneys go on producing it, and the bladder fills up. The urine in the bladder parts with some of its water content through the bladder walls as the night passes, and this concentrates the urine. When a test is needed to identify a substance that is present in only a small amount, a concentrated specimen is easier to work on. Such a test is the one which is used to diagnose a pregnancy.

After a blood test my doctor said I had anaemia and prescribed iron tablets for a few weeks. Now he says I need no more. But my friend had tests which also showed anaemia, but she has to have injections which she has been told she must have all her life. Why is there this difference?

There are many types of anaemia.

There is a simple anaemia, due to shortage of iron, the essential ingredient of the haemoglobin which carries oxygen round the body in red blood cells. This shortage can happen because of a faulty diet which does not provide enough essential iron, because of loss of blood due to injury or disease (for example, people with piles can become quite anaemic over a period of time), at times of heavy stress, and at times when extra demands are made on the body, for example during pregnancy.

In these cases the remedy is simple – replace the missing iron. In emergencies, for instance, after a heavy blood loss in an accident, iron replacement can be given by giving a blood transfusion. In other cases, it is enough to give the extra iron needed to make new red cells either as an injection or as tablets taken by mouth. Once the iron levels are up to normal, the patient is well again and all that is needed is to avoid lack of iron in the future, possibly by improving the iron content of the patient's general diet.

This was clearly the situation in your case.

But there are other kinds of anaemia, with many different causes. One is called pernicious anaemia (or Biermer's anaemia, after the Swiss doctor who described it in 1872). In this disease there is no shortage of iron in the diet, but the body is unable to use it to make new red cells. This is because of a lack of a vital substance which the body ought to make for itself in the stomach but in some cases fails to do. The disease can sometimes happen after stomach surgery. The vital substance is called the intrinsic factor and until just over 30 years ago, when doctors learned what it was, the only way to save the lives of people with this sort of anaemia was to feed them large quantities of the only known source of the factor – raw liver. It had to be raw, because cooking damaged the special factor in it, and this was repellent in the extreme. But then, happily, the substance was isolated in 1948 and was found to be Vitamin B12. Today, people with this sort of anaemia just need regular injections of B12 and they are fine. It has to be given by injection, by the way, because B12 is destroyed in the stomach if it is swallowed.

Clearly, this is the sort of anaemia which your friend has, but she will now have no further problems as long as she takes her treatment regularly.

Formed elements in the blood

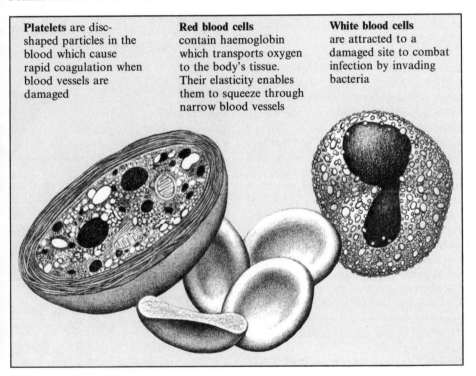

Platelets are disc-shaped particles in the blood which cause rapid coagulation when blood vessels are damaged

Red blood cells contain haemoglobin which transports oxygen to the body's tissue. Their elasticity enables them to squeeze through narrow blood vessels

White blood cells are attracted to a damaged site to combat infection by invading bacteria

Why did I have to have a catheter put in me to get urine for a test? Couldn't the doctor have used urine I passed in the normal way?

When a test has to be made to check for infection it needs to be uncontaminated, and urine passed in the ordinary manner picks up some germs on its way out of the bladder and through the vulva or penis. Passing a germ-free tube directly into the bladder will ensure that as clean as possible a specimen is collected.

Another way of collecting a virtually germ-free specimen is by means of the MSU (mid-stream urine). The patient is told to pass the first part of his bladderful into the lavatory, then to collect the next third or so into a sterilized specimen jar, and end by letting the remainder go into the lavatory. This method can give almost as uncontaminated a specimen as a catheter, and it is much simpler and pleasanter for a person to cope with.

My doctor told me to collect all the urine I passed for 24 hours for a test but usually all that is wanted is a small amount. Why was my test different?

The doctor was almost certainly investigating some aspect of your endocrine system. These glands produce their hormones in differing amounts over each 24 hours (or over the month, if they are the ovarian hormones) and an accurate estimation of what the glands are doing demands a check on the whole of the day's output.

Tests and checks

How many different kinds of X-rays are there? And what is the difference between X-rays used for tests and those used for treatments?

Certain body tissues are radio-opaque, that is, the X-rays cannot pass through them. Bones and teeth are good examples of tissues which show up clearly on X-rays. Other soft tissues can be seen as well, however, with varying degrees of clarity. A straight X-ray of the belly, for example, can show the outline of the large gut, and bubbles of air in it. Lungs, too, can be X-rayed, and expert radiologists become skilled at identifying tissue changes from these films.

But sometimes greater definition is needed, and one way of providing this is to outline the area to be studied with radio-opaque material. The gall bladder can be checked in this way and the bladder and kidneys and so can the gullet and stomach and intestines, by giving the patient barium. This is called a barium swallow (to check the gullet), or barium meal (to check the stomach and intestines), or barium enema (to check the rectum), in which case, of course, the barium is put in through the anus, rather than through the mouth.

It is also possible to X-ray the Fallopian tubes, using an opaque material introduced via the vagina (a salpingogram); the spinal column (a myelogram); the bladder (a cystogram); the bronchial tubes in the lungs (a bronchogram); different arteries around the body, but most particularly those supplying the heart and the brain (an arteriogram or angiogram); the spaces inside the brain (a ventriculogram); and indeed any body space into which either radio-opaque material or air can be put. Air, or a gas such as carbon dioxide, can be an effective material to use, because it leaves clearly defined areas on an X-ray.

A salpingogram is not always used for gynaecological examinations. A laparoscopy, which is a way of looking at the Fallopian tubes with a 'telescope' introduced through the abdominal walls, is frequently done now.

Sometimes real-time X-rays are used. That is, the doctor watches the patient's body through an X-ray screen while the body is actually functioning, rather than just taking a still picture. It is rather like the difference between a snapshot and a movie. Seeing how the heart beats, the lungs expand, or the barium goes down can be a great aid to the specialist who is making a diagnosis.

Nowadays, new technology has made it possible to take X-rays of layers of the body. For example, the exact point in the lungs where a growth of a tuberculous area has developed can be accurately pinpointed. The amount of X-rays needed to do these tests is carefully worked out to be the minimum needed to give a picture without damaging the tissues through which the rays pass. This is because X-rays are very powerful indeed and can destroy living cells. Sometimes this effect is needed for treatment of disease and then larger doses are used, with the site to which they are to be delivered extremely delicately worked out, so that only the sick tissue that needs to be destroyed is affected.

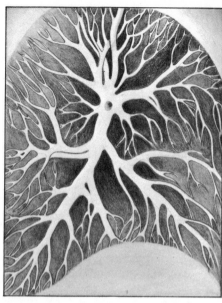

A **conventional X-ray** records shadows of varying density. In the bronchogram (*above*) radio-opaque material has outlined the right bronchial tree of the lung

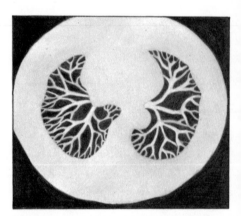

The **scan** of a cross-section of the chest looks down on the heart and aorta between the shapes of the lungs

When I got very thin and nervous, my doctor sent me for a test which involved breathing in and out of a tube. Why was that?

To do its work, the body burns up food and oxygen. This is called metabolism, and there is a basal metabolic rate (BMR) for each individual which can be measured by checking the amount of oxygen taken up by a person who is at total rest.

The thyroid, the endocrine gland at the root of the neck, is closely involved with metabolic rate. When the thyroid is overactive the rate is high. Since you were showing symptoms of an overactive thyroid – the loss of weight and nervousness – your doctor wanted the confirmation of a check on your BMR. This information will help him to make a firm diagnosis, although he may do other tests, such as blood checks, as well.

Incidentally, there is another test – the vital capacity test – which involves breathing in and out of a tube. Each person's lungs should expand enough to take in a certain amount of air. In people with impaired lungs or certain forms of heart disease this amount may be markedly reduced. In your case, the BMR was obviously being checked.

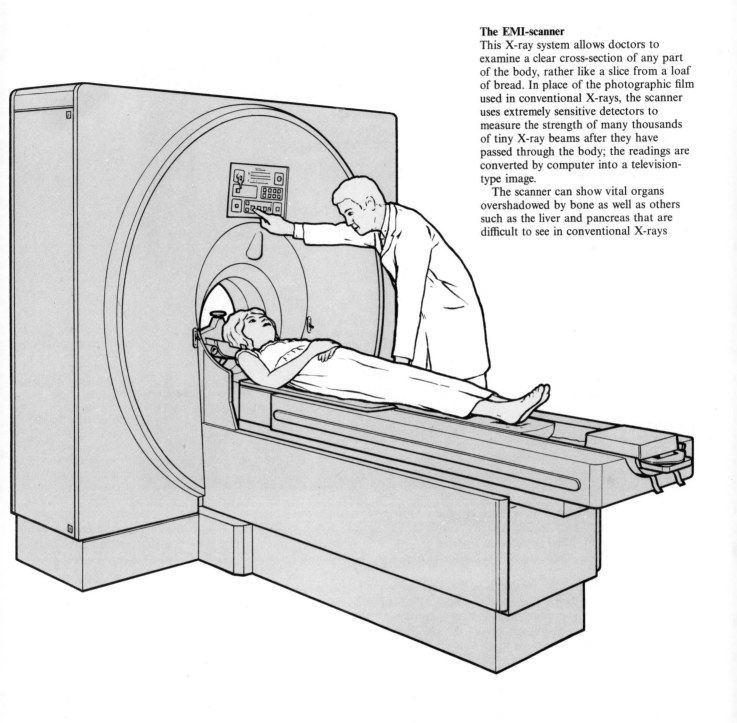

The EMI-scanner

This X-ray system allows doctors to examine a clear cross-section of any part of the body, rather like a slice from a loaf of bread. In place of the photographic film used in conventional X-rays, the scanner uses extremely sensitive detectors to measure the strength of many thousands of tiny X-ray beams after they have passed through the body; the readings are converted by computer into a television-type image.

The scanner can show vital organs overshadowed by bone as well as others such as the liver and pancreas that are difficult to see in conventional X-rays

When I had an X-ray for gall bladder trouble I was given a glass of very rich creamy milk to drink. It made me feel really nauseated. Why was this necessary, when the doctor knows that rich food disagrees with me?

The gall bladder releases its contents, bile, in response to the presence of fat in the diet. When a healthy person eats a piece of toast dripping with melted butter, out comes the bile, because it has the job of digesting fats. But when a person with gall bladder disease eats a fatty meal, the bile does not flow so freely and the result is discomfort and possibly nausea.

To prove that the problem that you were suffering from was gall bladder disease, you were first given a drug that is radio-opaque, and which is collected in the gall bladder as the liver makes bile, and then, 12 hours later, the first X-rays were taken to check on what your gall bladder was doing. The reason for the rich drink was to see what would happen when you swallowed extra fat. That can often clinch the diagnosis.

Tests and checks

When I went for an X-ray because of bladder trouble, a thick tube was put directly into my bladder. The second time I was given an injection into my arm. Why?

The first test was to check on the bladder itself. The tube (catheter) that was passed in carried a safe radio-opaque substance. When it filled your bladder, films were taken that showed its outline. As this did not give enough information, the second X-ray checked on your kidney function. The injection was again a radio-opaque substance carried, from the vein in your arm into which it was injected, to the kidneys. The substance was extracted by the kidneys, and X-ray films showed the way the urine passed out of them into the bladder. This test is called an IVP (intravenous pyelogram).

Sometimes doctors do a retrograde pyelogram. For this, two fine catheters are passed into the bladder, and on into the openings of the tubes that run from the kidneys, and radio-opaque material is put in. The X-rays show the shape of the pelvis of the kidney. This test is often done under a general anaesthetic because it can be uncomfortable.

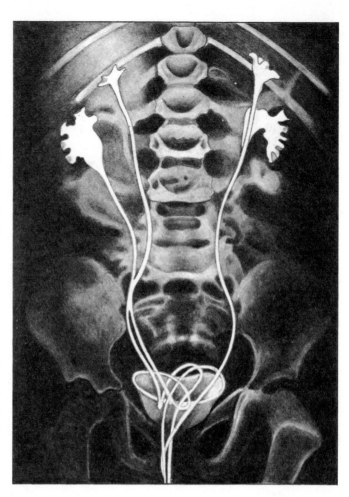

Retrograde pyelogram
A pyelogram – X-ray outline of the kidneys – is done under general anaesthetic by passing catheters up the ureters and injecting radio-opaque dye

My doctor says I have to have a test meal, because he thinks I may have an ulcer. What happens?

You will be told to fast for a number of hours, and then a fine tube will be passed through your nose, down the back of your throat and into your stomach. It is not as uncomfortable as it sounds when it is done by a skilful practitioner. A sample of your stomach juices will then be taken, and you will be given a drink of thin oatmeal porridge (for some people, this is the unpleasant bit – they don't like oatmeal), and specimens will be withdrawn from the tube from time to time. This test can show the different levels of gastric juices during a meal, and also demonstrates the rate at which the stomach empties – important factors in diagnosing stomach ailments such as ulcers.

When my little boy had a kidney infection, the doctor took throat swabs as well as checking his urine. Why did he do this?

One of the complications of scarlet fever (scarlatina) is a spread of infection from the throat, where the germs that cause the illness often enter the body, to the kidneys. Sometimes it is the kidney disorder that shows first because it is not always easy to diagnose scarlatina, or the similar condition of infectious sore throat, which is caused by a bacterium called the streptococcus. So your doctor took the throat swabs to check for the presence of these germs, because treatment to get rid of them, if they are present, is essential.

I had prolonged headaches after a feverish illness and my doctor said I should have a lumbar puncture. What is this, and why is it done?

The brain and the thick nerve trunk that goes from the brain, right through the spinal column, have a special circulation of their own, the cerebro-spinal fluid. In some disorders of the system the amount of fluid is increased, or it may contain extra white cells, or infecting organisms.

If a needle is passed into the space in the spine through which the fluid travels, its volume can be measured, and a specimen removed to check for signs of infection or other disease. In cases of severe and prolonged headache, a lumbar puncture can be a useful diagnostic tool, perhaps showing that the headaches are due to infection of the brain membranes. Once the cause is identified, the condition is much easier to treat, of course.

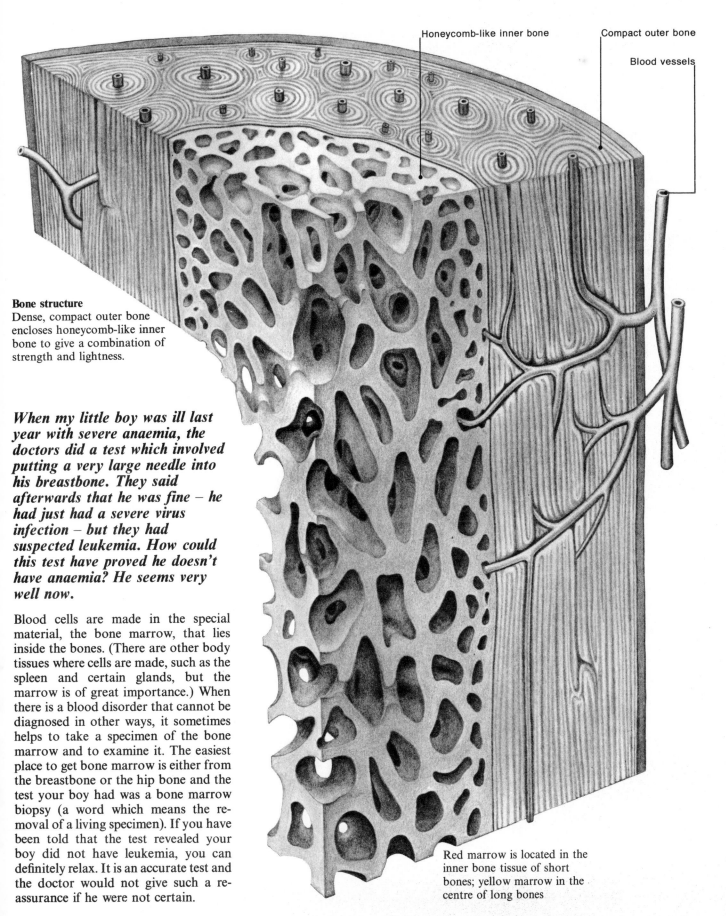

Honeycomb-like inner bone

Compact outer bone

Blood vessels

Bone structure
Dense, compact outer bone encloses honeycomb-like inner bone to give a combination of strength and lightness.

When my little boy was ill last year with severe anaemia, the doctors did a test which involved putting a very large needle into his breastbone. They said afterwards that he was fine – he had just had a severe virus infection – but they had suspected leukemia. How could this test have proved he doesn't have anaemia? He seems very well now.

Blood cells are made in the special material, the bone marrow, that lies inside the bones. (There are other body tissues where cells are made, such as the spleen and certain glands, but the marrow is of great importance.) When there is a blood disorder that cannot be diagnosed in other ways, it sometimes helps to take a specimen of the bone marrow and to examine it. The easiest place to get bone marrow is either from the breastbone or the hip bone and the test your boy had was a bone marrow biopsy (a word which means the removal of a living specimen). If you have been told that the test revealed your boy did not have leukemia, you can definitely relax. It is an accurate test and the doctor would not give such a reassurance if he were not certain.

Red marrow is located in the inner bone tissue of short bones; yellow marrow in the centre of long bones

Tests and checks

When a doctor gives a general physical check-up of the sort that you have to have when you take out insurance, what does he actually do?

Oddly enough, there can be no complete answer to this question. The sort of investigations doctors regard as essential vary greatly from country to country. In the USA, for example, a total physical check of a healthy person will include a great many blood tests and function tests that European doctors will not regard as necessary.

But most doctors in most countries will look at the heart function, checking on its beat, its regularity and its strength; the blood pressure; the body weight (almost everyone everywhere agrees that obesity is unhealthy); the kidneys (performing urine tests for colour, concentration, specific gravity and sugar and protein content); the lungs (checking breathing sounds and vital capacity); the blood (looking for signs of anaemia) and possibly the function of eyes and ears and the nervous system.

Beyond that basic set of physical examinations there can also be a battery of highly sophisticated tests. Some doctors will always do an ECG (EKG in the USA) – an electrocardiogram – which makes a tracing of the heart's action. Others may perform an EEG, an electroencephalogram, which traces brain impulses. There may be liver function tests, which involve taking blood and making a number of investigations on its contents. There may be blood tests for cholesterol, which is thought to play a part in coronary artery disease. There may be chest X-rays, especially in countries where tuberculosis is still a health problem and for patients who smoke, and other X-rays, depending on the individual patient and his doctor.

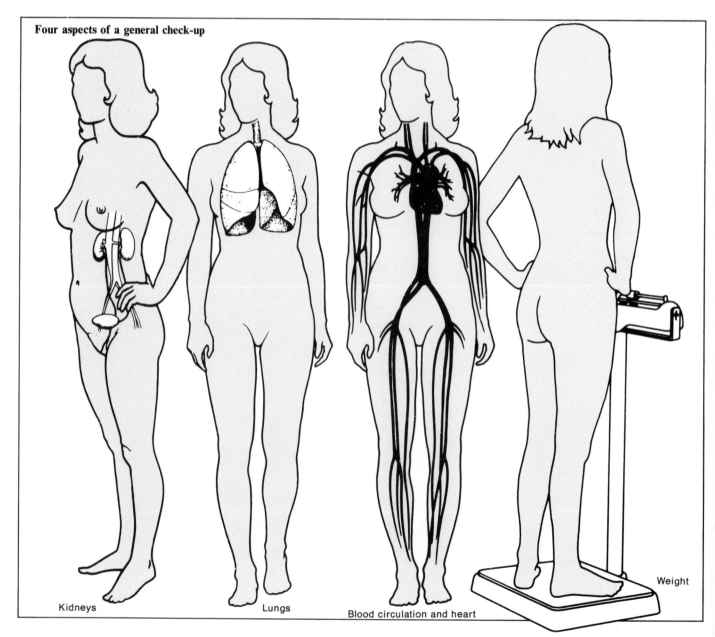

Four aspects of a general check-up

Kidneys   Lungs   Blood circulation and heart   Weight

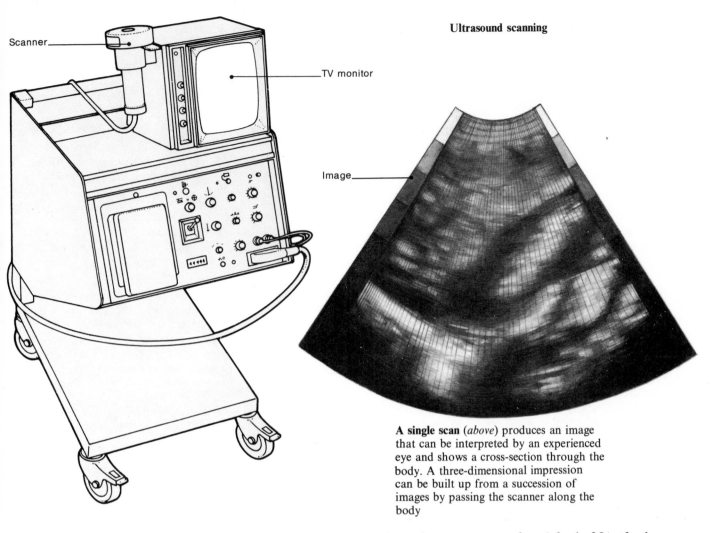

Ultrasound scanning

Scanner

TV monitor

Image

A single scan (*above*) produces an image that can be interpreted by an experienced eye and shows a cross-section through the body. A three-dimensional impression can be built up from a succession of images by passing the scanner along the body

My daughter is having a baby, and because she is older than the average mother (she is 39) she is to have a special test of the waters. I'm worried about this. What does it mean?

A developing baby floats inside the uterus, in a bag of membranes, containing a bath of water. This is called amniotic fluid, and study of a specimen of it can provide valuable information about the way the baby is developing. It can also reveal the baby's sex, because some of his or her body cells float in the water, and each body cell carries the evidence of gender differences. (It's all to do with tiny structures called chromosomes. Boys have XY chromosomes, girls XX.)

Taking a sample of this water used to be impossible because getting into the bag of membranes with a needle was as unpredictable and dangerous as pushing a sword into a small haystack in which a man is hiding, and hoping the sword will miss him. But a new technique – ultrasound scanning – now makes testing both safe and possible.

It was found during the World War II that it was possible to make accurate drawings of distant unseen objects by 'bouncing' sound off them and measuring the echo that came back. This was radar – and today a form of radar is used to 'bounce' sounds off the baby in the womb, and so make a picture of his position. It is even possible to watch him moving about, making breathing movements (which the unborn do, learning how to breathe after birth) and sucking his thumb.

This technique opened up a new world of investigation, because X-rays, if used to any excess, are not really safe – they can damage the baby. There is no evidence that sound can. Now the doctors have a tool that enables them to 'see' the unborn baby, and they can introduce a hollow needle into his bag of waters and withdraw a specimen with safety.

Such a specimen can show whether the baby is developing normally and can detect the presence of certain known handicaps. For example, Down's syndrome (it used to be called mongolism) can be detected via amniocentesis, as the water test is called, in time for the parents to choose whether or not they want to terminate the pregnancy. It is a test which is usually offered to older than average mothers, because the incidence of Down's syndrome is known to increase with parental age. Not all prebirth disorder can be detected in this way but more may be possible as the technique is developed.

The ultrasound scanning system is now being expanded to perform other investigations and whole body scanning to detect severe disease is a useful, though expensive, medical tool which is available in some special centres.

Medical puzzles

Although medicine has now divided itself into many different specialities, with expert doctors devoting their working lives to gaining more and more knowledge about one circumscribed area of the human body, it is not possible to put every question tidily into a category. Some are general, defying any form of pigeon-holing. This means that finding the right person to ask can be as big a puzzle as the original question. This section attempts to answer some of these questions.

Why does a blow cause a bruise?
And why do bruises go such different colours?
Are they more severe when they are purple?

A bruise is a loss of blood from the small capillaries into the surrounding tissues. The blood can get out if the skin is broken, but if not, it remains in the tissues, waiting to be absorbed.

The blood begins to change fairly soon, with the red pigment (haemoglobin) turning blue because it is deprived of oxygen. Then, the blueness turns green and yellow as the blood is broken down into bile pigments. Finally, it is all absorbed and the bruise disappears. The same process happens with bruising in deep tissues such as muscles. You can't actually see what is happening although you can feel it. Incidentally, it is not true that a bruise has to 'come out', that is, actually shows on the surface. Healing will take place whether you can see that a bruise is present or not.

A bruise hurts because of the swelling which is caused by the escaped blood pressing on adjacent nerves, and it will hurt more in the early stages, while it is still bluish-purple, than later on as the blood becomes absorbed. But the blue stage is no more 'severe' than the other stages.

Not all bruises are caused by blows. They may appear spontaneously in some blood or blood vessel disorders, which is why bruising that appears when there has been no injury to cause it should be reported to a doctor for diagnosis.

Why do I sometimes jump suddenly, just as I'm falling asleep?

This is called a myoclonic jerk, and it has been suggested that it is a throwback to our remotest ancestors who lived in trees, and that humans developed this reflex to prevent themselves falling off the branches as they dozed off.

But this is a romantic notion for which there seems to be no proof. What is known is that sleep occurs in four stages. There is the first very light, half-dozing state, then a light sleep stage, followed by a third somewhat deeper one which ends in the deepest of all which is stage four. These stages can be demonstrated on an EEG machine, because the brain's electrical impulses make different patterns as the sleeper passes through each stage.

Sometimes, as a person descends from stage three sleep to stage four there is a sudden upsurge of brain activity. This sends out a little burst of electrical impulses which go to all the muscles and make them contract in a sharp spasm.

Not everyone experiences this jerking although it happens to about two thirds of the population.

Why do I get shadows under my eyes when I'm tired?

The area surrounding the eyes is very active; there are a number of muscles there to control the movements of the eyelids and to produce the extremely wide range of expressions of which the human face is capable. This means there is a rich blood supply to the area, and that the skin around the eyes is thinner and a little less elastic than other skin.

A tired or ill person may have an increase of blood supply to the area, and this appears as puffing of the tissues beneath the eyes, and as shadowing as the blood shows through the thin skin.

In some conditions such as heart and kidney disease where there is marked fluid retention in the tissues, swelling around the eyes may be a significant sign of edema.

Some people have a family tendency to loose skin in this area, and to a bluish tint there. Little can or need be done to change this. Aging also causes stretching of the skin under the eyes.

I can swallow while I'm standing on my head. Why doesn't the food fall back down from my stomach?

When food gets into the gullet from the mouth, pushed there by the complex series of muscular movements called swallowing, a wave of peristalsis is set up. The gullet tightens and relaxes in successive sections, so pushing the food along at the rate of about an inch a minute. This movement is powerful enough to overcome the force of gravity.

Why is it that you can take things into your mouth which are too hot to touch?
If I put my finger in a cup of coffee it feels painfully hot, but I can drink the coffee comfortably.

There are several reasons for this. First of all, the mouth and gullet and stomach are lined with mucous membrane, and the membrane is covered by a layer of its own exudate (mucus). This acts in part as an insulator. The mucous lining of the stomach is particularly effective, being thicker than the lining of either the gullet or the mouth.

Also, the speed with which food and drink passes through the food tract comes into it. The hot .substance – especially if it is liquid – can pass over the mouth and throat area too quickly for heat to be transferred; you will find that if you try to take in a mouthful of hot coffee and keep it there without swallowing it you will experience discomfort and you might burn the tongue or mouth lining. Once it is in the stomach, however, it cannot harm the lining because of that extra heavy layer of mucus.

Also, it seems likely that because the blood supply to the whole area is particularly rich, excess heat is rapidly carried away into the general bloodstream, and is there dissipated.

Finally, habituation comes into it. There are people who train themselves to swallow food and drink that is exceedingly hot. They may do themselves a disservice because in some cases of malignant disease of the gut it is thought that the taking of excessively hot food has acted as a trigger.

Why do I get a lump in my throat when I'm sad?

There is no real lump, but there is a tightening of some of the muscles of the pharynx. Why this should happen in response to emotional stress is hard to say, but it seems to be an adrenalin response acting selectively on these particular muscles. The lump can become a chronic problem, instead of one that only happens at obvious times – when watching a sad movie for instance. People who are always under stress, suffering from constant low-level anxiety, may complain of a perpetual lump in the throat and fear that they have cancer there. But examination shows they have not. The problem is called globus hystericus. Dealing with the underlying anxiety gets rid of the lump.

Why do some people snore?

If there were one simple answer to this question, life would be much more tranquil for many people. Unfortunately there is not.

Snoring happens when the passages through which air passes in respiration are narrowed in any way, just as a sound is made in a tin whistle because the air is forced through a narrow space.

The causes of narrowing are many. A person who is sitting up and falls asleep stops exerting control on the muscles of the lower jaw and the palate. They relax, and this narrows the air entry. This is why so many people snore when they fall asleep in armchairs and on trains.

People lying down may also snore if they lie on their back because, again, the lower jaw drops and the muscles of the palate relax. If they lie on their sides with their heads thrown back the same effect may be noticed.

Obstructions of the airways, such as enlarged adenoids or tonsils may cause snoring. So may obstruction of the nose – the mouth has to be opened to allow air in and the jaw relaxes.

Swelling of the mucous membrane lining the airways will also act as an obstruction. This happens in a person with a cold, or some other upper respiratory infection. It also happens to women during pregnancy, and in some cases during the pre-menstrual period when there is a general tendency to fluid retention in the tissues which affects the membranes in the breathing passages together with all other tissues. And people suffering from allergies may develop congested mucous membranes.

The atmosphere in which a person sleeps can have an effect; a too-dry, centrally heated, or a too-moist, over-humidified atmosphere can lead to snoring in a susceptible individual.

In a few people there may be a tendency for the nostrils to flatten during sleep, which can lead to snoring. And people who are overweight also tend to snore more than thin people, but it is hard to be sure why this is. After all, there is rarely extra fat laid down in the area of the breathing passages. However, it is clearly a cause, because weight loss often leads to a reduction of noise during sleep.

Why do I get white fur on my tongue? Does it always mean I need a laxative?

It never means you need a laxative. It is a total myth that constipation causes furring of the tongue. It was probably invented by laxative manufacturers.

Tongue furring can occur for many reasons. The mouth is mildly alkaline in reaction – saliva, which washes it and moistens it, is an alkaline substance – and this maintains an essential disinfecting acid-alkaline balance which has the effect of keeping micro-organisms in check. Obviously, the mouth is vulnerable to a large number of such organisms, since it is in constant contact with the outside world. If the acid-alkaline balance changes for any reason then the micro-organisms can flourish, and it is they which create the white or yellowish furriness which may form a coating on the tongue.

The reason for a change in the balance may be local – infected teeth, or infection in the sinuses, draining into the mouth area – or the reason may be general, such as fever, which reduces the moisture in the mouth. Very debilitated people, in whom all the body processes are slowed down, are also prone to get furred tongues, and they may develop severe mouth sores and become even more ill unless they are carefully nursed and the tongue and mouth are regularly cleansed.

Medical puzzles

Why do some parts of the body keep on growing, such as the hair and nails, when other parts such as fingers and legs stay the same?

The way the body controls its growth processes still remains largely a mystery, although we do know that each cell carries in its genes – the fragments of material in the chromosomes which determine every aspect of the cell's activity – a control mechanism for growth.

How this is triggered and how switched off is still being investigated. We know that certain hormones are involved, and particularly the pituitary ones, but there are many other factors as well. What is clear is that certain tissues have a built-in 'stop' mechanism which, unless other factors intervene, makes growth cease at the right level.

An example of what can happen to change the growth control process is pituitary disease. In this, excess growth hormone is produced which overrides the cells' growth instructions and causes excess development. If the disease happens in a child whose bones are not yet fully formed, the result is gigantism and heights of over seven feet have been recorded. If it happens in a fully developed adult, the result is acromegaly in which heavy bony deposits on hands, feet and skull cause marked cragginess of appearance. The opposite can happen if there is a deficiency of growth hormone in a child. He becomes a dwarf if not treated.

Hair and nails are modified skin and, like skin, continue to replace themselves throughout life.

Why do people in some parts of the world live so much longer than others?

It is a remarkable fact that the Biblical estimation of a normal life span – three score years and 10 – is as true today as it was then, well over 5,000 years ago when all the diseases we have since learned to control ran rife. Most people given adequate food will live to be around 70. Women tend to live longer than men.

In some parts of the world it is claimed that these figures are greatly exceeded. Georgia in Russia seems to have a breed of long-lived people (and longevity undoubtedly runs in families; to live to a ripe old age yourself, choose ancestors who did). The Georgians have claimed citizens of 160 years. Ecuador and Tibet are also areas where claims of prolonged human life have been made.

If the claims are true, and they are rarely fully documented, the reasons could be, apart from the possession of the right genes, a low calorie diet (animal experiments have shown that limited feeding and long life go hand in hand) and a low-stress existence. Usually, a peaceable humdrum life will last much longer than one which is busy and exciting.

As the old joke says, perhaps these very old people who follow such regimes haven't actually lived longer – it just feels like it.

Why does some sweat smell, but not others? The sort you get on your forehead doesn't smell, but your armpits and feet do.

Sweat itself does not smell at all. However, it is an organic substance and so provides food and a growing medium for micro-organisms. It is the action of the latter on the sweat which creates odour. So, regular washing away of the sweat before it can become stale avoids smells.

Some sweat evaporates so fast that there is no time for invasion of micro-organisms. Facial sweat is like that. In protected areas of the body, however, the sweat can build up and the organisms can get to work happily and in peace. Armpits, the genitalia and the feet are examples of this. Feet also smell because of the way sweat acts on the materials used to clothe them; leather tends not to get odorous, but some plastics do.

Sweat in the armpits and round the genitals is different, however. There it is trapped in the hair, and may contain substances called pheromones – special attractants which arouse sexual desire. Many animals produce such substances which we take and use for perfumes. An example is civet, which comes from special sweat glands in a type of cat. Yet we deodorize away our own sweat.

When you cut yourself and it heals, how does the body know when to stop healing? Why doesn't a scar just get thicker and thicker?

Repair and growth are similar, in that each cell carries its own instructions about the growth that ought to happen, and switches off when it is complete. For example, fully seven-eighths of the liver can be removed surgically and the remaining stump will grow until the liver is back to full size again, and then stop. But loss of other tissue cannot be made good like this. For example, a broken bone will heal, but one shortened by amputation will not grow again (although some other animals can grow new limbs) and nerve tissue, once destroyed, will not be replaced. And we do not as yet fully understand why these differences should be.

Repair sometimes does go wrong, and there can be a too exuberant development of tissue where healing is taking place. There is a condition called 'proud flesh' in which granulation tissue appears over a healing site, and has to be removed. Similarly, a scar can overgrow and become keloid. There may be some connection between the likelihood of this developing and the amount of pigment in the skin. In fair-haired people a keloid scar is rare, but it is more common in brunettes and quite common in negroes. A keloid scar is harmless but disfiguring. This has been used by some black peoples as a source of adornment. Decorative cuts are made deliberately in the cheeks or over the body and substances are rubbed into them to encourage the appearance of wide keloid scars.

Why do I get gooseflesh when I'm cold and when I'm scared as well as when I see a sexually attractive person?

This is all part of the adrenalin response, and is a vestigial reaction. Animals with furry pelts have a mechanism for raising the individual hairs. This can be useful in cold conditions (trapping air in the fluffed out fur produces insulation) and also as a defence. A small animal can look remarkably large and menacing when all its hair is standing on end.

It is adrenalin which triggers this response by causing each tiny muscle alongside each hair, called the arrector pili muscle, to contract. Then the skin beneath the hair follicle is flattened, while that immediately round the hair itself is elevated. This creates the tiny bumps we call gooseflesh.

When it happens on hairy skin, all we see is the movement of the hair. On comparatively hairless skin we see the bumps because the follicles are still there even though the hairs are not.

When gooseflesh happens on the back of the neck it can feel rather odd, as the hairs do actually rise. A person who has experienced this might say, 'It made my hackles rise' meaning that he felt anger, or fear. And some people who get a rapid gooseflesh response may say, 'A goose walked over my grave', to explain the odd shuddering sensation which accompanies it.

The sexual response is also partly adrenalin-controlled, which is why a pretty girl can give a man gooseflesh.

Now I'm getting older it seems to take much longer for cuts and bruises and so on to clear up. Why is this?

Unfortunately almost everything slows up as age increases. Some of the slowing is due to actual changes in body responses, which is why cuts and injuries are slower to heal, but some of the slowing is also due to a tendency to expect slow-down, and to stop trying. For example, even though brain responses may be slower, and older people become less quick on the uptake than younger ones, they have a greater wealth of learned responses – experience – to draw on which more than makes up for the loss of speed of brain cells and other structures. But a person who tells himself that he is old and slow and useless becomes so, even though he need not. A slow-healing cut need hold no one back.

Why do some people sweat more than others?

Sweating is controlled by the parasympathetic nervous system, and happens in response to a need for cooling and also as a side effect of excitement.

The cooling effect is important. In hot climates a person would die if he did not sweat adequately. Sweating is triggered by a 'thermostat' centre in the brain. Interestingly, the sweating increases the longer a person is in hot conditions, rather than the reverse (most of us would expect a person in such conditions to sweat less as he got used to them). On his first day in hot conditions a person will sweat about one and a half litres of fluid an hour, and after 10 days or so, this will double. By the end of six weeks he will be sweating at the rate of about three and a half litres an hour. But, one important point, the sweat will become progressively less salty. This is an important protective point, because a person who has lost a lot of salt via sweat can feel very ill indeed (this is why the diets in most hot countries tend to be salty – anchovies and olives, for example).

People who have always lived in a temperate climate will have many of their sweat glands inactive, but people who live in the tropics tend to be much more efficient sweaters because all their glands operate fully.

The sweating of nervousness or excitement is due to the action of the parasympathetic nervous system, operating via a substance called acetylcholine which is similar to adrenalin. Control of anxiety by tranquillizers will reduce this sort of sweating, which is often very tiresome.

If sweating in some areas – notably the armpits – becomes a severe embarrassment, interruption of the sympathetic nerves which supply the area may give permanent relief.

Why do men have nipples?

Men and women are more alike than they are different. We all have the same sort of internal organs, brain structures and basic functions. It is only our sexual organs which differ, and even they don't differ all that much.

A man has a penis made of erectile tissue – tissue which can become engorged and enlarge and stiffen and which is very responsive. A woman has a clitoris, which is made of erectile tissue and which is also very responsive. We both have a pair of glands to produce our gametes (reproductive cells) and we both experience orgasm, sexual climax, though it differs a little.

Nipples are modified sweat glands; in women they have a function and respond early in puberty to hormonal stimulation and grow and change. The same thing can happen to men. About 50 per cent of boys at puberty develop a degree of gynaecomastia – swelling of the breasts and enlargement of the nipples. In most it regresses as the boy grows older.

The presence of vestigial, or useless, structures in the human body is not unusual. Some women, for example, develop a little row of nipples down the front of the abdomen as far as the groin, and these are distributed just like the nipples on mammals such as dogs and cats. (In the past, such women were regarded as witches by the superstitious because they were said to use their spare nipples for suckling the devil.)

Similarly, the appendix is thought to be a vestigial organ. Animals which eat a great deal of cellulose (grass eaters) need the extra length of gut to help digest it, and they have large appendices. Humans don't need appendices but still have the leftover remains of them. Men's nipples are also vestigial.

Medical puzzles

Why does your breath smell when you eat garlic? Does it come directly from your stomach?

No. The contents of the stomach smell unpleasant, even when food that is not particularly aromatic is eaten (if you have ever smelled vomit, you will know that) and the smell is held well inside the stomach, because the gullet is a potential tube rather than a constantly open one. (The trachea is always open – it has rings of cartilage round it to keep it so; the gullet, however, is collapsed like an empty toothpaste tube, except when there is food in it.)

The smell of garlic, curry spices, onions, alcohol and so on, gets to the breath from the only source it can – the lungs. What happens is that the molecules which create the aroma in these materials get through the stomach walls into the bloodstream, and are carried by it to the lungs. There they are picked up, together with the carbon dioxide which is to be exhaled, and carried out with it.

This is not the only way in which such substances escape from the body. They are picked up in sweat and in urine and, to a lesser extent, in stools.

This is why people who eat a particular diet as a regular thing may seem offensive to people who eat another sort of diet.

Some sociologists have said that a great deal of the prejudice that exists between different groups of people is due as much to the effects of diet as to the resentment of such obvious factors as their skin colour and different languages. A black man living in a white society and eating the local diet may be more acceptable than a white man who eats an 'alien' diet and who therefore smells different or 'wrong'.

Why do I yawn?

No one yet has been able fully to explain why we yawn. It is in part a reflex action – new-born babies do it, and so do animals – and partly an expression of feeling, since we do it when we are bored as well as when we are sleepy. One suggestion put forward is that it is a way of increasing the blood supply to the brain, since when we yawn we experience a temporary increase in heartbeat rate and also some constriction of peripheral blood vessels. But this is far from proven.

Oddly enough, yawning tends to be contagious. One yawner in a room can set everyone else off. Even reading about it can make it happen.

Why do people sigh when they are unhappy but also when they are content, for example after eating or making love?

Sighing is the opposite of yawning: it is an output of air, rather than an intake. Like yawning, it is something inexplicable, happening partly as a reflex, and partly as a means of expression.

Sighing is only significant when it happens to a person who has lost blood. Deep sighing respiration can show that a severe anaemia is present.

What damage does insomnia do?

Not so much as people imagine. In fact it is virtually impossible to keep awake a person who wants to sleep, unless, of course, it is being done by someone using dubious 'brainwashing' techniques. But the ordinary person cannot be kept awake – he or she will just fall asleep when it is necessary.

But many people complain of insomnia, and the reason is not that the actual insomnia makes them ill, but they feel deprived unless they have a full eight hours of uninterrupted slumber every night.

Yet the evidence is that many people try to sleep more than they actually need. Anxiety and depression may lead to extra sleeping, which is one way of keeping the bad feelings at bay, although the same feelings can also interfere with sleep. In such cases, treatment of the underlying causes helps to restore normal sleep rhythms.

A common cause for the complaint of insomnia is failure to realize that sleep needs change as life goes on. A child usually needs more sleep than an adult. Old people need less than the middle-aged. So, a man who sleeps his eight hours at 40 may need only six hours at 60, but will fret because of the 'lost' two hours. Yet he would be better off making real use of the time with reading and activity.

Also, there is a daily sleep 'ration' and a person who catnaps frequently, as many older people do, will need that much less sleep at night.

The ideal answer to insomnia in an otherwise healthy person is to be glad of it. It is a splendid conservation of time for, after all, we spend half of our lives sunk in slumber which is certainly dull.

Insomnia connected with illness needs treatment not because it is in itself a bad thing, but because it adds to the distress of the sick person. But it is the illness which matters, not the sleeplessness.

What is the difference between shivering and trembling?

Basically there is none at all. Both describe the situation in which muscles contract and relax rapidly and so give rise to a tremor.

Shivering is the word usually used to describe the reaction to cold. When the body temperature falls the thermostat in the brain triggers the muscles to work in order to make more heat. This is the teeth-chattering on an icy day which we cannot control until we have warmed up a little.

Trembling, on the other hand, usually means the shaking that comes from fear or excitement. Like so many other responses of this sort, it is due to the action of adrenalin and the parasympathetic nervous system.

I often faint, but my doctor says this is just because I'm tall. Can you explain this?

Any diminution of the vital blood supply to the brain can result in a loss of consciousness. Blood has to be pumped up to the brain, by the heart, against the force of gravity, and is helped on its way by the action of the muscles near the blood vessels carrying the blood upwards. If a person stands very still for a length of time, the action of the heart alone may not be enough to carry the blood up fast enough, and the result is a faint – an effective way of dealing with the problem because of course the lying-down posture ensures that blood can reach the brain swiftly and so causes consciousness to return.

Tall people are more likely to suffer such faints, because their blood has that much farther to go. This is why soldiers on parade are susceptible to faints; they tend to be tall, and they have to stand at attention. However, there is no need for them to faint; they can prevent it by frequent unobtrusive movements of the calf and upper arm muscles, which will encourage upward blood flow. British guardsmen who faint on parade are said to be punished for it rather than treated with sympathy.

Some people have a particularly sensitive vaso-vagal system. The nerve supply to a large area of the upper abdomen and lower chest – branches of the vagus nerve – can be stimulated and cause a constriction of blood vessels carrying blood up to the brain. People with this very sensitive system faint easily, and are particularly prone to do so as a result of emotional shock.

Victorian women were much given to fainting, largely, it is thought, because of the habit of tight lacing of corsets to provide a ridiculously small waist. Their blood had a dreadful job to get to the brain past the whalebone.

Why do we get high temperatures when we're ill?

This is part of the defensive mechanism against invasion by micro-organisms. The body marshals a number of different organism-fighting activities, including a rise in temperature. The extra heat may play a part in reducing the number of organisms (they operate most efficiently within a set temperature range) but may also be simply a side effect of the presence of the organisms and their poisons in the bloodstream. They irritate the centre in the brain which is responsible for temperature control, and it is this which causes the increase.

A high fever may also occur after an operation or an accident as a response to the insult the body has suffered, but not because of the presence of infection. And in some stress conditions there may be a small rise in temperature.

It is also known that the body's hormone status may be involved; people with an overactive thyroid tend to be hotter than other people (they are burning up body fuel more rapidly) and women often show a small temperature rise when they ovulate, a fact which can be used as part of birth control, or to start a pregnancy.

Why do I blush?

Again, it is because of adrenalin. When this busy hormone is pumped out, it affects blood vessel walls and causes some to contract and some to relax. Blushing happens when there is relaxation of surface blood vessels, and extra blood reaches the skin. It can happen because of fear (embarrassment is mild fear) and excitement of all kinds.

Other hormones are involved as well. Women may find at the menopause that they experience transient attacks of blood vessel activity which results in flushing of the face. It can also be a sexual arousal response. Not all people show a flush when they experience orgasm (sexual climax) but quite a number do.

Blushing is also a protective mechanism to prevent overheating. If we take in or produce too much heat, surface blood vessels relax, inner ones contract and extra blood is thus sent to the surface to be cooled by radiating its heat out through the skin. If the overheated surface of the skin is treated at the same time with cold air or ice, this will hurry the transfer of heat and allow the redness of the skin to recede.

There is also a phenomenon called a gustatory flush. Some people redden markedly when they eat any food. Others will do so if they eat extremely spicy food. Curry is one which will make most people red in the face.

Pitfalls of the thermometer
Taking somebody's temperature will not tell you much if you have no medical training. The body temperature is higher during the day than the night, and many people's daily average (measured in the mouth) differs from the standard value of 98.6°F. Feeling abnormally cold, or feverish symptoms, are warning signs

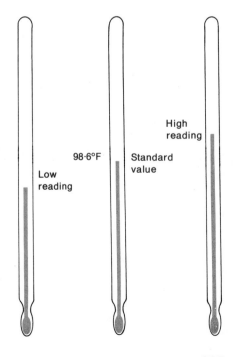

Medical puzzles

My grandmother who lived in the country used many old folk remedies. Are any of these proven to be of any use?

Some of them are indeed useful, and can be used safely now that we know what they do. For example, cobwebs wrapped around a cut will help to stop further bleeding because they contain fibrin, the substance that makes blood clot. Dock leaves contain a chemical that acts like an antihistamine and for this reason relieves the itching and rash caused by nettle stings.

Comfrey is a wild-growing plant for which a great many claims have been made. Country people advise, 'boil the leaves and use the water to soak aching feet, and use the pulp of the leaves as a dressing for cuts'; 'use the boiled leaves as a compress for an aching back'; 'comfrey leaves make a wonderful compress for sprained ankles'. The plant was called 'knitbone' in Cornwall and there they say that the grated root should be soaked in water, and then used to splint a broken bone. It has also been recommended for babies' nappy rashes.

There are three factors in comfrey which can be useful: allantoin, which is astringent, and is used in many modern ointments to stimulate tissue formation and hasten wound healing; tannin, which is present in strong tea, and which when applied to human tissue coagulates and forms a fairly hard tight 'skin'; and mucilage, a soft and sticky substance which can set to form a hardish crust and act as a protective support for an injury.

It will make a 'cast' for a broken bone, though not as strong as plaster of Paris. Applying it to cuts could help, too, as it would both provide a protective covering and would encourage healing.

However, tannin, when it dries, can cause contraction of tissue, and be more damaging than the original injury. Years ago cold, strong tea used to be applied to burns for the soothing effect of tannin, until it was realized that it made the area tighten and so caused greater deformity.

Marshmallow is a pretty plant with many uses. 'Stew it till tender, then use the liquid to bathe an abscess'; 'use leaves as a poultice for a boil or abscess'; 'use as a compress for sprains', are common pieces of country advice.

This plant contains mainly mucilage, which accounts for its use as a poultice and compress, and is also hygroscopic (in other words, it absorbs water easily). This means it will bring a boil or an abscess to a head by 'drawing' fluid out. However, it can only work when the boil or abscess is actually open, and not while it is 'blind' and building up to a head, so its use is fairly limited.

Elderberry, onions and **garlic, sage** and **rosemary**, are all popular and have been used for coughs and colds for many centuries. They have also been suggested for 'improving the digestion', 'relieving pain' (especially onions, which were put into ears to ease earache) and for 'kidney upsets'.

All of these plants contain, among other things, volatile oils, that is substances which produce powerful odours which can irritate the mucous membrane of the nose and throat and upper chest.

When this happens, the membrane responds by producing extra mucus, so that the nose runs more freely, and the chest secretions are softened and become easier to cough up. (It is the volatile oils in menthol chest rubs and in inhalants such as friar's balsam which make them so effective in the treatment of coughs and colds.) In addition, these oils are mildly antiseptic, so they reduce infection risk. They also encourage an increased supply of blood to any area with which they come into contact. This can be warming and soothing and can cut down on pain (it is this effect of the volatile oils in wintergreen that makes it so useful as a rub in some forms of rheumatic pain).

Raspberry is interesting, since the leaves contain a substance which is closely allied to ergot (which occurs in some cereal grains) and which has the effect of making the smooth muscle fibres of the uterus contract and therefore push out its contents. For this reason it has long been recommended as a treatment for painful periods. Also, regular use throughout pregnancy is said to ensure a more painfree childbirth. But there is no firm scientific evidence that using it all through pregnancy helps, though it might be useful during and immediately after labour. However, many doctors think raspberry should not be taken during pregnancy.

Blackcurrant is recommended by many country people for 'stomach upsets' – boil the stalks, and drink the cooled liquid. In fact, blackcurrants – the fruit – are rich in ascorbic acid, which is Vitamin C, and this is known to stimulate healing.

There are many other herbs and plants which have been recommended by rural people but it is not always possible to find out whether they do have any basis in scientific fact. However, one, plantain, is perhaps useful. Its seeds absorb a lot of water and become very plump, so 'swallow the seeds for a laxative' could be good advice; it works like bran, producing a high-bulk stool.

Other remedies that are interesting include the use of what are pretty obviously long-forgotten magical rites, many of which date back to Druidical times. For example, the 'cure' for female sterility advised by some old people is to eat, hard-boiled, an egg taken from a hen 'which has run with the cock'.

One particularly fascinating set of folk remedies involves the use of sugar and/or honey. It has been advised for poultices for varicose ulcers, for bedsores, for cuts and wounds of all sorts. A 'cut raisin applied to the stump of the umbilical cord of new-born babies', 'honey and pounded raisins' for a breast abscess, and 'sugar and soap' poultices for septic wounds are common folklore advice.

All these are perfectly sensible remedies, because in fact sugar is a powerful anti-bacterial agent. Organisms just cannot grow in it. That is why sugar is used to preserve fruit in jam-making. A pot of honey discovered in an Egyptian tomb was found to be as good as it ever had been though it had lain there for thousands of years.

There are lots of other remedies that have particularly lovely names – euphrasia, also called eyebright; camomile and mouse-ear; pettyspurge and tansy; celandine and dill. But there is little evidence that they actually work.

However, enough old cures have been proved to be effective to make us wonder whether tomorrow's great medical breakthroughs may not in fact be part of yesterday's wisdom.

I've never really put together a proper family medical chest.
What should be in one – and what is the best way to treat the problems that come up?

A good family medical chest should be simple, containing just the basics. Overloading it with fancy equipment will mean that you cannot find what you need in an emergency.

The following list provides the essential first-aid materials and simple medications that most families will need.

Individual adjustments will have to be made, of course. Some people will find, some items a little old fashioned, while others will find some a little too modern. Remember, by the way, that these items should be properly stored, ideally in a child-proof, lockable cabinet with a sloping top. A sloping top means that you will not be tempted to keep dangerous drugs on the outside of the cabinet where children can all too easily reach them. A child-proof cabinet is one which can be locked and can only be opened by an adult using both hands at once. There are several suitable ones for sale and they are worth looking for.

Family medical chest contents

1 Absorbent cotton – a small roll, rather than ready-made swabs.
2 Sterilized gauze squares.
3 A roll of white lint.
4 A large clean white handkerchief (useful for bleeding and burns).
5 Sticky dressings. Tastes differ in the use of these dressings, but as a general guide, Elastoplast or Band-aid is porous, stretchy, very adhesive and comfortable to wear, but not always waterproof; it can be obtained in a continuous roll for cutting off as needed, in addition to pre-cut packages.

Band-aids are waterproof and come in ready-cut dressings. There is also a ventilated type.

Zinc oxide plaster comes in rolls of varying widths, is not stretchy, is not completely waterproof and is, frankly, rather old-fashioned. However, it's useful for firm dressings (as, for example, when wound edges must be kept close together). It must always be used in conjunction with a dressing because it does not have a built-in dressing pad as do the previous two.

Sellotape or Scotch Tape makes useful dressing adhesive, especially for the face or for a temporary dressing in hairy areas – it is not so painful to remove.
6 Bandages. For infected nailbeds on fingers and small finger injuries, sticky dressings are not much use. So self-adhesive $\frac{1}{2}$-inch-wide bandage is better, or surgical gauze which makes a neat dressing, once you have learned the trick of applying it. It has to be used with a special applicator, but instructions are provided on the pack.
7 A sling, that is, a triangular calico bandage.
8 Paracetamol tablets and Paracetamol elixir for children, or aspirin. Always follow the instructions.
9 Indigestion mixture for occasional use. Certainly if indigestion is a common symptom that keeps recurring, medical help should be sought. However, most families will find that somebody over-indulges in food from time to time and needs a first-aid remedy. An excellent, fairly inexpensive one is magnesium trisilicate compound in powder form, which is taken dissolved in water. Keeps indefinitely if stored in a screwtop jar.
10 Kaodene or Kaopectate which is a proprietary kaolin sedative mixture for adults and children, to use for diarrhoea due to dietary indiscretion. This preparation has an indefinite shelf life. Of course, if diarrhoea is associated with illness, sickness, fretfulness, especially in childhood and old age, you should always call the doctor.
11 Tincture of Benzoin Compound (friar's balsam) – an old-fashioned but still effective treatment for colds and chest conditions. A teaspoonful dissolved in hot water will produce the fumes that can be inhaled to clear a sinus and relieve a tight chest. (It is also handy for removing heatmarks from polished furniture.)
12 Antiphlogistine poultice (kaolin). A time-honoured method of treating boils which still has much to commend it. The poultice is applied to lint, covered with a layer of gauze, and applied *not too hot* to infected areas. The boil should then come to a 'head' fairly rapidly, and open and drain.
13 Magnesium sulphate paste. This, too, is useful for boils and infections of this nature, but only after the lesion has started to drain. It will draw pus from open boils and resolve the condition quickly. It deteriorates in store, unfortunately, so check the jar every month or so if it is unused. It is cheap enough to discard and replace.
14 A surgical spirit (or rubbing alcohol) to clean skin round a wound.
15 Antihistamine cream for stings and sunburn and allergic hives or nettlerash.
16 Acriflavine in a watery base (not in spirit, because that stings as badly as iodine) to use as a local antiseptic for wounds and grazes.
17 A pair of scissors.
18 Safety pins for bandages or slings.

You will note that this list does not include any creams or lotions to be used for burns. The treatment for burns is the application of cold water. Nor does it include a thermometer. These are not easy to use properly and, anyway, a fever that is at all significant will show itself clearly. The sufferer will be hot to the touch, restless, dry-mouthed, obviously ill. Less obvious temperature variations are really not very important. Another essential part of being able to cope is to be fully prepared, not only with a first-aid kit and home nursing equipment, but with information. A great deal of valuable time can be lost if you can't find the telephone number of someone you need in a hurry. Here, then, is a list of vital phone numbers that you may require.

1 Your family doctor.
2 Your local police station, in case you need help to find a doctor in an emergency.
3 The local fire station, in case you need help to resuscitate someone who has had an electric shock, or in case some child or elderly person is locked in the bathroom.
4 The local hospital.

5 The local ambulance station.
6 Your nearest pharmacy and its opening hours.
7 Local authorities who provide information on health facilities and social services.
8 The address and telephone number of your family's place of work (it's amazing how often in emergencies people cannot be reached because no one knows where they work).
9 A neighbour who can be reached to hold the fort in an emergency.

In emergencies, lives can be saved if you have a little basic knowledge. Here is an account of what you should do when faced with a major problem.

Artificial respiration

Unless breathing of good air is continuous, vital centres in the brain can be dangerously damaged by lack of oxygen. A person can survive undamaged for only four to six minutes after breathing has stopped.

So, artificial respiration has to be started at the earliest possible moment after breathing has stopped; never waste time moving a person from one place to another when what he needs desperately is to get air into his lungs.

The most effective method of dealing with cessation of breath is the 'kiss of life' method. This is the easiest to do, and certainly works best.

First of all it's important to make *sure* that the patient is not breathing; look for movement of the chest or the upper part of the belly, or listen, putting your ear really close to the patient's nose and mouth.

Next, check for any obstruction. A person who has stopped breathing is unconscious, and this in itself may be the cause of the failure to breathe. In unconscious people the tongue may fall backwards and block the air passages. Very often this could be the only reason why the unconscious person can't breathe, and all that is needed is removal of this mechanical blockage.

This is quite easy to do. Lay the patient on his back. Pull the head back firmly as far as it will go, at the same time bringing the lower jaw upwards and forwards until the front teeth meet. The chin should be pointing directly at the ceiling. When it is in this position it is impossible for the tongue to fall back and block the airway. Don't be afraid to pull the head really well back – it's amazing how far back the neck can stretch. Sometimes it isn't just the tongue that is causing the blockage – there may be false teeth or blood or mucus or vomit. If this happens the contents of the mouth must be scooped out fast. Don't be squeamish – use bare fingers and hook it out.

If breathing doesn't then start again the 'kiss of life' must be given. For an adult patient, keep the head well back and the neck extended, kneel beside the patient's head and hold the chin with the right hand, and with the left hand pinch the patient's nostrils firmly together. Then seal your own mouth round his mouth with your lips and fill the lungs by blowing *gently*. Remove your mouth and turn your head slightly to the right and watch the chest fall before repeating the action again. It is sometimes easier to get a good seal round the mouth of a child by including the nose as well.

Whatever happens, continue the artificial respiration until the patient is really able to breathe by himself. It may be necessary to continue for as long as an hour or more, but whatever happens, the artificial respiration *must be continued*. If you get tired, then get someone else to take over if you possibly can.

Obviously, it is a great deal easier to give this sort of first aid if you have had a chance to practise the technique in non-emergency conditions. The Red Cross Society organizes classes in first aid and will teach the method. But if this isn't possible for you, there's no reason why you shouldn't practise now and again on members of your own family. In an ideal world, every individual should be taught this technique during schooldays.

Bleeding

Without rapid treatment of haemorrhage a patient can become so exsanguinated – that is, dangerously short of blood – that he can go into irreversible shock.

If bright red blood spurts from a wound it means an artery is damaged. Slow welling out of darker red blood means a vein is affected and the loss of blood will be slower. Both need to be dealt with rapidly.

Firm pressure applied directly on to the wound with a clean handkerchief knotted and pressed down hard will do, or bare fingers will serve perfectly well if nothing else is available. Never waste time looking for a dressing. Keep the pressure maintained until medical help comes.

If the bleeding decreases, apply a pressure dressing – a thick pad of dressing strapped on – and raise the injured limb to above head level. Thus, if it is a leg that is affected lay the patient flat on his back on the floor and rest the lower leg and foot on a chair.

Never disturb a blood clot if it forms on a wound. If a dressing is put on and gets blood-soaked, don't remove it; just add another one on top and keep on doing so until help comes.

Never, never attempt to apply a tourniquet. This is quite a skilled task, and more damage can be done with tourniquets than by the original injury.

Remember, *direct pressure is always the treatment to choose*.

If you suspect internal bleeding – and the symptoms of this are shock, pallor, raised pulse, rapid breathing, pain, anxiety – do not move the patient and do not handle him in any way. Keep him lying flat and send for urgent medical aid.

Burns and scalds

Burns can be caused by dry heat – that is, flame – or contact with electricity; wet heat such as boiling water (when it's called a scald), or chemicals.

The first essential is to remove the patient from the source of the burn.

If clothing is burning, wrap the individual immediately in a rug, or roll him across the floor as this will put the flames out rapidly. No attempt should ever be made to remove clothing or to investigate the injury.

If the burn or scald is fairly small and there is no apparent injury to the skin, home treatment is possible. But if a large area is affected – a whole foot or leg or an entire forearm, for example – then medical help should be sent for immediately. In addition, if there is severe blistering of the skin, medical help should be sent for.

If the face is affected, involving mouth, nose and/or eyes then, once again, immediate medical help is required.

The ideal treatment for a small burn or scald is to immediately plunge the affected area into cold water and keep it there until all pain stops. In the vast majority of cases, no further treatment is needed. Only if the skin later breaks will it be necessary to apply any sort of additional treatment.

It may be difficult to keep the injury in cold water for such a long period, but it is well worth persisting. It may be easier to sit a burnt person into a bath of cool water while waiting for medical help, rather than attempting to keep just one area cold. This is particularly so for children with burns on buttocks, legs or belly.

If a large area is affected, there may be considerable fluid loss. This is the most dangerous problem with a burn. The fluid must be replaced as fast as possible. So give the patient half a cupful of water to drink every 10 minutes until he goes to the hospital or a doctor arrives. But, of course, never attempt to give drinks to a patient who is unconscious.

If blisters appear, on no account should they be snipped. A blister has the function of protecting the underlying skin and it is much better to leave it alone. The doctor will prick it if it is really necessary.

Broken bones

If a bone breaks and adjacent soft tissues are injured, there may be severe haemorrhage which will, of course, need to be dealt with first. If the skull is injured and the patient becomes unconscious, then the important first-aid is to make sure that he goes on breathing.

In a fully conscious patient without any surface injury, the treatment is as follows:

First of all, look carefully for signs of bone injury. These include:
  deformity
  swelling
  local pain
  abnormally positioned limbs.

If any of these signs appear, *do not move the patient at all*. Leave him where he is until medical help arrives. If he absolutely must be moved, perhaps because he is lying in water or in the middle of the road or in a similarly dangerous position, then make sure that the injured limb is immobilized before the move is done. An arm can be supported by the uninjured arm, or held by the first-aider; an injured leg should be firmly bandaged to the other leg, which can thus provide an excellent splint. Never attempt to lift an injured person unaided. Always get help because unskilled carrying may result in further damage.

Even if you are sure there is no break in a bone, but suspect there is a dislocation of a joint, do not attempt to restore it. This is a highly skilled job, and unless you are a really experienced and well-trained person, you can cause much more severe damage by handling the joint.

If there is a blow on the head followed by even momentary unconsciousness, a doctor must be told immediately. If later on, there is any
  vomiting
  headache
  sleepiness
  bruising around the eyes
  bleeding from nose or ears,
then once again, a doctor must be told immediately.

Poisoning

This is the most preventable of all emergencies of course, but it still does occur.

If a child has swallowed a doubtful substance, such as berries from the garden or tablets which he has found lying around, make him sick by putting two fingers at the back of his throat. Do *not* give the traditional salt water or mustard-and-water emetic; if these fail to cause vomiting, they can complicate the treatment of the poisoning.

If a person has swallowed a liquid which causes burning of the mouth (such as bleach) *do not attempt to make him sick*. Get him to a hospital as fast as you possibly can.

If he has swallowed a petroleum product, such as paraffin, once again, *do not make him sick*. Paraffin is not poisonous if it is only swallowed, but it is poisonous if it is vomited and then inhaled. So, in this case, give ice-cream or a large tablespoon of oil (olive oil or cooking oil will do) which will help to prevent these further complications.

In the case of any other suspected poisoning, even if the patient seems perfectly fit, take him to a hospital as fast as possible and remember always to take with you, if possible, samples of what he has swallowed.

If at any point he should vomit, keep the vomit in a bowl to show the doctor. He will be able to decide whether or not any further treatment is then required.

More likely than these major emergencies are the day-to-day minor injuries. This chart will show you how to deal with them.

Arm sling which supports the arm

Triangular sling which is more suitable for a hand or rib injury

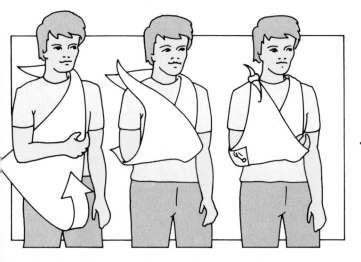

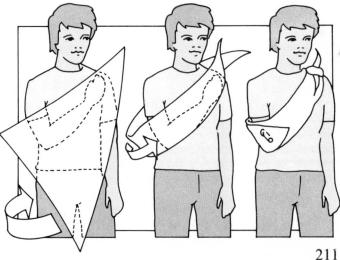

Medical puzzles

Condition	First aid	Medical help needed	Later treatment
Boils	Apply local heat (lint wrung out in hot water or kaolin poultice). If it opens by itself apply dressings of magnesium sulphate paste until all pus has drained away	If associated with raised temperature, yes. If one of a series, or if the sufferer has a general illness (especially diabetes), yes. If the sufferer is very young, or very old, yes	If local heat brings the boil to a head but it won't 'burst' by itself, a doctor will open it. Do not do it yourself. Thereafter, magnesium sulphate dressings
Animal bites and scratches	Wash well with ample water	Always wash the wound, however slight	As medically advised
Insect stings	Remove insect if still present. Lavishly apply antihistamine cream	If affecting mouth, throat, eyes, yes. If any pallor, sweating, shivering, faintness, yes	If infection appears, show doctor
Cuts	Stop bleeding by direct pressure on wound. If bright red spurts, maintain pressure; if darker red oozing, cease pressure after a few minutes and if no further bleeding, apply dressing. For a close union of the edges, apply dressing across cut. Do *not* remove any clots; these prevent further bleeding	If any foreign body (for example, glass) is present, yes. If bleeding will not stop, yes. If heavy blood loss, yes. If associated with head injury, yes. If suffered in the presence of well-manured earth, for example, in the garden, yes. If apparent further injury, for example, to bones, yes	Replace dressing as needed. If infection appears to have set in (local swellings, heat, pain in nearby areas, for example, under the arm in hand injuries, in the groin in leg injuries), see doctor. If pain persists, see doctor. Otherwise, remove dressings as soon as cut has united. When scab starts to separate do *not* pull at it but apply ventilated dressing until scab has come off completely. Thereafter rub in a little lanolin to soften scar
Bruises and bumps	Apply ice to reduce swelling and pain, and internal bleeding, which is cause of bruise	If associated with a head injury and there is any unconsciousness, headache, sickness, yes. If bruises appear in absence of any injury, yes. If any symptoms other than local pain, yes. Otherwise, no	Nil. But don't be alarmed by vivid colours in a resolving bruise – this is normal
Small burns and scalds	Immerse in cold water and keep there until all pain stops. *Never* apply any ointments or butter	If associated with shock (pallor, sweating, feelings of nausea and faintness), yes. If a large area is affected, yes	Do *not* snip blisters. If they break, cover with a dry dressing
Sunburn and associated heatstroke	Keep in cool place. If the sufferer is very hot and restless, a cool sponging will help. Lie him down in a shady place. Apply antihistamine cream to sunburned areas	If headache, sickness, giddiness, persists, yes. If a large area of skin is affected, yes. If any vomiting, yes. If infant less than one year old is affected, yes	Applications of antihistamine cream until all pain ceases. Never let it happen again!

Condition	First aid	Medical help needed	Later treatment
Cramp	If in leg, pull toes forwards and upwards. Elsewhere gentle massage	If frequent and persistent, yes. If associated with 'pins and needles', coldness, or numbness of area, yes. Otherwise, no	As medically advised
Grazes	Wash well with clean water. Remove obvious foreign bodies. Apply clean dry dressing after painting with acriflavine lotion	If associated with other injuries; if affecting a very large area; if affecting the face; if foreign bodies can't be easily removed, yes	Soak off old dressings if they stick, using warm water. Dry and redress. Report to doctor if infection appears
Styes	Bathe with hot water. Wrap absorbent cotton and gauze round bowl of wooden spoon to apply antibiotic eye ointment	If it does not get better in a week, yes. If one of a series, yes. If associated with general ill health, yes	As medically advised.
Foreign bodies (in ears, eyes, nose, throat)	If the object is easy to see and get hold of, remove gently (for eyes, pull upper lid forward and over lower lashes to 'sweep' out foreign body). If any difficulty or foreign body moves further in, *stop* at once. If corrosive liquid (e.g. acid) gets in eye, wash with lots of water	If unremovable yourself, obviously, yes. If in doubt that whole of object was removed (for example if pain persists in throat after fishbone was apparently removed), yes. If any associated damage experienced by eye, yes. If corrosive liquid damage to eye, yes	As medically advised.
Hysteria (that is, uncontrolled laughing and weeping)	Speak loudly and sharply; if this doesn't work, a firm slap followed at once by holding the person close to comfort her (or him – it happens to men too!)	If it is not possible in any way to stop the attack, yes. If associated with overdosage of alcohol, or any drugs, yes	As medically advised
Broken tooth	Plug with wet absorbent cotton or chewing gum (first chewing out all sugar, using other teeth). If plugging causes pain, do nothing	Yes. See dentist at once	As dentist advises
Toothache	Aspirin or paracetamol for pain. Local cold (ice wrapped in gauze) may relieve pain better than local heat which tends to increase throbbing	Ask dentist for urgent appointment	As dentist advises
Bleeding tooth socket	Make a plug of absorbent cotton bigger than socket and wet with clean water. Press hard into tooth socket for ten minutes	If bleeding persists, yes. If blood loss very heavy, yes	Return to dentist if any repetition. Otherwise, no further treatment needed

Patients' problems

Doctors have always been regarded as a special breed, ever since the days when they were priests and/or magicians as well as tenders of the sick. Most of us still feel that the doctor carries a special aura with him, which makes it difficult to talk to him as we would to other people like ourselves. It also makes it difficult to question his statements and his decisions. If he dismisses a particular form of treatment as 'quackery' it is hard to know whether one is justified in accepting or rejecting this statement. It is also difficult to know when it is reasonable and safe to treat one's own symptoms, and when one actually needs the care of an expert doctor. And then, of course, there are the difficulties of understanding the special language which doctors use. Indeed, patients do have problems.

I always seem to have trouble talking to my doctor. He never really understands what it is that worries me. How can I get things across to him?

It is almost impossible to have a 'normal' relationship with your doctor. You have to take yourself, your body and your mind, and probably a portion of your private life, and put it in front of him and say, 'help me'. This makes you feel subservient, and that may make you come across as hostile (many of us behave in precisely the opposite way to how we feel). You may also be frightened, which tends to make you less receptive to information because of the way adrenalin blocks concentrated thought. You may be deeply embarrassed and this can make you tongue-tied, or given to excessive chattering, depending on how this sort of feeling takes you. In other words, you don't behave normally.

Add to this the fact that many doctors tend to speak a special language of their own, and have as many problems in communicating with you as you have with them, and also that they may feel threatened and alarmed because of the trust you put in them (after all, it's an enormous responsibility) and it is clear that they don't behave all that normally either.

Once you can accept all these factors, it makes it easier to find a way to get across to your doctor what it is that worries you. Make allowances for your unease, fearfulness and loss of concentration, and circumnavigate them.

First, before you go to your doctor, *make a list of your symptoms*. You may not think it possible to forget a detail such as the way the pain wakes you in the middle of the night, but all too often patients do forget just such a point – and it can be a significant one.

Then, make an adjoining list of how long you have had the symptoms; what brings them on (eating? worry? sex? exercise?); what relieves them best? (pain-killers? eating? vomiting?); whether they are getting worse, or staying much the same, and how often you have them.

Then – and this is important but sometimes difficult – make a note of what has changed in your life recently (a failed exam or a love affair, a demotion at work, a financial loss, a bereavement). Good experiences can be just as stressful as bad ones, so list the good ones, too (a new job, new home, a raise in pay).

Finally, make a note of what it is that you are frightened of (cancer? heart disease?). Don't tell yourself that you are silly to fear these. Maybe you are silly in the sense that you haven't got them, but it is still not silly to feel that way. Admit the fear is there, and then your doctor can investigate whatever it is and calm your fears. Too many patients go to the doctor to talk earnestly about an in-growing toenail, when what they are longing for him to say is, 'You do not have cancer of the throat because you have a lump there when you swallow'. Unless you tell him, he is in the dark, and few doctors are psychic.

It is also important to show concern for the doctor himself. You may regard him as some sort of god – many patients do cast their doctors in this uncomfortable role – but he does not have divine patience, bottomless compassion or omnipotent vision. He or she is a man or woman like any other. He, too, likes to run his life according to his own schedule, to get regular meals, time to make love and a chance to relax. He, too, may have financial, sexual or health worries.

So treat him kindly. Don't suffer your agonizing pain for hours hoping it will go away, and then call him late at night or early on a Sunday morning. Don't get angry with him if his receptionist says he can't give you an appointment right away; he does have other patients, after all. If your symptoms really frighten you, and you tell her so, she should let you talk to him on the telephone so he can decide whether you can wait or not. If she will not let you talk to him at once, hold on to your temper, and then tell him calmly when you do get to him. If he has been instructing her to be so obstructive, and it has misfired, he needs you to tell him about it. And you may need to be helped to understand why your impatience was not really justified.

If you don't understand what he has told you, tell him. Words that are his stock-in-trade may be jargon to you, but if no one ever tells him that, he can't know about it. (There is a list of words opposite that will help you pick up some of the jargon.)

And don't be afraid to ask for a second opinion if you are not comfortable about what he has told you. No doctor worth his salt ever objects to such a request and certainly does not regard it as an insult. It is an intelligent response to a worrying situation; he will understand it and co-operate, because it is in his interest, too.

What help can I get from people who are not doctors, but who have specialist knowledge? You see them around hospitals and in private practice, but I'm never quite sure what they actually do.

The ancillary professions to medicine give an enormous range of skilled services and care to patients, and have played a large part in the worldwide improvement of health in this century. These aides are specially trained and pass qualifying examinations.

In some cases you may go directly to a practitioner, in other cases you are best referred to them by your own doctor. In all cases, a doctor will gladly advise.

Chiropodist (Podiatrist in US): a specialist in disorders of the feet who can treat and surgically remove corns, callouses, verrucae (plantar warts) and similar problems, advise on foot health and shoe design, but not perform major operations such as correction of a bunion. Patients are referred to orthopaedic surgeons for such help.

Dietician: a specialist in nutrition, able to plan a special diet for the treatment of disease, for example diabetes, cholecystitis, diverticulitis.

Health visitor (Specialist Physician's Assistant in US): a nurse primarily, with special training in preventive health care. She or he may work in clinics for mothers and babies, with the elderly, in school medical services and as part of general practice teams, and also may visit the homes of ill people to check on their care. Often, but not always, such aides are also midwives.

Laboratory technician: a person who is trained in the many techniques involved in performing blood tests and other laboratory investigations. He or she may collect blood from patients, and also carry out some tests on them.

Midwife: a practitioner in her own right with, in the UK, a legal right to deliver babies of normal pregnancies without the aid of a doctor, although in practice midwives usually work in close liaison with medical practitioners.

Occupational therapist: a specialist worker in rehabilitation, who helps people to return to normal life via structured activity. For example, a person who has had a stroke will be taught how to run her home again, and how to cook and clean and care for herself. The mentally ill in particular benefit greatly from the work of the occupational therapist, because the right sort of stimulation and distraction is extremely important in psychiatric illness.

Optician: a specialist in lenses used for the assistance of vision. An ophthalmic optician is trained to examines eyes, and prescribe and supply glasses. A dispensing optician may not examine or prescribe but may supply glasses. An orthoptist can provide exercise therapy for certain eye conditions, such as squint. An oculist is a medically qualified ophthalmologist.

Orthodontist: a specialist in treatment for the teeth involving realignment. A child who needs braces to prevent forward pushing of the teeth will be treated by an orthodontist.

Physiotherapist: a specialist who understands the action of muscles and the skeleton. Physiotherapists often work in hospitals arranging exercises for the bedfast, remedial exercise for patients suffering from damage to muscles or skeleton – for example, teaching a person with a fractured thigh to walk again – and they also provide some forms of electrical treatment to muscles (faradism) and heat treatments.

Psychologist: a person who has expert knowledge of the way the human mind works. Psychologists do not usually provide treatment for the mentally ill, although they may help in their care. Their function is to assess the way a mind is operating and to provide various forms of assistance. For example, behaviour therapy, in which an individual is taught how to overcome an unreasonable fear (a phobia) will be given by a psychologist. They also make assessments of intelligence and help in vocational selection. (They should not be confused with psychiatrists, who are medically qualified.

Psycho-analyst: some practitioners are medically qualified but not all. They attempt to relieve mental distress by means of discussion (psychotherapy), dream analysis and other interpretive techniques.

Radiographer: a person trained in the use of X-rays, both to take pictures and to give treatment, for example, X-ray therapy for cancer and some skin conditions.

Speech therapist: a person who helps people who have lost speech to regain it (for example, after a stroke or surgery on the larynx) and who also helps people with speech impediments.

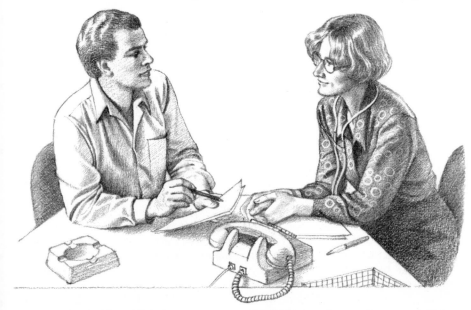

Doctor-patient understanding
Before you see your doctor you can help a great deal by making a full list of your symptoms and when they started. Don't be afraid to voice any fears you may have, and if you do not understand anything that your doctor says, ask for more explanation

Patients' problems

There are a lot of different treatments you can get these days apart from ordinary medical advice, such as homoeopathy, acupunture and so on. How can I tell which are safe to use?

A good doctor of medicine will never dismiss out of hand any therapy which may give a patient safe relief, whatever its source. Many doctors work in close liaison with spiritual healers, actively recommend osteopaths and are sympathetic to nature cure methods. Ask your doctor for his opinion before setting out to try a non-orthodox method of care. He may give you a valid warning, but he may also be able to suggest a good practitioner.

Once you go to a 'fringe' practitioner, don't lose touch with your doctor. Both disciplines will have something to offer you. Also, listen to what the fringe practitioner says. A good one, whatever his technique, never promises a 'cure' because that is the language of a quack. He will only offer the same thing that your doctor offers – an attempt to provide relief. Also, he will behave in a sensible professional way, treating you with quiet respect, and will not gossip about your symptoms to others (you can tell he does do this if he gossips about others to you) and, even if he is clearly in his activity to make money, he will not show an excessive interest in the cash side of your arrangement.

As for the rest of your queries, you can only use your commonsense.

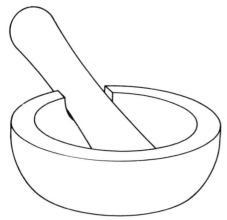

Homoeopathic medicine
What is it? A branch of medicine practised by people who have been trained in 'orthodox' medicine. A homoeopathic doctor may also use surgical and medical techniques similar to those used by any other ordinary doctor.

Homoeopathy is not an alternative to orthodox medicine, but an extension of it. It has been practised for over 150 years and has had some famous adherents – kings and queens and presidents. Homoeopathy makes a strong point of treating the whole patient, and being as interested in personality and life-style as the signs and symptoms of disease – an attitude shared by many non-homoeopathic doctors, of course.
How does it work? Homoeopathic remedies are natural ones, derived from minerals, plants and animal extracts, and they are prescribed on the principle of 'like treats like'. That means that if a medicine given in a largish dose can create certain symptoms in healthy people, the same medicine given in a minute dosage will relieve those symptoms when they arise from disease.

For example, in healthy people Gelsemium, a plant-derived medicine, causes depression, feelings of hot then cold, heaviness of the limbs, fever. An attack of influenza with these symptoms is treated homoeopathically by a small dose of Gelsemium. Belladonna can create symptoms like those of scarlet fever, so it is used in the treatment of that illness.

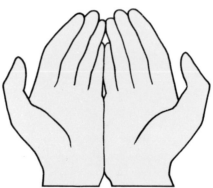

Spiritual healing
What is it? In the words of a spokesman for its adherents: 'A manifestation of God's love, intangible, working through the healer'.
How does it work? The spokesman could not say, except that the body gets out of touch with the rhythm of Nature, and the healer's hands bring God's power to correct this. 'We have had instances of growths dispersing in a matter of minutes, of locked joints with arthritic calcifications dissolved away. Doctors say it is not humanly possible to do this – it sounds like a fantasy – but it happens regularly.'

It does not always work. It may fail with a religious believer, yet succeed with a totally sceptic atheist. To be a believer in God is not necessary, although conversion may sometimes come after a successful treatment. Healers, the same spokesman explained, accept all patients, but they will always try to persuade patients to attend orthodox doctors as well. If a patient refuses to see a doctor, every effort will be made to persuade him to do so, 'although we can't force him. We never refuse any patient who comes for help.'

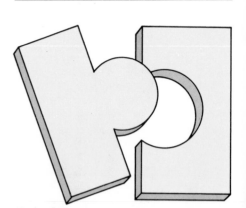

Osteopathy
What is it? Osteopathy is manipulative treatment directed at the skeleton and muscles, with the spine usually receiving most attention. Modern osteopathy derives from the English 'bone setters' of the 17th and 18th centuries, and also from the United States 'chiropractic', devised by one D.D. Palmer, which is similar to osteopathy. At one time it was claimed that spinal manipulation would give relief from a wide range of

disorders, including heart disease, diabetes and malignant growths. A modern and reputable osteopath does not make such claims; the bulk of his practice is with people who suffer from osteoarthritis, and the range of aches and pains that are labelled 'fibrositis' and 'rheumatism'.

If the good osteopath suspects his patient is suffering from diseases outside his scope, he will refer him back to orthodox medicine.

How does it work? Osteopaths believe that symptoms come from errors in the relation to each other of body structures – nerves, muscles, joints. Manipulation, they say, puts these errors right and allows normal function.

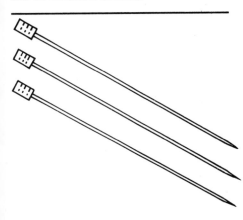

Acupuncture

What is it? The practice of a traditional form of a 4,000-year-old Chinese medicine, which still exists in that country side by side with modern orthodox medicine. Treatment involves the use of fine copper needles which are stuck into the body at various points often apparently unrelated to symptoms.

Thus, treatment of liver disease involves piercing the foot. Needle sticking can also achieve total anaesthesia – loss of feeling deep enough for major surgery in a conscious patient. This has been dramatically demonstrated by acupuncture practitioners in the Far East.

How does it work? The ancients talked about mysterious opposing forces, Yin and Yang, being involved in acupuncture, but recent work has suggested that complex brain chemistry may be involved.

When pain-carrying nerves are stimulated, the body produces its own natural pain-killing material, called endorphin, which 'locks' into special receptors in the brain to act like an opiate. It is now thought that acupuncture needles cause enough stimulation to increase endorphin supplies to effective levels.

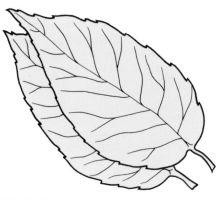

Herbalism

What is it? A method of treating illness using only plants and substances derived from plants.

How does it work? Where the plant substance contains an active principle, it works as any other medicine does, by acting on the diseased tissue, or on its function. Thus, to treat heart disorder, foxglove may be used, and it works well because the active principle in the plant, digitalin, affects the rate at which the heart beats. Similarly, rauwolfia affects blood pressure, and the opium poppy is a pain-killer and sedative. Herbalists use many other plant substances, though not all of them are of as proven efficacy as foxgloves and rauwolfia.

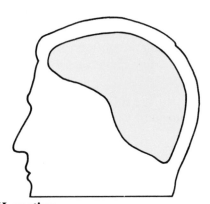

Hypnotism

What is it? A method of controlling the mind which enables a person to relax, and also to accept and act upon suggestions which will improve his sense of well-being. In some susceptible patients it has had remarkable results – removing warts, for example. It is often used to deal with obsessional states –

people who want to eat less or give up smoking or heavy drinking may find they can with the aid of hypnosis.

How does it work? No one really knows for sure, although the technique has been known for a long time and has been widely used, politically and religiously as well as medically. The patient is soothed and helped to relax until he or she goes into a trance-like state in which suggestions made by the hypnotist are planted, to be acted upon later after the trance is over. So, the smoker would be told that a cigarette would taste revolting – and it would – and make him want to put it out.

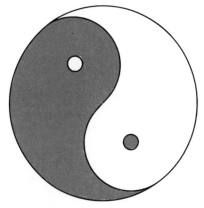

Naturopathy

What is it? Long popular in Europe, especially Germany, naturopaths say that disease is due to failure to observe natural laws of nutrition, breathing, posture, and so on. Treatment is aimed at correcting poor eating habits (and may include fasting and enemas), correcting mechanical faults (such as spinal misalignment) and giving psychological support.

It is said to be preventive first, curative second. However, naturopaths do accept for treatment people who are suffering from backaches, rheumatism, migraine and bronchitis. They do not claim to cure cancer but will accept cancer patients for treatment which is designed 'to improve the constitution'.

There are Health Farms run on naturopathic principles where treatment is given to improve nutrition, reduce weight and the symptoms due to obesity, and to manipulate the spine.

How does it work? By restoring to the body its natural functions through avoiding the build-up of toxic substances – mainly by diet control.

Patients' problems

*How can I tell whether a symptom
needs medical care or not?
This chart will show you.*

	Type	Associated with	Treatment
Headache	Occasional: mild	Lack of sleep. Over-eating. Over-drinking (alcohol). Working in a stuffy room. Periods. Anxiety. Head cold	A couple of pain-killing tablets and remove the cause
	Often: severe	A paticular food or other substance	Seek medical advice – it could be due to an allergy
	Involving one side of the head		Could be migraine – seek medical advice
	Severe	Reading. Being in a bright light. Visual disturbance – flashing, blurry	Seek medical advice – could be due to eyesight problems – you might need glasses
	Severe	Spots before the eyes	Seek medical advice – could be linked with illness
Indigestion	Occasional: dull pain under ribs	Unusual food. Eating too fast. Overwork and fatigue. Heavy smoking	A mild antacid. Avoid the cause in future
	Occasional to often: dull pain under ribs sometimes going through to the back	Hunger or eating (either can be involved)	Seek medical advice. Could be due to gastritis or ulcer
	Occasional to often	A particular food or drink, e.g. coffee or sugary foods	Stop taking suspect food – could be an allergy
Sickness	Occasional: returned food only	Over-eating/-drinking. Unusual foods	Stop eating. Drink water only until sickness stops. Avoid cause in future
	Occasional: returned food only	Diarrhoea and bellyache	Could be mild infection – if not better in 24 hours seek medical advice. Meanwhile take water only
	Occasional to often: looks like coffee grounds	Indigestion	Seek medical advice – could be due to gastric bleeding
	Frequent	Pregnancy	Seek medical advice for a simple remedy
	Occasional to frequent: in a child under two or a fragile old person		Can lead to dehydration – seek medical advice soon. Give water only to drink.

	Type	Associated with	Treatment
Constipation	Frequent	Soft sugary diet, low in fruits and vegetables	Take bran, extra water, *no* laxatives
	Occasional	Unusual foods. Fasting	Remove cause
	Occasional to frequent	Pregnancy	Discuss with doctor – also add bran to diet and more fluids
	Occasional to frequent	Attacks of diarrhoea. Pain	Seek medical advice – could be due to bowel disease. *No laxatives*
	Occasional to frequent	Bleeding from rectum	Seek medical advice – could be due to bowel disease, or be linked with piles (haemorrhoids)
	Occasional to frequent: in a baby	Breast-feeding	Could be normal low frequency of stools in breast-fed; discuss with doctor for reassurance
	Occasional to frequent: in a baby	Bottle-feeding	Could be due to errors in feeding. Extra sugar – very little – or fresh fruit juice and water may be needed – but discuss *first* with doctor
	Frequent: in older people	Heavy use of laxatives	Give up laxatives which can actually increase problem. Take more bran, fresh vegetables, more fluids in diet. Also discuss with doctor if this doesn't help
Diarrhoea	Occasional	Over-eating/-drinking. Unusual foods (e.g. green apples). Foreign holiday	Remove the cause. Take simple Kaolin mixture. If persistent (over 24 hours) seek medical advice
	Frequent: in a child under two or an old person. In pregnancy	Fretfulness. Sickness	Can lead to dehydration – get medical advice soon
Heartburn	Occasional: mild pain behind breast-bone	Over-eating. Unusual foods – especially spicy or fried	Drink water. Take a mild antacid. Avoid cause in future
	Occasional to frequent: mild pain behind breastbone	Pregnancy	Drink water. Take a mild antacid, as recommended by doctor or midwife
	Frequent: severe	Any food	Seek medical advice – could be gastric disorder
	Frequent	Lying flat	Seek medical advice – could be due to hiatus hernia (displacement of the stomach)

Patients' problems

	Type	Associated with	Treatment
Hoarseness	Occasional	Cold in the head	Wait till it cures itself
	Frequent	Anxiety	Seek medical advice for a diagnosis. If no physical cause found – could be due to tension – relaxation techniques will help
	Frequent	Smoking	Give up smoking
	Frequent	Pain in throat, loss of weight, difficulty in swallowing	Seek medical advice – could be due to disease in larynx
Sore throat	Occasional	Cold in the head	Wait until it cures itself. Take pain-killers
	Frequent	Smoking	Give up smoking
	Frequent	Anxiety	Discuss with doctor – could be tension problem needing treatment
	Constant	Hoarseness	Discuss with doctor – could be due to disease in larynx
Cough	Occasional: bubbly	Cold in the head	Wait till it cures itself. Hot drinks will comfort
	Occasional: dry	Time of year, certain foods or other substances, e.g. dust	Seek medical advice – could be an allergy
	Frequent: dry or bubbly	Smoking	Give up smoking
	Frequent: dry or bubbly	Breathlessness. Pain in chest. Pain in shoulders	Could be chest disease, e.g. chronic bronchitis. Seek medical advice
	Persistent: dry or bubbly	Nil else	Seek medical help – can be the only symptom of disease
Spots	Occasional: small, mildly infected		Most spots clear up alone in a few days. If persistent, seek medical advice
	Frequent: young person	Blackheads	Could be acne. Seek medical advice
	Frequent: slow to heal	General lethargy. Thirst. Weight loss. Itching around bottom (pruritis)	Seek medical advice – may be linked with diabetes
	Constant: getting bigger		Seek medical advice. Could be skin disease

What does it mean?

Many of the words used in medicines are built on Greek and Latin roots. This has produced a 'language' which can be used by doctors all over the world whatever their native language. In the past, all medical students needed a working knowledge of Latin and Greek before they could be accepted in a medical school. Nowadays, this is less commonly demanded even though many medical schools draw upon the classical language sources.

Hyper- at the beginning of a word means too much, that is, more than normal – thus, hypertension is high blood pressure.

Hypo- at the beginning of a word means too little, that is, less than normal – as hypothyroid in myxedema.

-itis any word ending thus indicates the presence of inflammation. (For example, appendicitis, tonsillitis.)

-oma a word ending so means a collection – as in haematoma – a blood collection. (A bruise is a haematoma.)

-ectomy a cutting off – as in appendectomy, tonsillectomy.

-ostomy an opening into – usually a permanent one. So, a colostomy is a permanent opening made into the large bowel (colon).

-otomy a temporary opening into; thus a tracheotomy is an opening made into the windpipe to allow air in, and later repaired when the normal air way is restored.

-ology means 'the study of'. So, biology is the study of life; psychology, the study of the way the human mind works.

Benign harmless. A wart is a benign tumour.

Tumour any sort of growth.

Virus a very small organism that may not be visible even under the new radio microscope. It can cause damage to the body by, *inter alia*, invading the individual cells.

Pathogen any harmful organism, either bacteria or virus.

Phobia an unreasonable fear. Thus agoraphobia, a fear of open spaces.

Coryza a cold in the head.

Rhinovirus a virus which causes a cold in the head.

Artefact a man-made object; a symptom which is an artefact is self-induced. Some people regard lung cancer caused by smoking as an artefact.

Prosthesis an artificial replacement for a living tissue. A prosthetic breast, or eye or hip, for example.

Psychosomatic any illness in which the emotional and psychological aspects are of at least as much, if not more, importance than the physical.

Epistaxis bleeding from the nose.

Neonatal pertaining to the new-born.

Puerperal pertaining to the period around childbirth, usually applied to the mother; thus puerperal fever is fever following childbirth.

Post partum after a birth.

Pre-partum before a birth.
(also auto-partum or ante-partum)

Primigravida a woman pregnant for the first time.

Primipara a woman giving birth for the first time.

Multigravida a woman who has had more than one birth.

Menarche the onset of periods in a girl.

Bacteria a micro-organism large enough to be seen under a microscope. It damages the body by, *inter alia*, producing poisons.

Patients' problems

What do the letters after my doctor's name mean?

This list is not complete; it would be almost impossible to provide one to cover the qualifications available in various parts of the world, but it is a fairly comprehensive one.

A.D.M.S.	Assistant Director Medical Services
A.H.A.	Associate Institute of Hospital Administrators or Area Health Authority
A.K.C.	Associate King's College, London
A.M.Q.	American Medical Qualification
A.M.S.	Army Medical Service
A.R.I.C.	Associate Royal Institute of Chemistry
B.A.O.	Bachelor of the Art of Obstetrics
B.C., B.Ch., B.Chir.	Bachelor of Surgery
B.Ch.D.	Bachelor of Dental Surgery
B.D.A.	British Dental Association
B.D.S.	Bachelor of Dental Surgery
B.D.Sc.	Bachelor of Dental Science
B.Hyg.	Bachelor of Hygiene
B.M.	Bachelor of Medicine
B.M.A.	British Medical Association
B.Med.Sc.	Bachelor of Medical Science
B.Pharm.	Bachelor of Pharmacology
B.Sc.	Bachelor of Science
B.S., Ch.B.	Bachelor of Surgery
C.C.F.P.	Certificate College of Family Physicians
C.M., Ch.M.	Master of Surgery
C.N.A.A.	Council of National Academic Awards
C.P.H.	Certificate in Public Health
C.R.C.P.	Certificate Royal College of Physicians
C.R.C.S.	Certificate Royal College of Surgeons
D.A.	Diploma in Anaesthetics
D.A.D.M.S.	Deputy Assistant Director Medical Services
D.A.P. & E.	Diploma in Applied Parasitology and Entomology
D.Av.Med.	Diploma in Aviation Medicine
D.C.D.	Diploma in Chest Diseases
D.C.H.	Diploma in Child Health
D.Ch.	Doctor of Surgery
D.C.M.T.	Diploma in Clinical Medicine of Tropics
D.C.P.	Diploma in Clinical Pathology
D.C. Path.	Diploma College of Pathologists
D.D.M.	Diploma in Dermatological Medicine
D.D.M.S.	Deputy Director Medical Services
D.D.O.	Diploma in Dental Orthopaedics
D.D.R.	Diploma in Diagnostic Radiology
D.D.S.	Doctor of Dental Surgery
D.F.Hom.	Diploma Faculty of Homoeopathy
D.G.M.S.	Director-General Medical Services
D.G.O.	Diploma in Gynaecology and Obstetrics
D.H.M.S.A.	Diploma in History of Medicine
D.Hyg.	Doctor of Hygiene
D.I.C.	Diploma of Membership of Imperial College of Science and Technology, London
D.I.H.	Diploma in Industrial Health
D.L.O.	Diploma in Laryngology and Otology
D.M.	Doctor of Medicine
D.M.D.	Doctor of Dental Medicine
D.M.H.S.	Director Medical and Health Services
D.M.J	Diploma in Medical Jurisprudence
D.M.R.	Diploma in Medical Radiology
D.M.R.D.	Diploma in Medical Radio-Diagnosis
D.M.R.E.	Diploma in Medical Radiology and Electrology
D.M.R.T.	Diploma in Medical Radio-Therapy
D.M.S.	Director Medical Services
D.M.S.A.	Diploma Medical Services Administration
D.M.S.S.	Director Medical and Sanitary Services
D.M.V.	Doctor of Veterinary Medicine
D.O.	Diploma in Ophthalmology
D.Obst. R.C.O.G.	Diploma Royal College of Obstetricians and Gynaecologists
D.O.M.S	Diploma in Ophthalmic Medicine and Surgery
D.Orth.	Diploma in Orthodontics
D.P.D.	Diploma in Public Dentistry
D.Phys.Med.	Diploma in Physical Medicine
D.P.H.	Diploma in Public Health
D.P.M.	Diploma in Psychological Medicine
D.R.	Diploma in Radiology
D.R.A.C.R.	Diploma of Royal Australasian College of Radiologists
D.R.C.Path.	Diploma Royal College of Pathologists
D.R.M.	Diploma in Radiation Medicine
D.S.	Doctor of Surgery
D.S.Sc.	Diploma in Sanitary Science
D.Sc.	Doctor of Science
D.S.M.	Diploma in Social Medicine

D.T.C.D.	Diploma in Tuberculosis and Chest Diseases
D.T.C.H.	Diploma in Tropical Child Health
D.T.D.	Diploma in Tuberculous Diseases
D.T.M. & H.	Diploma in Tropical Medicine and Hygiene
D.T.P.H.	Diploma in Tropical Public Health
E.D.	Efficiency Decoration
E.M.A.S.	Employment Medical Advisory Service
F.A.C.A.	Fellow American College of Anaesthetists
F.A.C.C.	Fellow American College of Cardiology
F.A.C.D.S.	Fellow Australasian College of Dental Surgeons
F.A.C.G.	Fellow American College of Gastro-enterology
F.A.C.M.A.	Fellow Australasian College Medical Administrators
F.A.C.O.	Fellow American College of Otolaryngology
F.A.C.O.G.	Fellow American College of Obstetricians and Gynaecologists
F.A.C.P.	Fellow American College of Physicians
F.A.C.R.	Fellow American College of Radiology
F.A.C.S.	Fellow American College of Surgeons
F.A.N.Z.C.P.	Fellow Australian and New Zealand College of Psychiatrists
F.B.Ps.S.	Fellow British Psychological Society
F.C.A.P.	Fellow College of American Pathologists
F.C.C.P.	Fellow American College of Chest Physicians
F.C.M.S.	Fellow College of Medicine and Surgery
F.C.Path.	Fellow College of Pathologists
F.C.P.S.	Fellow College of Physicians and Surgeons
F.C.S.	Fellow Chemical Society
F.R.C. Path.	Fellow Royal College of Pathologists
F.R.C. Psych.	Fellow Royal College of Psychiatrists
F.R.C.R.	Fellow Royal College of Radiologists
F.R.C.R.A.	Fellow Royal College of Radiologists, Australasia
F.R.C.S.	Fellow Royal College of Surgeons
F.R.E.S.	Fellow Royal Entomological Society
F.R.F.P.S.	Fellow Royal Faculty of Physicians and Surgeons
F.R.I.C.	Fellow Royal Institute of Chemistry
F.R.I.P.H.H.	Fellow Royal Institute of Public Health and Hygiene
F.R.M.S.	Fellow Royal Microscopical Society
F.R.S.	Fellow Royal Society
F.R.S.E.	Fellow Royal Society Edinburgh
F.R.S.H.	Fellow Royal Society of Health
F.R.S.S.	Fellow Royal Statistical Society
H.D.D.	Higher Dental Diploma
I.A.M.C.	Indian Army Medical Corps
I.L.E.A.	Inner London Education Authority
I.M.A.	Irish Medical Association
I.M.S.	Indian Medical Service
L.A.H.	Licentiate Apothecary's Hall, Dublin
L.C.P.S.	Licentiate College of Physicians and Surgeons
L.D.Sc.	Licentiate in Dental Science
L.D.S.	Licentiate in Dental Surgery
L.L.C.O.	Licentiate London College of Osteopathy
L.M.	Licentiate in Midwifery
L.M.C.C.	Licentiate Medical Council of Canada
L.M.S.	Licentiate in Medicine and Surgery
L.M.S.S.A.	Licentiate in Medicine and Surgery Society of Apothecaries, London
L.R.C.P.	Licentiate Royal College of Physicians
L.R.C.S.	Licentiate Royal College of Surgeons
L.R.F.P.S.	Licentiate Royal Faculty of Physicians and Surgeons
L.S.A.	Licentiate Society of Apothecaries, London
L.S.M.	Licentiate School of Medicine
M.A.C.D.	Member Australasian College of Dermatology
M.A.C.G.P.	Member Australasian College of General Practitioners
M.A.C.O.	Member Australian College of Ophthalmologists
M.A.C.R.	Member American College of Radiology
M.A.N.Z.C.P.	Member Australian and New Zealand College of Psychiatrists
M.A.O.	Master of the Art of Obstetrics
M.B.	Bachelor of Medicine

Acknowledgements
The author and publishers wish to
thank the following persons and
organizations for their assistance:

Sylvia Green   Dr John Mansell
Janet Bailes   Dr Adrian Pini
Toni Belfield   R J Russell
Dr P F Bolton   Stephen Thomas
Dr Colin Duncan   Dr Norma Williams
G H Linley   Dr Gillian Woods

Institutions
BUPA Medical Centre Ltd
EMI Ltd
The Family Planning Association
Guy's Hospital Medical School
The Health Education Council
King Edward's Hospital Fund for London
The London Foot Hospital
The Maudsley Hospital
The Royal Free Hospital
The Royal National Orthopaedic Hospital
University College Hospital
Westminster Hospital

Artists
Candida Amsden
Chris Bentley
Alan Cracknell (ACA)
Nigel Fradgley
Jane Hannath
Christine Howes
Ingrid Jacob
Diana Maclean (Linden Artists)
Mark Pearson
Bill Prosser (ACA)
Tess Stone
Bill Dawson Thompson (Artist Partners)
Michael Woods

Photographer
Michael St Maur Sheil

Studios
Arka Cartographics
Hayward and Martin Ltd
Summit Photography
Venner Artists Ltd

Illustrations on page 39
© Guttman Maclay Collection,
Institute of Psychiatry

Typesetting by Servis Filmsetting Ltd,
Manchester, England
Origination by Gilchrist Brothers Ltd,
Leeds, England

D. L. B. 37729–1979